Praise fc

MW01493582

"An excellent digest of all types of addiction, with a holistic, spiritual approach to healing."

– **Darlene Lancer**, licensed marriage and family therapist specializing in relationships, narcissism, and codependency and author of bestsellers *Codependency for Dummies*; *Dating, Loving, and Leaving a Narcissist*; *Conquering Shame and Codependency*; and many more

"Dr. Sanja Rozman's book *Serenity* is well-organized, immensely readable, relatable, and relational. Her language is personal and professional, vulnerable and compassionate. Her readers will appreciate her meaningful descriptions, definitions, diagrams, and summaries for various process and substance addictions, attachment, and the brain. Sanja respectfully regards her readers, never talking down and always rendering hope. Especially helpful are explanations and exercises for recovery; information [on] transformation, treatment, and recovery, and ways to take action for a personalized recovery plan. Readers will immediately feel her passion, sincerity, and warmth in this extremely accessible book. Her book is a welcome addition to the recovery community, including addicts, trauma survivors, family and friends, and also therapists. When it comes out in print, I will happily recommend it to my colleagues and clients. I might even give a copy to a few docs that I know."

– **Anna Valenti-Anderson**, LCSW, contributing expert to Making *Marriage a Success: Pearls of Wisdom from Experts Across the Nation* and *Making Advances: A Comprehensive Guide to the Treatment of Female Sex and Love Addicts*

"In this book, Dr. Sanja Rozman provides readers with a compassionate overview of the addictions and, more specifically, the oft misunderstood and misdiagnosed behavioral addictions. This insightful text offers compelling insight into the development of such addictions, as well as the similarities and differences between substance and behavioral issues. The book offers direction, insight, and hope toward healing these complex problems. Highly recommended for both therapists and the general public."

– **Dr. Rob Weiss**, digital-age intimacy and relationships expert, chief clinical officer for Seeking Integrity treatment centers, and author of bestsellers *Sex Addiction 101: A Basic Guide to Healing from Sex, Porn, and Love Addiction*; *Closer Together, Further Apart: The Effect of Technology and the Internet on Parenting, Work, and Relationships*; and *Prodependence: Moving Beyond Codependency*

"Recovery from addiction requires identifying and understanding how substances coexist within a constellation of behaviors. These accompanying behaviors involving food, work or relationships, are often addictions hiding in plain sight. *Serenity* is a **must-read guide** containing vital insights and exercises necessary to understand, identify, treat and recover from behavioral addictions."

– **Debra Kaplan**, MA, MBA, LPC, CSAT-S, and author of *For Love and Money: Exploring Sexual & Financial Betrayal in Relationships* and *Coupleship Inc: From Financial Conflict to Financial Intimacy*

"Dr. Rozman's *Serenity* is a **paradigm-shifting and compassionate approach** to addiction recovery showing her deep understanding of the emotional and psychological dynamics of compulsion and obsession, as well as their practical experience helping individuals overcome dependence. Rather than relying on sterile medical language or a judgmental lens, this book embraces a holistic and empathetic perspective that broadens the traditional definition of addiction—limited to substances—to include a range of behaviors motivated by the need to escape reality or soothe emotional pain.

"What sets *Serenity* apart is its compelling combination of insightful explanations, clear language, practical tools, deeply moving personal experiences, and real case examples. Dr. Rozman expertly guides readers through the complex landscape of addiction, illuminating its origins, impacts, and the intricate web of emotions that drive it. But understanding is just the first step. *Serenity* invites readers on a journey of self-discovery, empowering them with a structured path to healing and providing hope through actionable steps to break free from addiction's grasp and maintain recovery.

"*Serenity* is more than just a recovery guide; it is a catalyst for genuine transformation. For anyone seeking to step out of the darkness of addiction and step into a brighter, more empowered life, *Serenity* is a must-read. This book is also a powerful tool for anyone who wants to understand and support those on the path to recovery."

> **– Antonieta Contreras**, trauma therapist, supervisor,
> consultant, and author of the award-winning book
> *Traumatization and Its Aftermath*

"*Serenity* provides insight about what addiction is—and isn't. It also provides inspiration for those of us who struggle with addiction to continue on the path to 'better ourselves.' For those who love us, some insight on the nature of addiction and why we struggle to 'stop' what is so obvious to those who loved us as destructive to ourselves and relationships. The stories are relatable and provide a connection point to see ourselves and loved ones—through a lens that we can hopefully take hold of the inspiration to strive for Serenity. Thank you, Sanja, for your persistence in bringing this to reality."

> **– Tami VerHelst**, chief relationship officer for
> Seeking Integrity treatment resources

"Sanja Rozman wrote this extremely useful book with all the competence and the knowledge of a specialist with many years of experience helping patients with the difficult problem of addiction. In her book, together with the useful and updated scientific information, you can find many clinical examples of her work with patients including her own story. This makes this book unique as a valuable resource for both clinicians working in the field of addiction and also for patients suffering from it."

– **Dr. Vesna Bogdanovic**, MD, PhD, psychiatrist and psychotherapist specializing in analytical psychology and EMDR at San Raffaele Hospital in Milan, Italy; and supervisor, facilitator, accredited trainer, and member of the board of EMDR Europe

"Sanja Rozman is Slovenia's **leading specialist** in treating behavioral addictions. With *Serenity*, she is finally making her techniques and experience available to the anglophone world. Humans are humans, the world over. This book offers a chance to apply strategies and approaches that have worked wonders in one cultural setting to mental health professionals everywhere. Dr. Rozman takes an approach that will ring true to all trained psychologists, but adds her own elements that have led to so many positive outcomes in her practice. This is a great book for therapists, family members, and those who suffer from behavioral addictions."

– **Dr. Noah Charney**, bestselling author and professor of art

"*Serenity: How to Recognize, Understand, and Recover from Behavioral Addictions* is not just a book, but a **beacon of hope for anyone caught in the grip of addiction**. The book is characterized by a deep understanding of the human psyche and the complex nature of addiction, and offers an empathetic approach to recovery. Dr. Sanja Rozman draws on her extensive experience as a psychotherapist and survivor of addiction to write a story that is both psychoeducational and deeply personal.

"The book guides the reader through the intricate landscape of non-chemical addictions, examining a wide range of behavioral addictions with meticulous attention to detail. It explores the complexity of addiction on multiple levels—brain, behavior, family, and society—and offers insights from initial recognition through the nuanced journey to recovery. What makes this work particularly powerful is the inclusion of personal stories and testimonials that not only humanize the battle against addiction, but also provide the reader with real-life examples of resilience and hope. It addresses not only the individual struggles with addiction, but also addicts' families and friends, making it a comprehensive resource for anyone affected by this problem. The practical advice, exercises and strategies described in *Serenity* are presented in a compassionate tone and contain no moral judgments. Rozman invites readers on **a comprehensive journey of self-discovery and transformation where she emphasizes the critical importance of patience, self-care, community support, and a holistic approach to healing, addressing the interconnectedness of body, emotions, relationships, and spirituality in the recovery process.**

"In an academic landscape filled with technical and impersonal texts on addiction, *Serenity* stands out for its accessible language, warmth, and sincere desire to support others on their journey to recovery. It is a testament to the power of shared experience and the strength that lies in collective vulnerability. This book represents an invaluable contribution to the field of addiction recovery and offers indispensable insights for anyone seeking to understand the multifaceted nature of addiction, whether for personal healing and growth, educational purpose or professional reasons."

– **Metka Kuhar, PhD**, professor of psychology at University of Ljubljana, Slovenia and author of the Slovenian study *Adverse Childhood Experiences*

"Sanja Rozman, MD, is one of the most honest, approachable, down-to-earth, yet professional therapists and authors I have ever met. Her expertise and personal experience as a longtime practitioner give her a firm baseline for working with patients who suffer from different types of addiction and trauma, as well as people who are close to them. She has worked with some pioneers in this field and developed a unique method that has been successful for many sufferers. Therefore, it is no surprise that her books remain bestsellers even decades after their first publication, often being quoted and used by other authors.

"What makes Rozman so successful? Firstly, it is her great talent for storytelling. Her skillful intertwinement of expert knowledge, years of practice, and personal experience is catchy, easy to read, and relatable. Her honesty and openness are remarkable. Her optimism and belief that regardless of the trauma, one can always find a way out, are infectious and inspiring. Her methods are easily applicable, although not miraculously effective—the change in life is always a result of determination and hard work, with Rozman offering support and information on how to achieve both. Her books are practical and universal, yet not trivial. They help us recognize the bad patterns in our lives, which are mostly adopted in our childhood (and consolidated later on), and tell us how to replace them with healthier ones. Everyone can do that and start living a healthier and happier life, which is the main—and the most important—message of Sanja Rozman's books.

"The same is valid for *Serenity*, her latest book and the first on the international market. It is a result of decades of practical work, a lifetime of education, and an honest wish to help us overcome different types of addictions that prevent us from living authentically and building healthy relationships. We all have experience with addiction, whether we are addicts ourselves or care about a person who suffers from addiction. Thus, I am deeply convinced that anyone can benefit from this book, if not on personal level (which I find almost impossible to believe), but by giving us a deeper understanding of the modern society. Addictions are a major part of our reality, and we all suffer from different traumas, even those that seem tiny and insignificant. That is universal and deeply humane.

"I strongly believe that after reading this book, your life will change for the better. Rozman is a supporter of group therapies, and I agree with her that one plus one does not always make two, but sometimes it makes a hundred. Together we can achieve so much more [than we can] on our own, and when in trouble, there is no better company and support than Sanja Rozman and her book."

– **Urška Kaloper**, chief nonfiction editor at Mladinska knjiga, Rozman's publishing house in Slovenia

"*Serenity* not only raises awareness of addictions in the reader, but also draws road maps in diagnosis and treatment for themselves and their loved ones. I definitely recommend it to be read for business and private life as a relationship management training. It is a guide for all types of addiction whether you're aware of them or not."

– **Sema Erdem**, breast cancer survivor and advocate; and engineer with experience in education, systems engineering, complex projects management, and quality assurance in project management

"For the last couple of years, I have been working with Sanja to create live television shows and documentaries about trauma and addiction. The number of books she wrote, her education, and especially her hands-on practice is better witness to her expertise than my words. But last week, I noticed something that has escaped me during all our years of working together: her gaze . . .

"It was Tuesday, and she came to our studio to participate in our live show *The Unspoken Truths*. As usual, she was cheerful and full of expectations to have yet another opportunity to help people. This time, she noticed how exhausted I was, even though I was sure I had hidden it well, like a typical addict hiding emotions. As she sat in the studio to let the technician set her microphone and adjust the lighting, she was watching me carefully, saying something softly, looking at me deeply, and asking me something. And I knew that she actually cared. I was so touched that I didn't even remember the question.

"It was a moment of nonverbal communication, but it had a tremendous therapeutic effect on me. Later, I thought about it and noticed that her gaze softens when she speaks about the vulnerability of helpless children, getting decisive when the word is about the traps of addictive behaviors or the proven scientific facts. She never judges the patients, but looks at them with compassion."

– **Bojan Kodelja**, founder and owner of Independent TV, a network dedicated to educational and preventive programs for children, parents, and teachers

"I joined Sanja Rozman's program for non-chemical addictions because of problems in my marriage. More or less, I wanted to support my wife, who was already attending the group. Only later did I realize that the way I enter relationships stems from codependency, which was the result of many minor and major traumatic events from childhood. As a people pleaser, I never identified that my core problem was continuously scanning what other people need or want. I overlooked myself to the degree that I hardly existed at all.

"After three years of diligently following the program and using all the suggested means in the field of personal growth, physical health, and spirituality, I finally reawakened my inner feelings, which now dictate my direction in life from the awareness of who I really am. The most important thing I've learned is that I have to solve my problems as soon as they arise because there's no better time than right now. Everything you ignore gets bigger and heavier.

"All the acquired knowledge comes in very handy when I am working with clients. I now use this knowledge and see extraordinary insights in clients and strong shifts in the direction of improving self-image and self-confidence and overcoming various kinds of addictions. Knowledge in the field of non-chemical addictions is quite new in Slovenia, and it is difficult for me to imagine that I could have gained an understanding of the dynamics of complex post-traumatic stress disorder in the way that I experienced it right here, through my own personal experience."

– **Robert**, family and marriage therapist, intern under supervision, and former client

SERENITY

SERENITY

HOW TO RECOGNIZE, UNDERSTAND, AND RECOVER FROM BEHAVIORAL ADDICTIONS

SANJA ROZMAN

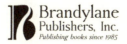
Brandylane
Publishers, Inc.
Publishing books since 1985

ISBN: 978-1-962416-78-8
Library of Congress Control Number: 2024923254

Images and cover design by Katja Rozman.

The Twelve Steps are reprinted with permission of Alcoholics Anonymous World Services, Inc. ("A.A.W.S."). Permission to reprint the Twelve Steps does not mean that A.A.W.S. has reviewed or approved the contents of this publication, or that A.A. necessarily agrees with the views expressed herein. A.A. is a program of recovery from alcoholism only—use of the Twelve Steps in connection with programs and activities which are patterned after A.A., but which address other problems, or in any other non-A.A. context, does not imply otherwise. Printed in the United States of America.

All the stories in this book are based on real people's experiences. Names and details have been changed to protect the privacy of those involved.

Published by
Brandylane Publishers, Inc.
5 S. 1st Street
Richmond, Virginia 23219

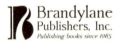
Brandylane
Publishers, Inc.
Publishing books since 1985

brandylanepublishers.com

*To all those who are struggling to find
your path towards sobriety, serenity, and a
better tomorrow.*

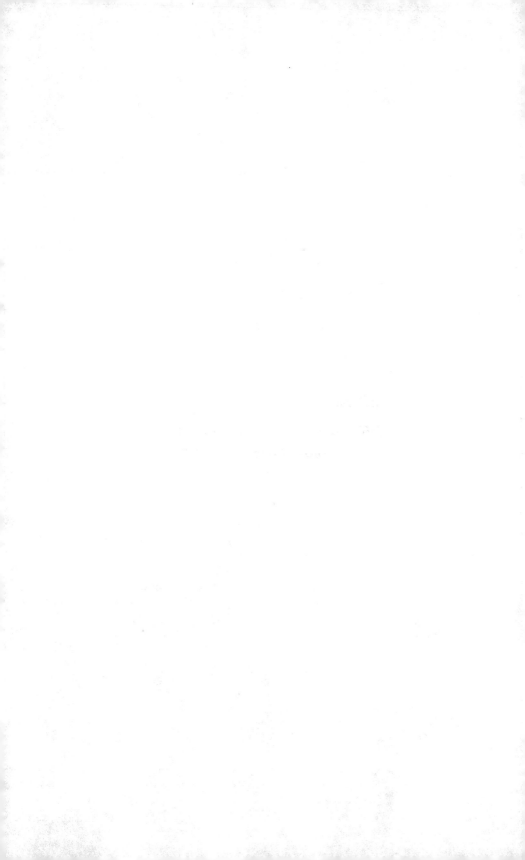

TABLE OF CONTENTS

*God, grant me the **SERENITY** to accept the things I cannot change,*

***COURAGE** to change the things I can,*

*and **WISDOM** to know the difference.*[1]

---

[1] The Serenity Prayer has been used at meetings of Alcoholics Anonymous and other twelve-step fellowships from the very beginning of the twelve-step movement in the 1940s. It describes the recovery process, and hundreds of thousands of recovering addicts recite it daily at their meetings.

How to Use This Book

Addiction! What comes to mind when you hear that word?

Perhaps you first think of drug addicts who inject themselves with their daily dose of addictive death, sticking dirty needles into their swollen veins in dark and gloomy places. Or perhaps you think of alcoholics who stagger around deserted streets late at night, talking or singing out loud, making fools of themselves and disturbing the peace. Perhaps you think of smokers, lighting up one cigarette after another in hazy bars, coughing and risking a terrible death of lung cancer.

Maybe you remember more personal experiences—how you waited for your father to come home, trying to guess whether today would be one of those rare good days or one of those when you, your mother, and your sister would need to hide in the barn to weather his rage, waiting for him to fall asleep before you could come back into the house. Maybe your body remembers the tension, anxiety, and icelike numbness and emptiness that followed his outbursts.

Addictions of all kinds, whether substance- or behavior-based, are responsible for a lot of pain and destruction, especially in families. That is why we tend to blame addicts for their actions, and resent their out-of-control behavior. *They could have prevented all the misery,* we think, *if only they had tried harder!*

But when an addicted person comes to me asking for help, approaching them with such a blaming attitude would only create a chasm of misunderstanding between us, preventing me from doing them any good. So, despite my recognition of the mistakes these addicts are making, I have learned to look past the obvious—their bad behavior—to the core of their problems, and recognize that their struggles are not just reflections of a lack of character or morality, but rather misdirected efforts to overcome the pain in their lives. If you take the time to really listen to these people, you'll uncover a story that makes a lot of sense!

This book is not only for those who are beginning to realize their out-of-control, repetitive, and adverse behaviors might be signs of an addiction. Rather, addiction concerns all of us. You might worry about the destructive behavior of a family member or someone you love. If you are a parent, a teacher, or just a concerned citizen conscious of the situation in which our young people are growing up, there is a lot you need to learn about the traps of modern addictions. Over the past ten years, groundbreaking new information has come to light, and it's hard to keep up with it all, let alone the new kinds of addiction that seem to emerge daily. In any case, you need to understand addictive behaviors in order to help yourself or your loved ones to stop engaging in them; and if you have children, to prevent the passing on of addictive traits to the next generation.

Usually, when someone talks about addictions, they group them into two categories: substance addictions and behavioral addictions. That makes sense, as substances and behaviors can be easily observed. When someone repetitively abuses mind-altering substances such as alcohol, nicotine, drugs, or prescription medications, they are said to have a **substance addiction.** But people can behave like addicts even when they are not abusing any substances. When people abuse relationships, sex, money, risk, food, the Internet, and other behaviors to escape reality or numb their pain, we say they have a **process** or **behavioral addiction.**

Serenity is divided into four sections:

Part One: How to Recognize Addiction starts with the true story of one of my clients, followed by my personal experience of behavioral addictions. It addresses old, outdated concepts of addiction and explains the contemporary view of addiction as a disease—a consequence of traumatic insecure attachment and a dysfunctional attempt at affect regulation. Exercises at the end of this section help the reader check his or her own dysfunctional behaviors for signs of potential addiction.

Part Two: How to Understand Addiction explains addiction on different levels: what happens in the brain, at the level of thinking and feeling, when an addiction is present; how addiction is expressed in a person's behavior; what effects addiction can have on a family; and what effects it can have on society as a whole. The exercises accompanying this section deal with the shame and consequences of addiction, and encourage readers to construct their own addiction and trauma timelines to enable them to begin to understand and forgive themselves.

Part Three: Behavioral Addictions explains each of the most common behavioral addictions: addictions to food, work, money, risk (including gambling), modern electronic media (including cyber addictions), and relationship and sex addictions. This section defines the behaviors typical of these specific addictions, discusses some important features of those behaviors, and assesses the scope of each addiction. A real-life example illustrates the theory. This part of the work also offers tips on how addicts can maintain their abstinence, as well as ways their family members can cope and help the addict. The exercises in this section are about achieving and maintaining abstinence and identifying resources that can help in this endeavor.

Part Four: How to Recover from Addiction is about the process of recovery. It explains the tools an addict needs to recover, the stages of recovery, and the problems addicts can encounter at each stage. It also helps the reader create their own personal recovery plan across the four dimensions of human experience: the body, the mind, relationships, and spirituality.

Different people can use this book in different ways:

- Suppose you are a concerned person—a teacher, a psychotherapist, or a doctor—who wants to be informed about the perils of modern lifestyles and their effect on the youth. You need general information about behavioral addictions, and you'll find it in Parts One and Two. For thorough, up-to-date information about behavioral addictions, I suggest you read the whole book.

- Suppose you are a friend or family member—a spouse, mother, father, sibling, or child—of someone you suspect has problems with a behavioral addiction. In that case, you should read Parts One, Two, and Four, as well as the chapter about your relative's specific addiction in Part Three. You should also be conscious of the boundary between helping and enabling an addict. The chapter on codependency will alert you to possible mistakes. Finally, you will find advice on how family members of addicts can deal with the crisis of addiction throughout Part Three.

- If you think or know that *you* might be addicted to a substance or a behavior, you should read Parts One, Two, and Four—as well as the chapter about your specific addiction in Part Three—and complete all the exercises, which will help you take active control of your addiction and internalize what you have learned. Several of these exercises will help you devise your own **personalized recovery plan**—a process thoroughly explained in Part Four of this book—and make the decision to pursue abstinence and step onto the path to recovery. As part of this plan, reading this book will be the first—but hopefully not the last!—step you take along that path toward freedom from addiction.

The Stories Worth Telling

For thirty years, I have worked as a psychotherapist for people recovering from behavioral addictions. Once I gained their trust, many of them told me about their shame; feelings of worthlessness, powerlessness, and despair; and memories so terrible, they had to be removed from awareness. Their need to numb these painful feelings is why these clients acted out and pursued their addictions—not to fulfill feelings of lust or greed, nor out of a lack of morality.

As a therapist, I do not focus on how my clients try to

escape reality, but on how their attempts to do so transform their inner worlds. I'm interested in learning about how it feels to be addicted.

Between our sessions, my clients often send me letters as a means of allowing me to track their recovery. In these letters, they share what they feel in language spoken from the heart. Nobody can describe their experiences better than they can. That is why I've included some of my clients' personal testimonies in my book, separated from the rest of the text by *italic font*. I use these testimonies to help readers understand the lived experience behind the dry and difficult-to-understand theory of addiction.[2] Their shared experiences are a powerful tool that can help you, the reader, connect emotionally to the subject matter. As you read their words, you might even realize you have been struggling with similar problems. After all, I have found that under the surface of many out-of-control behaviors is the same pain and helplessness we all share, regardless of what each of us uses to block it from awareness. It is always easier to see what is wrong with others than to find fault within yourself, but in naming the problem you are facing, you have taken the first step toward correcting it.

I am so very grateful to my clients for gifting me with their truths. They mustered the courage to overcome the shame they felt—the worst feeling for an addict—so that their explanations of their experiences could help others.

In addition to my academic knowledge and the knowledge of addiction I've acquired over the course of my career, I also have personal experience with addiction and what it means to be a partner of an addict. Like everyone else, I initially tried to find love by following the old patterns of behavior I learned during childhood—but they led me astray. Frustrated by the elusiveness of what I so desperately needed, I kept trying to paint over reality with fantasy pictures I thought better and prettier. But one day, the illusions disappeared, and all I was left with was the pain hidden behind them.

---

[2] All the stories and letters in the book are true stories of my clients, but names and personal information have been changed to protect their identities.

So I surrendered. I stopped trying to convince the people I loved to star in the drama of my life. I decided to stop lying to myself and others, and—for once in my life—to start trying to see what reality was all about.

Looking at all the mess in my life, I found the best word for it was **addiction**. I did not feel ashamed or humiliated to use that word, for it helped me understand the reasons for some of my harmful behavior, find help, and take back control over my life. As a person who has walked the walk, I have a great deal of respect for people in recovery from addiction, for I know that changing one's life in pursuit of becoming a better person is one of the most demanding and important tasks one can accomplish.

Thanks to my profession, I have met many others who have also taken that walk, inspired by the love of their children and driven by their determination to avoid passing the disease of addiction on to them. I have seen them changed by that experience, becoming aware of their responsibility to life, love, and spiritual growth. I believe they are the bearers of a new awareness of life's meaning, the importance of love, and the divine spark in all of us. To them, I dedicate this book.

A Note for Readers

This book started as an idea. In the long hours of sitting with my clients, I was inspired by their efforts to better themselves, and decided that helping them and others through their most challenging times was my purpose in life. As a witness to their transformations, I wished I could share their stories with others, so their experiences might serve as a road map for those still struggling to find their own ways out of addiction.

It took longer than I expected, and the joint effort of many people, to arrange these ideas in the form of a book. As you hold this book in your hands, dear reader, you are looking at our collective endeavor to express something meaningful. The creative circle will be complete when you read the book and it inspires new ideas in you. Feel free to highlight the passages that speak to you, write notes on its pages, and make it your own. You can also visit my website,[3] Instagram,[4] Facebook,[5] or YouTube channel[6] to find out more about my work and life. Please feel free to contact me with any questions you may have.

---

[3] https://www.sanjarozman.com
[4] https://www.instagram.com/sanjarozman.author
[5] https://www.facebook.com/rozmansanja
[6] https://www.youtube.com/channel/UCEKIMymK99vaAI7V5R7UuLw

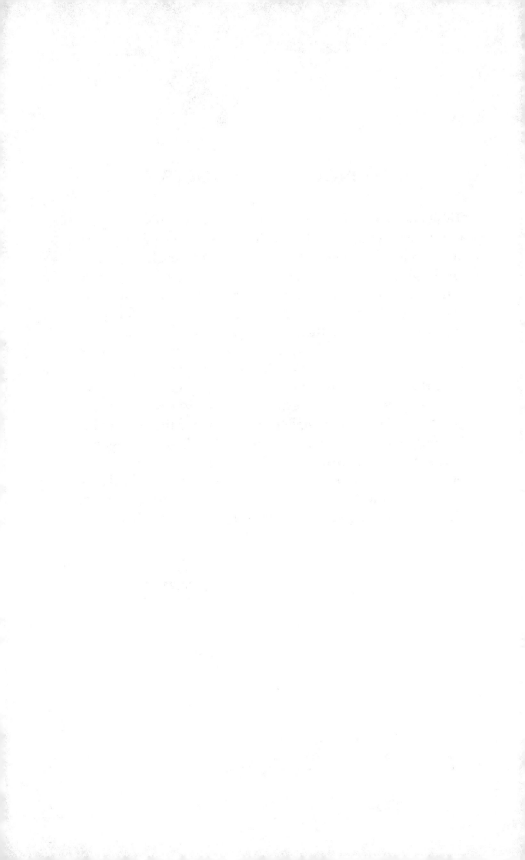

PART ONE:

HOW TO RECOGNIZE ADDICTION

Addiction is
the only prison
where the locks are
on the inside!

1

Sara's Story

Sara was a lively little girl with curly brown hair and big dark eyes. She lived with her parents on her grandmother's old farm. Having no brothers or sisters and no friends to keep her company, she spent most of her time playing with chickens in the yard. Her mother and father were often away working, managing the farm and striving to amass enough money to one day build a house of their own—leaving Sara in the care of her old grandmother, who was convinced children didn't need much adult attention and should be left to fend for themselves. Sara longed for someone to be close to, and dreamed of the day when her family would be together in their new home.

One day, one of Sara's neighbors noticed how lonely she was. He started coming by, talking to her, and bringing her candy. Sara loved helping him work in his garden. When she was only five, he began telling her stories about men and women and what they do behind closed doors.

One day, while playing with some roses, Sara hurt her finger. The neighbor invited her into his kitchen to put a Band-Aid on her wound. Thus gaining her trust, he showed her an adult magazine he kept under his bed. Then he asked her to touch him in the same way the women in the pictures touched the men. Sara hated it, but was convinced she had to comply. He told her what they were doing was okay and that everyone did it—but also that she shouldn't tell anyone about it, or something terrible would happen.

After this incident, something did not feel right to Sara—but seeing that her parents said nothing about her interaction with her neighbor, she kept visiting him. And at the end of the day, what went on between the two of them was the only genuine contact and intimacy she had with anyone—something she desperately wanted.

These secret meetings continued for three years, during which time Sara began attending school. She felt somehow different from her classmates. All they seemed to want to do was read comic books or play video games; but she, on the other hand, was trying to make sense of her odd experiences. She was far too young to feel lust, but her neighbor's actions stirred in her a combination of arousal, fear, and disgust. With no one to explain these feelings to her, she didn't understand that she could have refused her neighbor's advances or told someone else what was happening. When she tried to win over her peers with talk of the "forbidden things" she'd learned about, they thought she was weird and began avoiding her.

When Sara was eight, it finally happened: her father came to pick her up from their neighbor's house unannounced, and caught them in the act. For a moment, he stood at the door, frozen. Then he grabbed Sara and pushed her out the door.

"Go home and get yourself washed up!" he ordered.

Scared to death, Sara obeyed, running to the bathroom. There, she scrubbed her skin to wash the neighbor's touch and smell from her body, scraping so hard that blood began to ooze from her skin. Then she lay in her bed and listened, waiting for that terrible thing the neighbor had promised her would happen if someone found out what they did together. Perhaps her father would kill her, and the neighbor too. She heard screaming coming from downstairs. Then everything went quiet.

Sara waited for someone to come into her room to punish her, or to tell her what she should do. She shivered from the cold and her own crippling fear. But nobody ever came. In the early hours of the morning, she finally fell asleep, exhausted.

When Sara entered the kitchen the following day to

prepare for school, her father directed a stern look at her. "We will never speak another word about what happened. You are not to tell anyone!" he said. Then her mother and father left for work and let her find her own way to school.

Sara drifted off to class as if she were sleepwalking, feeling nothing but confusion. Somehow, she survived the following days; but her grades fell dramatically. Her teachers began thinking about putting her in a special program for children with learning disabilities. At home, the family obeyed her father's order and never spoke about what had gone on—nor much else. The neighbor left her alone, even going so far as to avoid her. He was, however, still invited to family events, and they even celebrated his birthday together, expecting Sara to be polite to him as if he were a family member.

What could Sara have made of all of that? Without guidance, she could only conclude she was to blame for what had happened between them—that she was bad, abandoned, dirty, and helpless. She felt shame, fear, and hopelessness, as well as frightful loneliness.

In time, Sara discovered how to ease the pain a little. Eating helped—but only if she ate so much that her whole body ached. She put on a lot of weight—yet no one said anything, even though entire boxes of chocolates went missing. Sara desperately wanted her parents to notice her and help her understand what happened. In her desperation, she tried to get attention the only way the adults in her life had taught her: she sexually provoked her classmates. But this also didn't work, and her peers distanced themselves from her even more fervently.

Sara struggled through school, trying to think about nothing and shutting herself off from everybody and everything. Years passed, she developed into a beautiful young girl. Suddenly, other men began to notice her, sweet-talk her, and offer her candy and drinks in return for sexual favors. It was usually older men who were interested in her—men similar to her father, whose attention she wanted so badly. Their advances were familiar; this, she knew. Here, she had power.

Of course, older men who try to seduce young teenage girls

don't have innocent things on their minds. They often forced Sara into perverse acts, passed her around like an object, and sometimes even beat her. She repeatedly ran away from home, often spending the night in some rundown shed; and cruised the bars where men went to pick up women.

Somehow, Sara finished middle school, and enrolled in an educational program with the goal of becoming a hairdresser. This program was not available in her hometown, so she had to leave home to stay in a rental. After that, her parents lost all control over her behavior. At sixteen, she supported herself financially by waitressing at a dump of a bar. The owner expected her to be nice to the male clientele, who talked dirty and felt her up. She lived with an older man who beat her and "lent" her to his friends. Drugs and alcohol became a part of their routine, enabling Sara to shut out her pain and awareness of what she was doing.

By this time, Sara's feelings of self-worth were far less than nonexistent. Alcohol, drugs, sex, violence, and danger had become her way of life. She obliged whoever wanted her, and was convinced she was obligated to satisfy them sexually if they showed any kind of interest. Over time, she became more and more attracted to rough and violent men. Their combination of violence and eroticism seemed to be the most effective drug, extinguishing the wild tornado of emotion raging within her—at least for a night.

Infatuation proved even more potent. Whenever Sara fell in love, she forgot about everything, and became convinced her newest boyfriend was a knight in shining armor who would finally take her away from her hellish life. When she finally found the man she thought of as her Mr. Right, at the age of twenty-four, he was like her—profoundly wounded and without boundaries. At first, their romance felt like heaven—but only two months later, the relationship turned violent, and she realized she was living with a terribly dangerous man. She tried to understand and excuse his beatings, hoping he would change, but after he broke her arm one night, she finally decided to seek help.

Sara's story tells us how and why addictions begin. When she came to me searching for help, she was addicted to sex and relationships, food, nicotine, and alcohol; by contrast, her abuse of illegal drugs, while problematic, proved relatively easy for her to give up. It would have been easy to judge her as simply irresponsible—but knowing her entire story, who could blame her for trying to ease her pain? The substances, and her behavior, helped her survive both her sexual abuse and the betrayal she suffered at the hands of her own family, who had left her to deal with her trauma alone.

2

How My Addiction
Shaped My Life

When Sara came to me asking for help, I was working as a therapist, helping people recover from behavioral addictions. In addition to my expertise as a medical doctor and a psychotherapist, I was well equipped to understand and empathize with her—because I had my own experiences with addiction in my life.

I first encountered addiction as a problem that would significantly influence my life more than thirty years ago, when my husband, whom I thought I knew very well, came home one night looking like he had suffered a beating. He refused to seek help for his bruises or explain what had happened. After a lot of persuading, he finally confessed he had a gambling problem. He had gambled away everything we had at the slot machines, and gotten into a fight with some of the people he owed.

I was floored. I'd had no idea this was happening, when it had started, or how far he had gone. When he explained that he couldn't resist gambling, describing the urge to gamble as stronger than his own will, I was convinced he was lying. It made no sense to me that a person could do such a stupid thing. I couldn't understand why he wasn't able to simply stop himself from acting on his urges. Certainly, he was clever and intelligent enough to have foreseen the consequences of his behavior—consequences so harmful that, in my opinion, *anyone* would have stopped and "sobered up." To me, my husband's betrayal meant he just didn't love me enough to stop—and this thought triggered terrible anxiety within me.

Overwhelmed by feelings of rejection, I began to lash out. I could no longer see him as my partner—only as a stranger and an enemy. I wasn't able to understand that he was also hurting. Though we both attempted to explain our pain, we each thought it was the other who needed to change. We had lost trust in one another.

In my case, I was lucky enough to get help right away. (Not everybody is!) I knew a fellow doctor, a therapist who specialized in treating addictions. I wanted to persuade my husband to see the doctor so he could fix his "bad habit" and we could go on living as before—but the therapist insisted we both come to treatment. Desperate to return to the way things were, I obliged.

But when we went to our first meeting, I found my assessment of the problem completely upended. As we sat together in the therapist's office, he explained that my husband's addiction was in fact a disease, and that pressure, blackmail, verbal inducement, or outbursts of rage on my part would only hinder his recovery. To remove any of that negative influence, he told me to leave my husband's treatment in his hands and concentrate on what was wrong with my own worldview.

I was shocked. I had walked into the therapist's office convinced that my husband's behavior was the only bad thing in my life—even though I had been experiencing health problems for years, and often felt inexplicable dissatisfaction and tension whose source I didn't even want to know. I had thought I needed to compromise to make my marriage work, and was offended that my husband's behavior seemed to indicate all my sacrifices had been in vain—but as we spoke, I slowly realized that over time, the many small compromises had taken their toll, generating a deep-seated anger within me. I had tried to ignore it, but at times, I lost control and lashed out with outbursts so violent and unstoppable, they made me fear my own reactions.

Furthermore, whenever this happened and the emotional upheaval became too much, I retreated into a fantasy world of my own creation. I had always been a dreamer. As far back as I could remember, daydreaming had been my primary defense mechanism in times of stress. It had started as an innocent pastime, but I now realized that over the years, it had developed into an impassable jungle of romantic fiction continually bubbling away in the back of my mind. While daydreaming, I was in my own world—emotionally inaccessible.

I hadn't been aware how far from reality my fantasy life had taken me. What brought me back to earth was my therapist's revelation that my fantasies and outbursts of rage were also symptoms of addiction—**relationship addiction, or codependence**. I'd really needed somebody to tell me that—though at the time, I felt disappointed that the therapist did not praise me for my heroic role in saving my family, but rather loaded upon me a significant share of the blame that I thought should have been placed on my husband. Nevertheless, for the first time, I clearly saw how far the consequences of my daydreaming and the compromises I'd made had taken me.

From then on, my problem had a name and a form—and as such, I had the opportunity to deal with it. It no longer seemed an inseparable part of me, but rather some kind of colossal defense mechanism that had attached itself to me and grew in size whenever I agreed to a harmful compromise. Equipped with this new knowledge, I resolved to follow the therapist's advice and work on my own issues of codependence and relationship addiction.

This was easier said than done. At the time, in the 1990s, information about codependence was almost impossible to find—especially in Slovenia, where I lived. The only available resource in my native language was a translated version of the popular book *Women Who Love Too Much* by Robin Norwood.[7] Reading this book helped me conceptualize my own behavior. Despite my initial resistance to being blamed for my husband's terrible conduct, my new perspective allowed me to realize that

---

[7] Robin Norwood, *Women Who Love Too Much: When You Keep Wishing and Hoping He'll Change* (New York: Pocket Books, 2008).

I was nevertheless partially responsible for it—in large part thanks to my lack of reaction when I'd felt us drifting apart.

Now aware of the symptoms of addiction and codependence, I began to see addictive and codependent traits in the people around me. Suddenly, they were everywhere—and those who were aware of my pursuit of therapy seemed very interested in what I had to say. Many of them wanted to know more about relationship addiction.

My curiosity was piqued, and I knew I needed to learn more. Inspired, I expanded my research to texts from other languages and began to read other books on addiction and codependence by English and American authors, devouring every scrap of information I could get my hands on. Before the advent of the Internet, finding the right books was a challenge; but I was determined to get to the bottom of my problem. I felt I must do so to help not only myself, but also my fellow codependents, who desperately needed this information—but who did not speak English and could not read those books.

Three years into treatment, I wrote a book about my recovery from codependence, *Stronger Than Love*.[8] In this book, I described the profound personal changes I had gone through in therapy. The book struck a chord in many people who were unused to such sincere disclosure, and I was praised for my candidness. Being completely honest about my behaviors—especially those I wasn't proud of—seemed to have opened a channel of communication directly to people's hearts.

To bridge the information gap and make it easier for people to understand and talk about behavioral addictions, I swiftly wrote six more books on the subject. Not only were these books widely read, but my public appearances sold out, and people started turning to me to help them with their addictions and codependency. I accepted this challenge, and began devoting most of my time, energy, and even money to educating myself further, enrolling in many educational programs for psychotherapists and obtaining licenses that would

---

[8] *Stronger Than Love* was published in Slovenia under the title *Sanje o rdečem oblaku* in 1993.

allow me to treat people. I gave many lectures, and appeared in the media on many occasions. Since my husband's diagnosis, my life had entirely changed.

In the beginning, this new life was very painful. Despite all our efforts at therapy, my marriage had fallen apart. My husband's addiction seemed stronger than he was. I was left alone to raise our two small children, and had to face up to my worst nightmare: that I might never find love again. But at the same time, my recovery from relationship addiction made it possible for me to hold onto healthier convictions: that I was good and worthy of love, and that there is enough love in this world for everyone.

Eventually, I found new love, gave birth to a third daughter, was there for all three of my children as they journeyed into adulthood, and even survived cancer. My life is now far more beautiful and far more profound than I had ever imagined, even in my wildest dreams.

When I think back to the first years of my recovery, as difficult as they were, I am thankful for everything that happened. I know I am still on the path of recovery, and always will be. The disease of addiction—or rather, my recovery from it—has shaped me mercilessly, transforming me from a daydreaming, people-pleasing codependent into a strong but compassionate person. My life now has a far deeper meaning than it did before I entered recovery. All the people I have met, and their stories, inspired a creative spark to evolve within me. It has now matured. May it be a light for you in dark places, when all other lights go out.[9]

---

[9] J.R.R. Tolkien, *The Fellowship of the Ring* (London: HarperCollins, 1995), 367.

3

What Is Addiction?

Nowadays, addictions seem so common that we have learned to tolerate them—believing their existence is "just the way things are," that nothing can be done about them, and that others' addictions are none of our business anyway. However, none of this is true. We are all interconnected participants in creating this world—so others' misery touches all of us, even if we look the other way.

Just like me when I first encountered the issue so many years ago, everyone has a personal concept of addiction—but this concept is likely to change when addiction strikes close to home, affecting a member of their family or even themselves. From this closer perspective, everything changes, and so the affected person, too, must change.

Not so long ago, addiction was thought to be caused by substances: alcohol, nicotine, or prescription drugs. It was believed that these substances had such an effect on people, some found it difficult to control their use. Nevertheless, the fact that addicts continued to use them was attributed to a series of incorrect choices or a bad habit on their part, as in general, people thought everybody always did what they believed was best for themselves. As a result, the fact that addicts did things that hurt their families or themselves was considered the result of a flaw in their very personhood, and they were deemed stupid or morally impaired—or so full of themselves that they would choose their own pleasure over their duties and responsibilities to others. According to this understanding, they should be forced by the threat of punishment to respect the rules we must all obey!

It was addicts in recovery who initially challenged these false concepts. They argued that something had happened to them when they became addicted, and that after that, they had lost the ability to freely choose to indulge their addictions or not. Most of the time, they could still control their behavior. But when they were caught off guard, or faced challenges like conflicts, fatigue, anger, stress, and loneliness, their ability to prevent themselves from acting out was compromised. Their wishes became wants; their wants grew into needs, desires, and cravings to indulge; and before they knew it, they succumbed to this inner drive, feeling they would die if they abstained. This *inability to control the adverse behavior, despite their awareness of the consequences*, is one of the main characteristics of addiction.

Some people still think addicts are simply unwilling to stop indulging in their addictions—and that if they only really wanted to, they could. This is what I used to think about my husband's gambling. *He doesn't care about the children or me, and prefers to indulge in his own pleasure. Insensitive idiot,* I thought—*choosing a stupid slot machine over us!* On the other hand, I rationalized my own out-of-control outbursts of codependent rage and fantasies as normal responses to the situation. But in both cases, I had to learn I was wrong. Both my husband's gambling and my emotional outbursts were indicative of a *loss of control*—the same feeling addicts experience.

Along with a loss of control, addicts also experience the *loss of the ability to enjoy what they do*. What has become a necessity is no longer pleasurable. Rather, it is just as necessary as breathing—or so the addict's brain suggests.

Over the years, it has become increasingly accepted that addiction is a disease—a *chronic* one. And like most diseases, if left untreated, it will only get worse. It will have *consequences in various dimensions of an addict's life*, causing physical ailments and psychological problems that lead to a loss of contact with reality, problems in relationships, and impaired personal and spiritual growth. But addiction differs from other diseases in the fact that addicts create these consequences themselves as they pursue the object of their addiction. This is why it took so long for the medical community, and society in general, to acknowledge addiction as a disease.

When I studied medicine, I was taught that addictions of all sorts were merely a result of drinking or of taking too many drugs—mind-altering substances that affect the brain in ways that induce an altered state of consciousness, inebriation, or a "high." After a while, the effect wears off, and the person experiences **withdrawal**—a really unpleasant physical and emotional feeling—along with a sense of guilt. At the time, people generally considered moderate use of these various substances acceptable. Only if you crossed some indeterminate threshold, they believed, could the substance somehow enslave you, causing you to become addicted. Only when this happened would addicts crave the substance all the time, even at the grave cost of their social fluency.

This theory explained substance addictions well enough—but how could someone develop an addiction when no mind-altering substance was involved? At the time, the medical community considered the behaviors we now know as symptoms of behavioral addictions to be symptoms of personality disorders instead—but failed to explain what caused them. However, some addicts recovering from alcohol addiction recognized that their gambling, sexual acting out, activities in relationships, and other behaviors had the same obsessive and compulsive characteristics as the behaviors they exhibited when addicted to substances. Furthermore, they noticed that the only way they could stop themselves from engaging in these behaviors was by adhering to the same principles that had helped them remain sober. And so, it was recovering addicts who birthed the idea that one can become addicted to certain behaviors as well as substances.

It was difficult to convince the doctors, however. They resisted the idea that activities in which everyone takes part could become a disease in some. Only in the last decade has scientific advancement proved the truth of this theory, as brain scanning techniques have captured comparable changes in the brains of substance addicts, gamblers, and other patients with behavior-based addictions. As a result, the doctors' denial has slowly started to vanish, and efforts to include behavioral addictions in the list of recognized diseases related to addiction are underway.

But now we need a new definition of addiction—one that includes both substance and behavioral addictions; and clearly describes the difference between mere bad behaviors that could be stopped anytime by an act of free will, and a disease that should be taken care of in quite a different way, with expert guidance and a structured program.[10]

The Contemporary Definition of Addiction

In 2001, the American Society of Addiction Medicine[11] adopted a contemporary definition of addiction based on the newest research into the disease. Their definition, which takes into account both substance and behavioral addictions, now forms the basis of our modern understanding of addiction. Its main features are:

1. Addiction is a **disease**. It takes a long time to develop, worsens over time, and exhibits periods of deterioration, improvement, and relapses. Once an addiction forms, the addict's ability to control the behavior associated with it is impaired—if not permanently, then at least much longer than the addict would hope.

[10] In English, "addiction" and "dependence" are used as synonyms. Related expressions such as *addictive* or *addict* are less common, and have a slightly stronger meaning. *Dependent* and *dependency* are used more frequently, and their connotations are a little softer. As expressions connected with the word *dependence* describe a form of relationship, *addiction* and related expressions relate directly to the disease of addiction, which I describe in this book; and so I decided to use the word *addiction*. Therefore, we are all *dependent* (in the context of lacking independence) on someone or something, while some of us are also *addicted*.

[11] The American Society of Addiction Medicine is a professional society representing over five thousand physicians, clinicians, and associated professionals who work in the field of addiction medicine.

2. Addicts become **obsessed** and **preoccupied** with a substance or behavior, and think, plan, and talk about it all the time.

3. An addict's behavior is both **compulsive**—driven, the result of an irresistible urge—and **impulsive**—undertaken without thought.

4. **Triggers**—emotionally stressful states such as hunger, anger, loneliness, or tiredness—can affect an addict by weakening their willpower or prompting them to engage in addictive behavior. (Notice that the first letters of these states spell HALT!)

5. **Cues** are situations that remind the addict of times when they have indulged their addiction, like meeting a friend in the same bar where they used to drink. Both triggers and cues activate the memory of the bad old times of acting out, and the affected areas of the brain reawaken.

6. When addicts stop using an addictive substance or indulging in an addictive behavior, they experience a set of very unpleasant and sometimes dangerous physical and psychological symptoms like nausea, vomiting, severe headaches, drowsiness, and shivering. These are collectively known as **withdrawal symptoms**, and all of them can be alleviated almost immediately with just a small dose of the addictive substance—or in the case of behavioral addictions, by undertaking an action related to the addiction, such as receiving phone call from a lover who abandoned them.

7. As their disease progresses, addicts require more and more of a substance or indulgence in a behavior to achieve the same effect: the numbing of anxiety. They develop an **increased tolerance** for the substance or behavior.

There is a lot of debate on whether and when it can be safe for addicts to engage with the focus of their addictions again and whether they should be taught to do so moderately; but if you ask me, such a course is much too risky. I know of a case of an alcoholic who had been sober for twenty years and decided to celebrate his anniversary with a shot of whiskey, fooling himself into believing the danger was long past. In only a couple of days, all was lost: his nearly adult children, who had never seen him drunk before, met the worst monster of a father; and his wife decided she was not taking it anymore. After this relapse, he wasn't able to stop again for a long time. The problem of control is even more complex in behavioral addictions since people cannot completely stop eating, using money, being in relationships, or even denying themselves access to the Internet. In most cases, behavioral addicts are therefore forced to stick to relative boundaries—which make it even easier for them to fool themselves into thinking they have their addiction under control, and to accidentally slide back into their old ways.

But despite all the temptations a recovering addict may face throughout the rest of their life, we should not forget that recovery from addiction is possible. We'll discuss aspects of recovery in Part Four of the book—and develop a plan that will help you resist the temptation to fall back into addiction whenever it rears its head.

4

Why Did It Happen?: The Origins of Addiction

No one begins to drink or indulge in bad behavior with the intent of becoming an addict. Addictions take time to develop—and in the beginning, when someone is merely misusing a substance or develops a bad habit of acting in a certain negative way, they may not believe it will become an addiction at all.

Psychotherapists rarely talk about good or bad habits. Instead, we use the word **adaptive** for behavior that helps the person survive difficult and dangerous times. Behaviors that are detrimental to a person's survival, on the other hand, are labeled **maladaptive**.

From Sara's story, you can see that her **acting out**[12] as a child was, at the time, definitely adaptive. She tried to come to terms with her confused sexual feelings and her craving for intimacy by seducing boys and men; and to ease her emotional pain by stuffing herself with food. Later, when she got her hands on addictive substances, she turned to drinking and taking drugs. These actions numbed her pain and helped her cope emotionally—but at the cost of many negative consequences. When Sara was just a child, she could not have known what she did to survive each day would have such grave consequences later. When she was mature enough to

---

[12] **Acting out** is a term in psychology meaning *to perform an action, usually in a destructive way, in order to gain relief from tension or anxiety.*

understand those consequences, the addiction had already taken hold, robbing her of the ability to choose how she behaved.

Every day, I am confronted by parents who come to me complaining that their child was fine and had no problems until new friends entered the scene—friends who dragged them out into the streets and taught them to drink and take drugs. I find it difficult to explain to these parents that the seeds of addiction can be sown as early as the first few years of childhood, as they were in Sara's case. I am not looking to excuse their children's behavior when I say this, nor to blame the parents for it. Indeed, unlike Sara, many addicts are born into good, solid families, and will tell you they had ideal childhoods—on the surface, that is! After all, who knows what goes on in the soul of a child too young to speak?

Life is tough for everyone, and it need not be as tough as Sara's to be intolerable. Indeed, everybody experiences painful events at some point in their lives. This is normal. We are all born immature, totally dependent on our caretakers; and we are meant to grow and learn to be independent. Growing up is all about letting go of every familiar thing that brings you safety and learning to keep yourself safe instead. Eventually, everyone must let go of parental care—but this can be painful, and can provoke feelings of abandonment that psychologists call **separation anxiety**.

To mature and develop the inner strength they will use to keep themselves safe when they've grown up, all children need safety, structure, support, and some challenge. If such development takes place within a loving family that offers adequate support and encouragement, along with some limitations and exposure to frustrations, children learn important life lessons step by step. In small enough doses, poison acts like medicine, and the difficult experience of separation drives development and growth.

However, not all families are safe enough to provide opportunities for optimal growth. Sometimes things get complicated, and obstacles arise that impair a child's development. A family may, for instance, be either too cold or too distant, or it may not offer enough support to a growing child. On the other hand, a family may be far too close, **enmeshed**, with unclear boundaries that do not offer enough challenge as the child matures. Children from such families cannot learn how to react healthily to the outside world. And sometimes, even in the best of families, things happen that are just too difficult to bear. We use the word **trauma** to refer to a person's response to a situation so grave, it cannot be endured, and the traumatized person can only give up and prepare to die. There is no definitive measure that distinguishes how difficult a person's circumstances must be for that to happen; instead, a person's response is determined by the largely unquantifiable ratio between their capabilities at that time and the magnitude of the problem.

When trauma occurs, a psychological program is triggered to prepare the person for a life-or-death struggle. Unfortunately, it is not unusual for adults around a traumatized child to ignore the child's distress, leaving the child alone to manage his or her emotions. Let's say, for example, that a three-year-old child is left in the care of her father, who gets drunk and passes out on the kitchen floor. When crying and other efforts at communication fail, the child, experiencing abandonment for the first time in her life, sits in the dark, frozen with terror. She realizes there is no one to take care of her. But by the time the girl's mother comes home from the night shift, things are seemingly back to normal, and everybody pretends nothing was wrong.

As previously noted, almost everyone faces potentially traumatic events while growing up. However, even if that trauma is not extreme, it is important to bear in mind that not all people are equally **resilient** in the face of unpleasant or traumatic events, and that some people may thus react more negatively to certain events than others might. This is the case even among children from "normal" families in "normal" life circumstances—to say nothing of children from families that are outright hurtful and abusive, which increases the likelihood that those children will engage in extreme behaviors as a way to cope with their pain.

The fact is, no matter who you are, life hurts—and if you're a small child without emotional support, like the children from abusive families, there is little you can do to rid yourself of the causes of your pain, or to distance yourself from it. You're simply there, small and vulnerable, dealing with things as best you can. Indeed, it makes sense in those circumstances to do whatever you can to reduce the pain.

But what can a very young child do to numb pain? Dreaming of someone who will come and "save" them is one of the first avenues children have at their disposal. Or they may dream of being the hero who will "save" their mother, and that she will then take care of them, and everything will turn out alright. Beyond daydreaming, stuffing themselves with food, especially sweets, is also possible for children. Older children may discover the soothing effects of masturbation, while some children are sadly victims of sexual abuse, and learn that violence and sexual pleasure can override their anxiety.

What is common to all these behaviors? They are far "too" good. They give pleasure without demanding much effort. We feel pleasure with our brains—the most sophisticated objects in the known universe, meant to help us understand the world around us. The human brain wants us to remember things that feel good, so it takes special note of them, just as we might add a particular website to our list of "favorites" to find it later. This takes place in the part of the brain that deals with emotional experiences by releasing the chemical **dopamine**. If we repeat such pleasant behavior too often, our brains will create a special "shortcut" to prompt this pleasurable behavior, and engaging in the behavior will no longer be a matter of choice—it will become automatic.

We'll discuss this process in more detail later, but at this stage, let us just acknowledge that the basis for addiction is typically formed in childhood. In fact, the problems that later lead to addiction can be present in a child as young as three or four, and be first noticed in the later years of elementary school. However, these problems do not yet constitute addiction; rather, they are a weakness, a source of constant inner pain.

To ignore the things that hurt them, people—including children—often choose to engage in their favorite behavior, temporarily suppressing their pain but leaving its cause intact. As a result, the hurt underneath becomes worse and worse, and they tend to try more and more ways to ease the pain, leading to a vicious cycle. The beginnings of addiction often go unnoticed, as they develop slowly, with the future addict adjusting to small changes along the way until finally, full addiction results.

When an addict finally decides to go to therapy after decades of acting out, it's because the pleasurable behavior can no longer override the pain caused by the consequences of their addiction. Unfortunately, it usually takes a long time for them to come to that conclusion, because even in the throes of addiction, they have formed efficient systems of fooling themselves and others. They underestimate the consequences of their behavior and overestimate their family's patience until they reach a point some call "rock bottom." Before then, there is no point discussing their childhood and the causes of their addiction—it simply doesn't help. To begin correcting their mistaken ways of thinking, they must first sober up, literally— by abstaining not just from alcohol, but from everything that influences their minds.

5

Exercises to Recognize Addiction

People say talk is cheap—and that the road to hell is paved with good intentions. To make lasting positive changes in our lives, we must move beyond merely having good intentions and start working toward becoming autonomous and independent, keeping our promises, and reaching our goals—acting on our intentions, instead of acting out.

Yes, it's difficult! But choosing only the easiest paths in life will get you nowhere. There is no easy way out of addiction. If you want to get out, you need to stop looking for shortcuts and start taking the right paths—those that will get you where you need to be.

So . . . let's go! The following exercises are designed to further your understanding of the role addiction may have in your life and help you pave your way to a better and healthier future. Don't skip them, for they are the first part of the important work we all must do to improve our lives, whether we prove to be addicted to these harmful behaviors or not. Instead, try to embrace the change—after all, it's the only constant in life!

Exercise 1: What are the harmful behaviors I keep repeating?

This exercise lists behaviors typical of people suffering from various substance-based and behavioral addictions. As you read these lists, check the boxes corresponding to *all the behaviors you have ever repeated.*[13] Be sure to check acting out (overindulgent) as well as acting in (restrictive) behaviors, along with the typical beliefs commonly present alongside these addictions. Actions, after all, follow beliefs. The *belief* that one is worthless, flawed, or powerless can make someone feel bad, but if they discover drinking a shot of whiskey helps them feel better, they'll be motivated to repeat that *behavior* often—transforming their harmful habit into a full-blown addiction.

SUBSTANCE ADDICTIONS

Addiction to Alcohol

- Constantly drinking alcoholic beverages; getting drunk; or just sipping one drink after another, never really getting drunk, nor sobering up

- Trying and failing to control your drinking over certain periods

- Drinking more than you originally intended, especially as a result of a loss of control

- Unsuccessfully attempting to stop drinking

- Experiencing emotional outbursts when you are unable to drink

- Drinking to feel "normal"

- Experiencing hangovers the day after drinking, or losing your memory of what happened while you were drinking

- Developing a tolerance and needing to drink more to achieve the same effect

---

[13] You can also list the behaviors you used to have problems with, but managed to stop. Even these behaviors are important in creating a complete list of possible addictions you might face, so that you can be aware of any vulnerable areas in your psyche.

- Working or driving while under the influence

- Continuing to drink despite partners' or family members' threats to leave if you do not stop

- Continuing to drink despite health problems caused by alcohol consumption

- Appearing drunk in inappropriate situations (e.g., a parent-teacher meeting or hospital visit)

- Lying to yourself and others about how much you drink

- Spending a lot of time getting alcohol or recovering from drinking

- Other: ....

Addiction to Psychoactive Drugs[14]

- Regularly using psychoactive drugs in an attempt to feel better emotionally

- Experiencing distress if you are unable to obtain the drugs you want

- Experiencing withdrawal symptoms if you are unable to obtain the drugs you want

- Developing a tolerance and needing to increase the quantity of drugs taken to achieve the same effects

- Continuing to take drugs or engage in drug-seeking behavior despite partners' or family members' threats to leave if you do not stop

- Continuing to take drugs or engage in drug-seeking behavior despite threats of losing your job or reputation

---

[14] **Psychoactive drugs,** whether prescribed by a doctor or provided illegally, are those that act on the nervous system to alter consciousness, modify perceptions, and change moods.

- Hanging out with dangerous people in order to obtain drugs

- Acquiring drugs illegally

- Other: ....

Addiction to a Legal Substance (e.g., Sugar, Chocolate, Nicotine, or Caffeine)

- Consuming the substance despite previously having decided to give it up

- Consuming more and more of the substance more and more often

- Being unable to stop after having, for example, "just one" piece of cake or one cigarette

- Continuing to consume the substance despite developing health problems (e.g., obesity) as a result

- Experiencing withdrawal symptoms such as headaches, inability to concentrate, and restlessness if you avoid consuming the substance

- Going to disproportionate trouble to obtain the substance (e.g., driving twenty miles in the middle of the night to get chocolate or cigarettes)

- Hiding your supply of the substance from others, or worrying about not having enough

- Other: ....

BEHAVIORAL ADDICTIONS

Addictions to Food: Bulimia Nervosa and Compulsive Overeating

- Constantly thinking about or obsessing over food

- Devoting a lot of time and effort to maintaining a certain diet, and being extremely upset if you are unable to do so

- Obsessing over maintaining a certain body type

- Obsessing over your and others' body weight

- Constantly commenting on or controlling your own or others' eating habits

- Constantly comparing your body and eating habits to others'

- Planning meals well in advance, and becoming irritable if you are unable to stick to the plan

- Wolfing down food while alone, but eating little or nothing in public

- Eating enormous quantities of food in a short time, and even feeling unable to stop eating (**bingeing**)

- Purging by inducing vomiting after meals or abusing large quantities of laxatives

- Trying the latest "wonder diets" to lose weight or achieve some other goal, but abandoning them after a few weeks or months to start another diet

- Becoming ashamed and angry at yourself for overeating

- Losing control over your consumption of food (e.g., being unable to stop after only one piece of candy)

- Comforting yourself with food (**emotional eating**)

- Gaining and losing weight rapidly (e.g., fluctuating up to twenty pounds per month)

- Obsessing over exercise and becoming extremely rest-less if you are unable to work out

- Other: ....

Addictions to Food: Anorexia Nervosa and Orthorexia

- Rapidly losing weight or failing to gain weight when your weight drops below 15 percent of that expected for a person of your age and height, or when your BMI is less than 17.5

- Constantly thinking about or obsessing over food

- Experiencing extreme dread at the thought of gaining weight

- Devoting a lot of time and effort to maintaining a certain diet, and being extremely upset if you are unable to do so

- Bingeing and purging

- Sticking to an extremely restrictive diet, refusing to eat certain types of food (e.g., carbs or fats), or eating only certain foods

- Having an unrealistic perception of your body (e.g., viewing yourself as overweight even if you are danger-ously underweight)

- Obsessing over maintaining a certain body type

- Obsessing over your and others' body weight

- Constantly commenting on or controlling your own or others' eating habits

- Constantly comparing your body and eating habits to others'

- Planning meals well in advance, and becoming irritable

if you are unable to stick to the plan

- Fasting to the point of experiencing extreme fatigue, dizziness, or faintness

- Experiencing **amenorrhea**—the absence of a menstrual period in women, or failure to begin a menstrual cycle in girls—in combination with low body weight

- Constantly feeling cold

- Exercising to an extreme degree in order to "burn calories"

- Experiencing suicidal thoughts

- Undertaking extreme or unbalanced diets, or fasting to "cleanse" your body

- Being afraid of food

- Other: ....

Addiction to Work

- Constantly working overtime despite health problems, conflicts in the family, and signs that your children are being neglected

- Feeling anxious if you cannot control what is going on at work (e.g., during your vacation time)

- Losing your sense of time while working

- Working even when you are sick out of the belief something terrible might happen if you stay at home and rest (e.g., that you'll be laid off or demoted)

- Experiencing rage-fueled outbursts, irritation, sleeplessness, tension, impatience, forgetfulness, problems with concentration, and changing moods if you are unable to work

- Feeling extremely anxious if you cannot achieve perfection at work

- Constantly thinking about what else needs to be done at work

- Burning out and being unable to do any professional work for a long period

- Alternating between working too much and being unable to work at all

- Believing you are irreplaceable in your work role

- Believing work is the most important thing in life

- Other: ....

Addictions to Money (Spending, Shopping, Debt) and Risk

- Believing your happiness depends on how much money you have

- Obsessing over earning money

- Hoarding money or luxury items

- Obtaining money in unfair or illegal ways (e.g., fraud, scams, selling useless or stolen objects)

- Shopping to improve your mood

- Being "in the red" most of the time

- Taking out loans to cover loans

- Investing in risky businesses, lending money to unreliable people or gamblers, or investing in money chains or cryptocurrencies

- Refusing to spend money you have saved for important

things, like buying or renting a place to stay; or preferring to live in poor conditions so you can save

- Spending your partner's money as revenge when they neglect you (**financial infidelity**)

- Being constantly in debt to people who are emotionally important to you as a means of maintaining a connection to them, or using money as a measure of how important you are to loved ones (**financial dependence**)

- Taking responsibility for paying off the debts of addicted family members (e.g., gamblers or drug addicts) so they do not leave you (**financial enabling**)

- Taking excessive financial risks

- Borrowing from dangerous or unreliable people

- Making risky business decisions

- Ignoring and violating financial regulations

- Driving dangerously, engaging in high-risk sports, or otherwise living "on the edge"

- Other: ....

Addiction to Gambling
- Gambling with the purpose of "earning" money

- Experiencing conflicts with family members due to gambling

- Being absent from work or school because of gambling

- Spending more money gambling than you can afford

- Gambling or "staying in the game" longer than you originally intended

- Going into debt as a result of gambling

- Committing fraud or theft to obtain money you can use to gamble

- Attempting to recoup your losses by doubling down and increasing your bets (**chasing losses**)

- Alternating between periods of obsessive gambling and periods of compulsively working to try to cover your debts

- Being convinced there exists a method for overcoming "the machine" or "the house"

- Believing fortune or luck is on your side and the next big win is just around the corner

- Being convinced fortune will come your way if you always play your favorite machine, and feeling that if someone else plays "your" machine, they may get away with "your" money

- Other: ....

Addiction to Video Games

- Obsessively playing video games at the expense of other important activities (e.g., school, work, dating, friends, family, etc.)

- Losing track of time while playing video games, or playing longer than you originally intended

- Spending a lot of time thinking about video games, even when you are not playing them (e.g., reliving past experiences or planning your next game session)

- Needing to play longer to achieve your original level of satisfaction

- Seeking ever more stimulating (i.e., exciting, new, or

more challenging) video games, or using more powerful equipment, to achieve the same level of satisfaction

- Feeling restless, moody, angry, anxious, bored, sad, or
  irritable when you are unable to play video games, or
  attempt (or are forced) to cut down on the time you
  spend playing video games

- Playing video games as a way to escape or forget about
  personal problems or reduce negative feelings (e.g.,
  boredom, frustration, anxiety, anger, shame, depression,
  etc.)

- Lying to family members, therapists, or others to hide
  the extent of your gaming

- Committing illegal or maladaptive acts related to the
  use of video games

- Losing work, educational opportunities, and relationships as a direct or indirect result of playing video
  games

- Performing poorly in school as a direct or indirect result of playing video games

- Experiencing health problems as a direct or indirect result of playing video games, and continuing to game despite these problems

- Feeling intense anger if parents or friends take away
  your computer, tablet, smartphone, or gaming console

- Neglecting sleep or recreational activities, such as
  friendships or hobbies you previously enjoyed, to play
  video games

- Getting angry at and insulting players who play poorly
  or make mistakes while playing a video game

- Other: ....

Addictions to the Internet and Social Media

- Spending time scrolling through social media and news at the expense of other important activities like performing your job, completing schoolwork, visiting family, or going out with friends

- Feeling unable to stop scrolling through social media despite the problems it creates (lack of sleep, isolation, etc.)

- Obsessively thinking about social media even when you are not online

- Feeling the need to post every trivial detail of your life online in anticipation of receiving reactions in the form of "likes"

- Feeling pressure to compete with and compare yourself to other users

- Feeling depressed and envious if you believe your life and achievements are not as impressive as those of other social media users

- Feeling the urge to check your news feed regularly each day, and feeling anxious if you are unable to do so

- Frequently arguing with others over your use of social media

- Hiding your use of social media—especially dating sites—from your partner or family

- Using the Internet, email, or social media to send intimidating or threatening messages (**cyberbullying**)

- Procrastinating or wasting time by checking your news feed instead of working

- Anticipating "likes" and notifications to the degree that

it interferes with your normal functioning

- Experiencing fatigue and stress, including sleep disorders, due to your use of social media

- Using social media despite the potential for severe consequences (e.g., checking your messages while driving or while logged into a work computer)

- Experiencing health issues such as headaches, blurry vision due to strained eyes as a result of long hours spent staring at a screen, back and neck pain due to consistent bending of the neck to look at your phone, or carpal tunnel syndrome[15] as a result of your use of electronics

- Other: ....

Addiction to Romance

- Constantly thinking about your romantic relationship

- Feeling desperate and alone when not in a relationship

- Using sex, seduction, or manipulation to attract or hold onto a partner

- Feigning interest in activities you don't enjoy as a way of meeting someone new or holding onto an existing partner

- Being unable to enjoy close relationships, even if you want to

- Constantly being in love, but changing partners, immediately entering a new relationship after a breakup, or even having several partners at once

---

[15] **Carpal tunnel syndrome** is a medical condition caused by compression of the median nerve as it travels through the wrist, which occurs due to long hours of repeating the same movement with one's hands and arms.

- Using multiple dating sites to hook up with new lovers, or just to feel the rush of excitement when someone chooses you—even when you are already in a committed relationship

- Obsessively considering every person of your preferred sex as a potential love partner, regardless of their personal attributes

- Feeling worthless without a partner

- Missing out on important commitments (to family, your job, etc.) to search for a new partner or fix an existing relationship

- Repeatedly swearing to give up hunting for new relationships, but not following through

- Other: ....

Addiction to "Love"

- Constantly thinking about your love relationship

- Expecting your partner to change or make your life perfect

- Feeling a loss of identity if a partner leaves you

- Feeling desperate and alone when you are not in a relationship

- Staying in destructive relationships out of a fear of abandonment

- Trying to control or change your partner to improve the relationship

- Giving up important hobbies, friendships, or activities you don't share with your partner

- Missing out on important commitments (to family, your job, etc.) to fix an existing relationship

- Stalking or blackmailing an ex-partner to convince them to return to you

- Constantly struggling to maintain the sexual or romantic intensity in your relationship

- Using sex, seduction, or manipulation to attract or hold onto a partner

- Repeatedly swearing to end the relationship and focus on yourself, but not following through

- Other: ....

Codependence and Addiction to Destructive Relationships

- Constantly thinking about your romantic relationship

- Expecting your partner to change or make your life perfect

- Feeling a loss of identity if a partner leaves you

- Feeling desperate and alone when not in a relationship

- Staying in destructive relationships out of a fear of abandonment

- Trying to control or change your partner to improve the relationship

- Giving up important hobbies, friendships, or activities you don't share with your partner

- Missing out on important commitments (to family, your job, etc.) to fix an existing relationship

- Taking care of your partner, but not yourself

- Choosing emotionally unavailable, married, sociopathic, narcissistic, or addicted partners

- Staying with a partner who abuses you physically, psychologically, or sexually

- Taking pride in staying in a destructive relationship because you feel your partner needs you

- Constantly struggling to maintain the sexual or romantic intensity in your relationship

- Using sex, seduction, or manipulation to attract or hold onto a partner

- Feigning interest in activities you don't enjoy in order to hold onto a partner

- Being unable to enjoy close relationships, even if you want to

- Repeatedly swearing to end the relationship and focus on yourself, but not following through

- Other: ....

Addiction to Sex[16]

- Constantly thinking about sex, fantasizing about past sexual encounters, or planning future sexual encounters

- Masturbating excessively or compulsively

- Frequently and obsessively consuming pornography in any form

- Engaging in frequent and compulsive sex with prostitutes of any gender

- Engaging in frequent and compulsive anonymous sex with multiple partners to achieve a sexual high

---

[16] Adapted from Patrick Carnes, *Facing the Shadow: Starting Sexual and Relationship Recovery* (Carefree, AZ: Gentle Path Press, 2010), 76–78.

- Being sexual without genuinely intending to have a relationship, and without being truthful about your intentions (**seductive sex**)

- Engaging in multiple affairs while in a committed relationship

- Obtaining sexual pleasure from exposing your private parts and performing sexual acts in front of other people (**exhibitionism**)

- Obtaining sexual pleasure from watching others when they are naked or engaging in sexual activity (**voyeurism**)

- Obtaining sexual pleasure from rubbing against another person while in a crowd (**frotteurism**)

- Being aroused by sadistic activities, such as hurting or degrading another sexually (**sadism**)

- Being aroused by masochistic activities, such as being hurt or degraded (**masochism**)

- Exploiting children, the disabled, or otherwise vulnerable persons for your own sexual pleasure

- Other: ....

Co-sex Addiction (Sexual Codependence)

- Dressing and behaving seductively, even if you do not want to, out of a belief your partner is being unfaithful because you are not attractive or sexually proactive enough

- Trying to get revenge on a cheating sex-addicted partner by being unfaithful yourself

- Believing you must behave or dress in a certain way to control your sex-addicted partner's sexual drive

- Withdrawing sexually as a way to control your partner's sexuality

- Believing the sex addict's promises that "it won't happen again"

- Ignoring your friends when they tell you of the sex addict's acting out

- Lying about, rationalizing, or covering up the sex addict's behavior

- Obsessing over the sex addict (e.g., constantly looking for clues to their acting out, checking their spending habits or where they have been and for how long, etc.)

- Experiencing memory loss, unpredictable behavior, or destructive acts against yourself or others, produced by preoccupation with the sex addict

- Experiencing accidents, destructive acts perpetrated against yourself or others, or other dangerous situations produced by preoccupation with the sex addict

- Experiencing severe mood changes—from hope to fear, from grief to self-pity, from anger to guilt, and back to hope again—in progressive cycles, leading to a state of numbness

- Ignoring your own sense of sexual boundaries, morals, or ethics to please your sexually addicted partner and prevent abandonment—for example, agreeing to a threesome, swinging, or imitating a porn scene when you don't actually enjoy these acts

- Being afraid to admit you don't enjoy certain sex acts

- Other: ....

Sexual Anorexia

- Avoiding situations where sexual proposals may happen

- Feeling shame and disgust at nudity and provocative pictures, situations, or words in the context of normal social situations (e.g., on billboards or in movies)

- Dressing "down" to avoid being seen as sexually provocative

- Considering yourself sexually unappealing and rejecting any sexual interest from others as a result

- Choosing jobs that allow you to avoid public interaction out of anxiety and fear of embarrassing yourself in front of others

- Feeling unworthy of the relationships you desire, and refraining from ever attempting to enter into one

- Missing out on important commitments to family, work, and other important areas of your life in order to avoid exposure to sexual topics

- Being unable to enjoy intimate relationships, even if you want to

- Spending a great deal of time anxiously studying others for signs of approval or rejection

- Other: ....

List your thoughts while working on this exercise:

....

Discuss your answers with a trusted friend, and take notes on your conversation:

....

....

....

Exercise 2: What problems do I have as a result of these behaviors?

The behaviors you checked in the previous exercise have negative consequences. Addicts often do not want to admit that—and if they do, they will not admit their problems have anything to do with their behaviors. Of course, if they did, that would be a reason to stop engaging in those behaviors—which they do not want to do. But if you really want to live free of addiction, you need to take responsibility for your actions and their consequences. Ultimately, addicts only decide to stop engaging in these harmful behaviors and take control of their addictions when they admit the consequences of those addictions are ruining their lives.

Consider the categories from the previous exercise. Which listed behaviors did you recognize as your own? Copy those behaviors into the list below, and then write down the troubles you have in life because of them. This list of the negative consequences of your behaviors will help you stay motivated to avoid those behaviors when your conviction to remain sober starts fading. Be sincere and thorough as you consider those consequences, and remember that even though you may easily be able to find people with more significant problems than you, that does not necessarily mean you are doing well.

Example:

Harmful Behavior #1: Choosing emotionally unavailable, married, sociopathic, narcissistic, or addicted partners (a sign of **relationship addiction***)*

Resulting problems: My adult children refuse to contact me because they do not want to witness my partner humiliating me.

Harmful Behavior #1:

....

Resulting Problems:

....

....

....

Harmful Behavior #2:

....

Resulting Problems:

....

....

....

Harmful Behavior #3:

....

Resulting Problems:

....

....

....

Harmful Behavior #4:

....

Resulting Problems:

....

....

....

Harmful Behavior #5:

....

Resulting Problems:

....

....

....

List your thoughts while working on this exercise:

....

....

....

Discuss your answers with a trusted friend, and take notes on your conversation:

....

....

....

Exercise 3: Is it an addiction or not?

The moment of truth! As many a psychotherapist will tell you, a diagnosis of addiction does not depend on *what* you do, nor on *how much* or *how often* you do it. Other criteria exist to help you decide whether your repetitive, harmful behavior constitutes an addiction or not. These are the same criteria doctors use, so if you consider them honestly, the result will be as reliable as their diagnosis—maybe even more so, because there is no point in lying to yourself. As such, you may have a clearer picture of your addiction than your doctor, to whom you may be ashamed to admit certain truths about your life.

In this exercise, consider the behaviors you identified in Exercise 1 that you assessed as the *most harmful* in Exercise 2. Choose one behavior and see if it fits the eleven criteria listed below. *Note that for a person to be diagnosed with addiction, they must display at least two of the following eleven criteria within twelve months.* The presence of two or three criteria indicates a mild problem, the presence of four or five indicates a moderate problem, and the presence of six or more is indicative of severe addiction.

*Example: You suspect you might have a **sex addiction**—an obsessive interest in sexual activities and porn. You consider the following list, and discover your experience is consistent with criteria 1, 2, 5, 8, and 10. This is an addiction!*

The Criteria for Addiction

1. Engaging in the behavior longer than you originally meant to

2. Wanting to cut down on or stop engaging in the behavior, but not managing to

3. Spending a lot of time engaging in, or recovering after engaging in, the behavior

4. Feeling cravings and urges to engage in the behavior

5. Failing to meet obligations at work, home, or school because of the behavior

6. Continuing to engage in the behavior even when it causes problems in your relationships

7. Giving up important social, occupational, or recreational activities to engage in the behavior, or as a result of its consequences

8. Continuing to engage in the behavior even when it puts you in danger

9. Continuing to engage in the behavior even when you know it may be causing or worsening a physical or psychological problem from which you suffer

10. Developing a tolerance—needing to engage in the behavior more often to achieve the effect you want

11. Developing withdrawal symptoms when you do not engage in the behavior

List your thoughts while working on this exercise:

....

....

....

Discuss your answers with a trusted friend, and take notes on your conversation:

....

....

....

PART TWO:

HOW TO UNDERSTAND ADDICTION

"Human beings have a deep need to bond and form connections.
If we can't connect with each other, we will connect with
whatever we can find . . .
It is disconnection that drives addiction."

— Christopher Kennedy Lawford

6

Know Your Enemy!

"I can stop whenever I really want to."

That's what they all say, don't they? But for addicts, this no longer holds true.

After finishing the first set of exercises, you may have concluded that the behaviors ruining your life are simply bad habits. After all, habits can be changed if one only wants to change them. But with addiction, this is not the case. In cases of addiction, something more profound, operating at an unconscious level, seemingly hijacks the addict's ability to stick to their good intentions to change their harmful habits and behaviors. What is it? Know your enemy!

There is a lot of confusion and misunderstanding surrounding addiction. Since almost everyone has some experience with it, many people believe they understand it when in actuality, their understanding consists only of common prejudices and incorrect, outdated "facts." **Denial** and **projection**—both the addict's and their families' and friends'—add to the mess,[17] along with an unbelievable social tolerance for the misery an addict's family experiences. Often, the addict's acting out and its consequences for their families remain hidden from the rest of society for years—until an invisible line is crossed. Then the

---

[17] **Denial** and **projection** are common psychological strategies people unconsciously use to protect themselves from anxiety arising from unacceptable thoughts or feelings.

tables turn, and the addicts are blamed and punished for both what they did and did not do while in the grip of their addiction.

Many of the misunderstandings surrounding addiction stem from the fact that most people consider only one aspect of the disease. They say, for example: "John drinks too much and is difficult at times, but he is a good worker and a devoted father, and his children need him"—ignoring the proven fact that so many children of alcoholics will suffer complex post-traumatic consequences. These will become evident only after decades, when the said children have formed their own partnerships, and their impaired ability to bond becomes evident.

However, addiction has consequences on many other levels as well. Doctors are interested in how addiction may cause impairment at the level of the *brain* and other organs. Meanwhile, psychotherapists talk about controlling the *behaviors* associated with addiction, only rarely delving deeper to determine their causes. Social workers, family therapists, and legislators are concerned with addressing problems addiction may cause within the *family*, while sociologists debate the *culture* of addiction.

All of these professionals engage in valuable pursuits, for addiction reaches and affects all levels of the human experience. Let's first take a quick look at these different levels, as an overview. Then, in separate chapters, we will explore them in more detail.

Addiction at Different Levels of the Human Experience

- **Problems at the level of the brain**

  Scientists are just beginning to understand the processes in the human brain that enable us to feel, think, love, and judge aspects of the world around us. However, they already know that addiction changes the brain's neural pathways, which convey and control emotion, pleasure, risk, motivation, memory, and related aspects of the human experience. Different addictions affect these same pathways in different proportions, but the addictive process works similarly in all cases. And while the brain cannot be cured of neurological diseases like addiction, once the damaging behavior has ceased, the brain will slowly and independently recover its normal functioning.

- **Problems at the level of thinking, feeling, judgment, and belief**

   Addicts often possess a set of thoughts and beliefs that help maintain their disease. Typically, these thoughts and beliefs consist of toxic shame, feelings of low self-esteem, cravings, the **addiction cycle**, and the **addictive system**.[18] Three years is an optimistic assessment of the time it takes a recovering addict to permanently change such beliefs.

- **Problems at the level of behavior**

   To look inside the brain, we need the latest medical equipment; to learn about feeling and thinking, we rely on what addicts tell us. But an addict's behavior can be seen with our own eyes, and we can trust it to tell us the truth about that person.

   As you completed the first exercise in this book, you were confronted with a long list of adverse behaviors addicts cannot cease on their own. Unfortunately, to stop engaging in unwanted behavior, one must do more than merely *want* to stop. Changes at deeper levels are necessary.

- **Problems at the level of the family**

   Addiction often runs in families. A family is a complex organism composed of many people, each contributing to the whole and all interdependent. As the older family members take care of the younger family members, they also transfer their systems of thinking and values to the younger generation, teaching them what life is supposed to be like—and passing down their addictive systems of thinking as well.

- **Problems at the level of society**

   In general, most people seem able to accept that addiction exists, and that people can suffer and even die of it—as long as it stays away from their own families! As a society, how-

---

[18] See Chapter 8 for an explanation of the addiction cycle and the addictive system.

ever, we seem unaware of how addiction—which is essentially a quest for eternal happiness, free of all pain and suffering—can spring from modern consumerist values, which afford praise and admiration to those with the most money or belongings. We have a pill or a diet for every minor ailment that befalls us, and often strive to make pleasure and happiness the center of our lives. Can you see where such thinking may lead?

Whether you are worried you may be an addict yourself, or are concerned for a loved one who exhibits problematic behaviors like those listed in Exercise 1, addiction may affect your life on many levels—and to battle it, you must arm yourself with knowledge. You must do away with prejudices and misunderstandings about addiction that might cause you to fail. You must update your understanding of addiction. To do this, let's look at the effects of addiction at each of the levels of the human experience more thoroughly.

7

Problems at the Level of the Brain

When I started working as a physician almost forty years ago, most professionals and laypeople believed addiction was primarily an issue of loose morals and irresponsible self-indulgence, and that substances like alcohol or drugs were responsible for turning people into addicts. But a decade later, when I started working with recovering addicts, they taught me there is an underlying pathological change in addicts' thinking that makes them resistant to change for the better. At the time, we assumed this change occurred at the level of the brain, and believed it was what made addiction a disease. But we weren't yet able to prove it.

In the last ten years or so, exciting new discoveries have led to the development of **brain scanning techniques** that directly or indirectly image the structure, function, and pharmacology of the nervous system. Now we can actually observe the parts of the brain as they function. When the brain's neural pathways are active, what we used to observe as merely "gray" and "white" matter can now be illuminated. We can observe the differences between the brain scans of healthy people, addicts, and those with other brain diseases. As a result of this research, we can speculate that a change in the perceived functioning of the brain—which can be shown in a brain scan—is connected to a change in behavior.

As it turns out, the brain scans of people with substance addictions look excitingly similar to those of persons with behavioral addictions, suggesting both types of addiction involve the same underlying pathological change. This is something doctors and research scientists suspected for a long time—but now, we can prove it!

Ultimately, observation of brain scans has taught us *addiction is a chronic brain disease affecting the connected circuits—the systems—of the brain responsible for reward, motivation, memory, and related processes.* Our brains are made up of thousands of **neurons**, nerve cells that connect with thousands of other nerve cells in an intricate web that conducts electrical and chemical impulses. The brain's primary function is to learn. When a person engages in learning, new connections are forged in the brain, and some old ones are eliminated. This is how the things we learn become physically engraved in our brains. It takes a lot of repetition to change a neural pathway, but once it is changed—that is, when a piece of information is encoded, or learned—that pathway can persist throughout a person's life—unless it is changed again.

IMAGE 1: A simple model of the brain anatomy

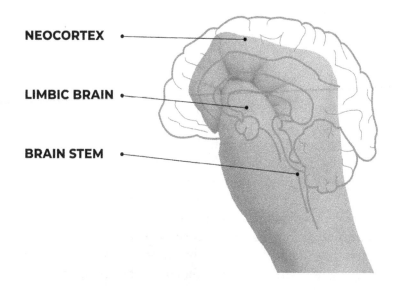

NEOCORTEX

LIMBIC BRAIN

BRAIN STEM

Dr. Daniel J. Siegel, a clinical professor of psychiatry at the UCLA School of Medicine and executive director of the Mindsight Institute, developed this very simple model of brain anatomy comparing each hemisphere of the brain to a fist. The brain is made up of two "fists," representing the left and right hemispheres and mirroring each other. In this model, the fingers represent the part of the brain right behind the forehead. We call this the **neocortex**, and it is the seat of thinking, judgment, and reason. The area in the center of the fist—the palm of the hand and the thumb—represent the **limbic brain**, the part of the brain that allows us to feel emotions. We sometimes call this the reptilian or "lizard" brain, partly because it looks just like a lizard curled up in the brain, and partly because it is the seat of instinct. It doesn't consciously think; it feels. Its function is to warn us of pending danger and see that we get away in time. Meanwhile, the wrist represents the **brain stem**, which takes care of the body's automatic functions, such as breathing and digesting.

In normal circumstances, the neocortex has authority over most other parts of the brain, and allows us to check whether our plans make sense before we act. If the lower centers of the brain want to eat, play, or have sex, the thinking brain checks whether these actions are appropriate, and if they are not, it can decide not to undertake them. However, it has been proven that in addicts, the baser parts of the brain take command, hijacking the neocortex. This means that though an addict may well know an action they take is wrong and inappropriate, they do it anyway. (Sound familiar?)

But how does this hijacking happen? It happens because the brain learns. Indeed, addiction is different from most other diseases because it is learned. While learning, the brain sorts experiences into good and bad ones, marking memories of pleasant experiences with **dopamine** and other chemicals to allow us to remember and return to them later. This is how we experience pleasure. A sense of pleasure may be so great, it can even override the experience of pain—which is a good solution, provided the pain is only temporary. But if the pain is chronic, as it is when a child suffers neglect because of his parents' drinking, that emergency measure will be used too often, and become habitual. The brain will adapt, releasing more and more dopamine in an effort to mask the pain—and eventually driving the child to seek substances that deliver the same effect, rather than solutions that may resolve the problem. At the same time, the brain will develop resistance to the dopamine, meaning progressively more of it is necessary to trigger the pleasurable reaction. Soon, the unfortunate child may seek a shot of dopamine just to weather a lousy day, or if they are tormented by an unpleasant memory. It's like taking a shot of heroin every time you feel uneasy, for dopamine is a thousand times more potent than heroin!

Our brain is the source of potent chemicals that change how we think and feel. This explains how behavioral addictions can have the same effects and consequences as substance addictions, even though no drugs are involved: the brain itself produces these addictive substances, and can be trained to do so through engaging in certain pleasurable behaviors!

Humans spend almost twenty years maturing, during which time the brain undergoes dramatic changes. Between the ages of eleven and twenty, the brain is especially vulnerable to ingested, inhaled, or injected mind-altering substances, including nicotine and alcohol. However, we all know teens often experiment with drinking and drugs. Recent research has proven that preventing children from getting drunk or using drugs before they fully mature could be an essential factor in preventing them from becoming addicted to those substances later. Parents, teachers, and others who work with teens can use this research to support their warnings against drinking and using drugs before adulthood. In this way, we can see how learning about addiction can directly improve your ability to cope with it.

When it comes to addiction, problems at the level of the brain manifest themselves as addictive cravings and increased tolerance. We'll discuss both below.

Addictive cravings

For healthy people, food is just food, and sex is just sex. A healthy person can want these things, but choose not to partake of them—since, if they want something, they first check with their thinking brain to determine whether indulging their want is socially and personally acceptable, or not. But instead of merely wanting these or other experiences, addicts experience **cravings**. These feelings consist of more than merely wanting something very badly, and they are much worse. When we crave something, it is our primitive "lizard" brain that wants it. The object of desire feels not like a want, but like a need, required for our very survival—and no amount of reasoning can convince us otherwise. When they experience cravings, addicts genuinely feel as if they may die if they do not indulge in the focus of their craving—immediately.

Increased tolerance

After using alcohol or other mind-altering substances consistently, often over an extended period, a person must partake of more and more of the substance to achieve the same effect. Their body has begun adapting to the chemicals associated with that substance, and they have developed an **increased tolerance** to it. This increased tolerance is one of the signs of addiction.

The body's ability to respond by adaptation is one of its most wonderful features. But if the brain is overwhelmed with too many pleasurable events, as an addict's is, it responds by becoming less sensitive to them. That means events that would be pleasurable for most people become neutral for an addict.

Increased tolerance is also a feature of behavioral addictions. A typical example can be seen in sex addicts who abuse online pornography to arouse themselves sexually. Like online search engines, pornographic websites can "learn" users' preferences. If a user frequently visits such sites, as addicts do, the algorithms soon decipher their sexual arousal templates and guide them toward further examples of their "perfect," tailor-made erotic image. Bombarded by thousands of these images, the addicts' bodies respond by heightening their response threshold. Now, if the stimulation is not intense enough, their brains will not secrete dopamine, and they will feel no pleasure. As a result, porn addicts soon find that normal human sexual behaviors no longer arouse them—which usually leads to impotence when faced with their partners. After all, how can an ordinary, imperfect mortal woman compete with such idealized images? Some studies have even found that teenagers who use porn become incapable of sexual intercourse, able to react only to extreme pornographic imagery obtained from the Internet.

To overcome this problem, addicts seek progressively more intense experiences. Here, dopamine has a mighty helper: adrenaline. *Danger, violence,* and *forbidden or disgusting images or scenarios* release all kinds of chemicals into the brain, enhancing the experience. When the addiction progresses, the addict must use more and more of the drug/behavior to achieve the same result. Proceeding in this direction leads the addict to feel terrible in the absence of their chosen stimulus, but only a little better in its presence. They now use the substance or engage in the behavior just to feel normal, and the initial sensation of pleasure is almost entirely lost.

Along with this change, the consequences of not adequately dealing with the psychological root of their addiction arise. The negative consequences of their addictive behaviors pile up, leading to more bad feelings, and a vicious circle is formed. Soon, they need to use substances or engage in addictive behaviors just to feel and perform *normally,* and to weather the bad feelings derived from the substance or behavior itself. As the old saying goes: *"First a man takes a drink; then the drink takes a drink; then the drink takes a man!"*

Adriana's Story

Adriana's letter is an excellent example of how danger can begin to appear attractive due to changes in brain chemistry:

> *I was walking my dog when . . . I came into contact with the part of me that drags me down into this cave of shame. That part is so hurtful, and makes me feel so impoverished! I felt so small, worthless, dirty, and ugly. There was nothing good or sincere there. Just pain and the screaming for more pain. "Longing" for abuse because the abuse was the only*

thing it knew, the only thing that made me feel anything at all.

When this part of me comes alive, everything else shuts down. Everything that meant something before loses its meaning. There's only a wish for danger, to be a captive— even more, to be threatened! To be able to feel everything I'm not able or allowed to feel. This is a terrible, terrible world, where everything is so dark, dangerous, and dirty; but I have to go there because there's a part of me inside that is nonexistent outside. It is a part to which the physical doesn't matter, the pain doesn't matter, tomorrow doesn't matter. . . . All that matters is just feeling the feelings I'm not allowed to feel, even just for a moment. It's just like a magnet, pulling me toward it, only much stronger. It feels like it's my only means of survival. If I don't do it, I'll die. I want it NOW! It's so powerful! I have no limits. I feel no remorse or empathy. I go all the way. Alone! This is the part of me that comes alive when I drink. Alcohol is the key to that door, it's the point of entry, and then . . . it's sex. And both of them combined . . . wow!

8

Problems at the Level of Thinking, Feeling, Judgment, and Beliefs

Addiction is a disease of the brain's reward, motivation, memory, and related systems. It changes the way people think and feel, how they judge themselves and the world around them, and even what they believe. And although we cannot observe it directly at first, it eventually shows itself in persistent changed behavior. *An addict's inability to stop engaging in a certain behavior despite negative consequences in the family, at work, with money, to their reputation, and in other aspects of their lives is so typical that this inability is one of the diagnostic criteria for addiction.*

As an addict's behavior changes, becoming more and more illogical, the addict must gradually change the way they think and reason in an attempt to make sense of their new behavior. Denial and other defense mechanisms take over the addict's mind, changing their interpretation of what is happening and providing them with excuses for doing what they know is not right—thus taking them even further from the solid ground of truth. Eventually, their systems of beliefs change as well, solidifying into a new form that enables their addiction.

In his book *Out of the Shadows: Understanding Sexual*

Addiction, Patrick Carnes, PhD, asserts most addicts believe these statements:[19]

- I am basically a very bad person.

- No one will love me as I am.

- If I had to rely on others, my needs would never be met.

- My drug/behavior is my most important need.

In addition, addicts report changes in how they feel emotions. They experience:

- Increased anxiety, depression, and emotional pain;

- Increased sensitivity to stress as a result of overstimulation of their stress system, combined with decreased sensitivity to normal pleasure; and

- Difficulty experiencing emotions and understanding what they mean.

They also experience problems at the level of thinking, feeling, judgment, and belief, including:

- Loss of control over their own actions,

- Toxic shame, and

- The addiction cycle and addictive system, defined later in this chapter.

Loss of control—operating on autopilot

As we have discussed, the brain's function is to learn. We have all experienced what happens when we repeat an action many times: we become more and more fluent and confident in what we do, until eventually, we have learned to do it so thoroughly, we can do it without effort. For example, when we first get into a car to learn to drive, we struggle to remember how to operate

---

[19] Patrick Carnes, *Out of the Shadows: Understanding Sexual Addiction* (Center City, MN: Hazelden, 2001), 152.

all the levers and buttons, and try to look in the rearview mirror and at the road ahead at the same time. But after a while, we become used to the steps and actions required to drive, and can do so for hours without much active thinking. Our bodies and brains have learned to operate the vehicle without our conscious input, and we can chat or listen to music and still drive without any problems.

In a way, being able to perform on autopilot is useful: it allows us to save energy and accomplish many tasks simultaneously. But it can backfire when we realize we just wolfed down that piece of cake from the fridge without being aware of doing so—even though we consciously knew we shouldn't eat it—because we were on "autopilot." When an addict engages in a negative behavior too often, their brain eventually learns to conduct that behavior so easily, it becomes hard for the addict to notice they're doing it—and hard for them to stop.

Toxic shame

Everybody feels shame sometimes. It is an **adaptive emotion**,[20] because it helps us behave in a way that allows us to be accepted in society. When we break some social rule by, for example, not being appropriately dressed for a certain occasion, a feeling of shame makes us aware of others' disapproval so we can correct our mistake. But some people feel **toxic shame**—meaning they are ashamed of *who they are*, not just *what they do*. Since our sense of self is not an action that can be corrected, toxic shame is much more painful than typical shame.

I was surprised to hear a client say she was ashamed her father was a drunk. Her father's behavior was not her fault, and there was nothing she could do to change it. Her shame, therefore, was not about anything she was doing, but rather derived from her relationship to an embarrassing family member. Nevertheless, that shame hurt her, so it made perfect sense to her to try to numb those feelings through any means that worked. And ultimately, it led her down the path to addiction.

---

[20] **Adaptive emotions** are those that enable an individual to adjust to their environment appropriately and effectively.

Addiction cycles and the addictive system

All the changes to an addict's behavior and thinking operate together in a special cycle that soon takes on a life of its own. We call this the **addiction cycle**.

IMAGE 2: The addiction cycle

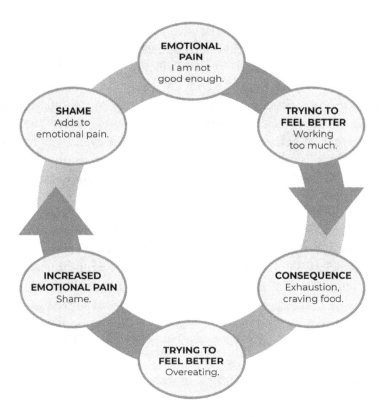

The addiction cycle starts with a feeling that you are not good enough. Feeling shame for who you are, you try to do something to feel better. But when this fails to rid you of your shame in the long term, you feel additional shame for failing—so you feel a little worse off than you did before. To get rid of the initial shame as well as the new, additional shame, you engage in the same behavior you used to attempt to make yourself feel better the first time, ultimately failing again—and on and on, feeling worse and worse at the end of each cycle.

Such cycles can repeat themselves many times a day, resulting in added shame that sucks you down into the deep, desperate hole of helplessness. With each turn, you go deeper. This is how an addiction forms. We call this "tornado" of multiple addiction cycles the **addictive system.**

IMAGE 3: The "tornado" of addiction

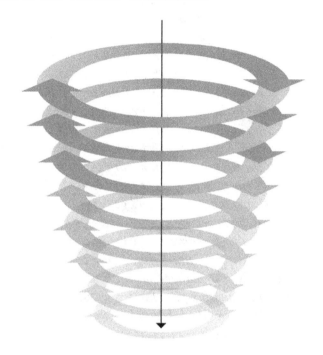

Karen's Story

Let's see how the addiction cycle plays out in Karen's case:

> *When I start my day, I'm all enthusiastic and confident that today will be the day I finally start my new life—that I'll no longer waste my life by trying to change what cannot be changed. I exercise, meditate, and prepare myself a good breakfast. I'm sure I'm in control of my life, and looking forward to the good times ahead.*
>
> *I get on my bike and feel proud of getting some exercise on the way to work. Everything seems fine. But I've*

set off a little too late, and the traffic is heavy, so I'm fif-
teen minutes late for work, again. My boss meets me at the
door, looking at his watch with his eyebrows raised. If only
I could disappear into a great big hole in the ground! All the
good feeling is now gone. I see him talking to his secretary,
and I'm sure they're discussing my dismissal. In my chest,
I feel a painful emptiness. I cannot work; I'm too stressed.
Then the secretary comes in, carrying a pile of papers I fin-
ished the day before, telling me I got them all wrong. They
need to be redone by lunchtime.

I put away the work I just started and dive into the
pile of papers. I feel humiliated and angry. I'll never be able
to do this by lunchtime. Everybody goes to lunch, laughing
and chatting in a friendly manner, but I've got no choice
but to skip it and stay so I can finish what I have to do.
When they're gone, I open my drawer to find some leftover
cookies from yesterday. I eat them while typing, feeling be-
trayed and abandoned. Then I go to the vending machine in
the hallway to get some coffee, and—to hell with it—some
chocolate too. Goodbye to all my good intentions! I work
without stopping until five, when everybody goes home,
and I only just manage to finish yesterday's pile of mail.
After that, another pile of letters waits to be answered and
sent. Of course, it all has to be done today. I'm exhausted!
I feel like a victim, angry at everybody and abandoned by
everybody. How come everyone else can have a life while
I'm left alone in the dark office, typing angrily and hating
them all?

At eight, I've finally finished most of the work and head
home. It starts raining. I'm cold and wet. I don't have the
energy left to prepare a proper meal. I stop at the gas station
and buy a loaf of fresh bread and a large bowl of ice cream.
I eat the bread while riding my bike, almost hitting an old
lady on the pavement. She yells at me, calling me names.
As soon as I get home, I get into bed with the ice cream
and eat it all. After that, I go for the box of chocolates I had
bought for my mom's birthday. To hell with it! I'm entitled

to some pampering after such a bad day. I turn on the TV and watch it while finishing off the last chocolates from my secret stash. I feel bloated and disgusting. It's been a bad day, again. But tomorrow, tomorrow will be different . . .

9

Problems at the Level of Behavior

The first of the exercises in this book listed many behaviors in which addicts may engage as part of their addiction. In fact, most of us behave in these ways on occasion—but that does not mean we are all addicts. To diagnose addiction, an addiction cycle must be present. To be indicative of an addiction, a person's behavior must have the following characteristics:

- The behavior must be **harmful.** There is no such thing as a good addiction.

- The behavior must **change the person's mood** or level of consciousness; **numb their feelings**; or **bring relief**, pleasure, satiation, self-oblivion, or a measure of escape from reality.

- The behavior must be **repeated** very often.

- The person must experience a **loss of control** over the behavior, indicating that this behavior operates at an unconscious level—that is, automatically.

In general, people behave in a way that makes sense to them. Initially, *addiction seems to be an exception to the rule*, because we know addicts repeat their harmful behavior, although they know it may have negative consequences for themselves.

But we have already proven this behavior helps numb their bad feelings about themselves, so it makes sense for them to engage in it—at least initially. Once the more negative consequences of that behavior begin to pile up, the addictive system has already taken hold, and the person's ability to stop engaging in these behaviors has been compromised.

Thus far, we have spoken of substance addictions and behavioral addictions. In a way, however, substance addictions are behaviors, too. The difference between alcoholics and "social drinkers," who have a glass or two after dinner, for example, does not lie in the quantity or quality of liquor they consume. After all, the substance is neutral. People are not addicted to alcohol; instead, they are addicted to *the process of getting drunk,* or to *getting high on drugs. Alcoholics drink to get drunk—to have some relief from the gnawing sense of guilt and shame generated by the addiction cycle.* I remember hearing Christopher Lawford Kennedy, an elite actor and well-known speaker at addiction conferences, tell an audience, "When I first got drunk at the age of twelve, I knew that God had given me the answer to all my problems!" The difference between alcoholics and social drinkers is not in the act of drinking, though alcoholics do so much more often. Rather, it is in the *purpose* behind the action.

Similarly, we can understand the difference between occasional players and problem gamblers in this way: the latter go to the casino to "earn" money, while occasional players gamble merely to play and have some fun. Food addicts don't eat to satisfy hunger; rather, their **emotional eating**—stuffing themselves with food until they are full—helps numb their negative feelings. Sex addicts are not hypersexual in the sense that they have a greater sex drive than others; what drives them to engage in sexual acts is the resulting oblivion that temporarily shuts down the angry, shaming voices in their heads. And codependents or relationship addicts don't "love too much"—rather, believing they must sacrifice themselves to earn love, they try to ensure their lovers won't leave by doing their best to please their partners.

Jane's Story

Jane, 32, is addicted to shopping—something that, for most, is a neutral behavior. Let's see how this addiction works in her case:

> When I'm stressed or feeling abandoned, I go shopping. I mean, I go to the store every day to buy groceries and stuff; but this is different. Shopping for groceries is not particularly exciting. It just needs to be done. No big deal.
>
> But when I go shopping as part of my addiction, it's different. I prepare myself in an almost ritual manner: I dress well; put my makeup on; wear perfume, jewelry, and high heels. I go to the costly boutiques, fooling myself that I'm only going to try some clothes on, just for the fun of it. I seek out the sexiest and the most expensive items and take them to the dressing room. I feel pride when the salesgirl looks at me in admiration, and I know I smell of wealth and prestige. I look down at her, and she looks up at me. I try the dresses on, imagining how I would enter the room dressed like that, and everyone would stop talking and gaze at me. In such a dress, I would be the center of attention. All the men would instantly be attracted to me. How could they resist me? And my boyfriend, who has not been returning my calls lately, would see how gorgeous I am and be sorry. He'd come back to me, and we'd make up.
>
> I look at myself in the mirror and think, I've got to have this dress. I can't afford it, but it doesn't really matter. When my boyfriend and I are back together, it'll be worth it.
>
> I come out of the dressing room in the new outfit, and the saleswoman says, "Wow!" With an elegant movement of my manicured hand, I take out my credit card.
>
> As soon as I step out of the store, I'm overcome with guilt. What have I done? I promised the kids I'd take them to the seaside next month, but now the money's gone. I'm just like my father, who gambled away every dime he could lay his hands on, leaving us penniless and in debt. How I hated my mother saying, "No, dear, we can't! We don't have the money!" every time I had any kind of wish at all. Now

I'm doing it to my kids. Like father, like daughter!

I decide to wait until tomorrow, when another saleswoman will be working, and return the dress, saying my friend bought it, not me. Just the thought of doing that makes me ashamed. But until tomorrow, I can still try it on in my bedroom and enjoy the sense of power it gives me. . . .

10

Problems at the Level of the Family

At their best, families are often thought of as sacred, providing us with a peaceful home: a safe place where we can share our lives with those we love. A space where everyone is supposed to be accepted and loved just as they are, without the need to pretend or wear a mask, and where shared love weaves a warm nest in which children can safely grow into adults. An abode where kids learn what love really means. A peaceful haven.

But that's not always the case! In fact, most violence and abuse occur between family members. **Domestic abuse**, also called **domestic violence**, which the United Nations (UN) defines as "a pattern of behavior in any relationship that is used to gain or maintain power and control over an intimate partner,"[21] is a major epidemic in the United States. As the UN describes, this type of abuse consists of "physical, sexual, emotional, economic or psychological actions or threats of actions that influence another person. This includes any behaviors that frighten, intimidate, terrorize, manipulate, hurt, humiliate, blame, injure, or wound someone. Domestic abuse can happen to anyone of any race, age, sexual orientation, religion, or gender. It can occur within a range of relationships including

---

[21] United Nations, "What Is Domestic Abuse?," United Nations, United Nations, 2020, https://www.un.org/en/coronavirus/what-is-domestic-abuse.

couples who are married, living together or dating. Domestic violence affects people of all socioeconomic backgrounds and education levels."[22] Indeed, in the US, more than ten million adults experience domestic abuse annually, and the devastating consequences of domestic violence can last a lifetime and affect multiple generations.

Unfortunately, domestic abuse is just one of the terrible effects addiction can have on a family. In this chapter, we'll discuss the problem of addiction at the level of the family. In the process, we'll examine:

- Addiction's origins as an attachment disorder,

- Dysfunctional rules and roles in families affected by addiction,

- The "games" played in families wherein one or more family members suffers from addiction, and

- Traumatic events and their consequences, which can often arise from addiction.

Addiction as an attachment disorder

When addiction strikes, the intricate web of attachment between family members is tainted. Love transforms into its opposite: fear. Addiction corrupts feelings of safety into the need to control, longing for peace into a desire for numbness, feelings of intimacy into feelings of intensity, striving for competence into struggling for perfection. Nothing is as it is supposed to be—and yet, family members still think what they experience is love!

Members of a family affected by addiction learn that love is based on fear. Later in life, they may look for love where there is none—in addiction! This may lead them to ruin their own lives.

---

[22] Ibid.

TABLE 1: The differences between love and addiction

When love is present in the family, its members feel and experience ...	When addiction is present in the family, its members feel and experience ...
Love	Fear
Safety	Control
Peace	Numbness
Intimacy in relationships	Intensity in relationships
Feelings of competence	Demand for perfection
Secure attachment	Insecure dependence

People start learning what love is as soon as they are born. No words are necessary to teach them about this aspect of the human experience, for *a child's primary instinct is to attach to the person who cares for them.* When a baby is one year old, it has learned the basic facts that will later influence all its decisions: whether the world is safe and friendly and the people in it loving—or not. For those who are **securely attached**, the foundation is rock solid because their caretakers are consistently present, loving, and caring. When they later encounter hardships in their lives, as everyone does eventually, they will be able to draw strength from their core beliefs, find solutions, and know how to get help.

But those who are **insecurely attached** have foundations built on quicksand—foundations that can be shaken by life's ordeals. Love is a basic human need, and they still need it, although it would bring them pain; but they look for love in the wrong places. Trying to resolve why love hurts, they look for solutions that will become problems themselves. Some of them—those who have mostly been neglected as infants—become **loners.** Believing it is impossible to have your needs met by other people, they strive to be self-sufficient. Others, who received some of the love they needed, but inconsistently, may become convinced there is not enough love in the world to go around. They **cling** to the people they love, constantly fearing abandonment. And then there are those whose understanding of love and fear gets mixed up because their caregivers were abusive. They look for love, but find only **violence** and **betrayal**.

TABLE 2: Secure and insecure attachment

Secure attachment	I am okay; others are okay; the world is safe.	
Insecure attachment	Parents were distant or neglectful	Loners: "I don't need love!"
	Parents were loving, but inconsistently so	Clingers, relationship addicts: "Love is my most important need!"
	Parents were abusive	Those who confuse love and violence: "Love hurts!"

Maybe you think this explanation sounds too simple to be accurate—but it has been scientifically proven,[23] and is proven every day in clinical practice. *Attachment and the way we love formulate the core of our personality.* A family in which one or more of the members are addicts is not safe. Maybe it doesn't look unsafe on the outside because, for example, the father and mother are respectable members of society and hide their drinking—but the infant child feels as if her parents are wrapped in shields of ice. She runs into her mother's arms,

---

[23] Wikipedia provides a brief overview of **attachment theory,** "a psychological, evolutionary, and ethological theory concerning relationships between humans." This theory, formulated by psychiatrist and psychoanalyst John Bowlby and further augmented by developmental psychologist Mary Ainsworth in the 1960s and '70s, states as its most important tenet that to achieve normal social and emotional development, young children must develop a relationship with at least one primary caregiver. "Attachment theory," Wikipedia, Wikipedia Foundation, Inc., August 29, 2023, https://en.wikipedia.org/wiki/Attachment_theory.

only to meet her cold, glassy gaze; and for the baby, this is a shocking, traumatic event.

Iris's Story

Iris, 36, told me this story:

> *I was maybe five years old when my mother and my brother went to see our grandparents while Dad watched over me. I was playing, and he was drinking. He called me, and I saw that something was very wrong. He was pale, unable to walk. He asked me to go to the bathroom, fetch a bucket, and put it beside his bed. Then he threw up into it. The vomit was all red from the wine, and I thought it was blood. I was terrified, thinking he might die. I would be left alone. How would I survive?*
>
> *I don't remember much of what happened afterward. I think he asked me to lie on the bed next to him. I don't know if I did. I don't remember where I slept that night—if I even did. Or did I go away when I thought it was "safe" and he didn't need me anymore? "Need" me—I was five! I know I felt fear for my own survival, realizing there was nobody anywhere to protect me or help me. In a room, in the middle of a summer night, I and an unconscious drunk man, my father, asking me for help. Asking me to lie down next to him to help him fall asleep. I felt it was wrong. But I had nobody to be my witness. Nobody whom I could tell. It was just him and me.*
>
> *The following day, too. I couldn't tell him what had happened because he was the one doing it to me. I couldn't rely on him. I didn't dare so much as blink an eye. I was the only one who knew. It was too risky to tell, so I kept it to myself. I endured it. I knew it would make me special in his eyes. A silent promise to stay silent in exchange for a thank you in his eyes. I felt sorry for him. I was ashamed someone might find out. I didn't feel telling my mother would be safe. I forgot that I was a child, and took responsibility for the situation . . .*

It may surprise you to learn that at its core, *addiction is an attachment disorder*. It's a disorder of the ability to love, first formed in an unsafe family and later played out in most relationships in the addict's life. Again, we can see that the root of addiction does not arise as late as adolescence, when the first acting out with drinking and drugs begins, but rather that its seeds are sown at the very beginning of an infant's life in the addicted family. That is why it is so important to consider the whole family in recovery: even if they don't (yet) show signs of addiction themselves, all the members are likely to be affected and need help.

Dysfunctional family rules and roles

Those who live with an alcoholic or another kind of addict must constantly deal with a wide range of issues that are brought on by the addict's disease and subsequently passed on to all family members. They must tolerate the addict's:

- anger,

- criminal acts,

- broken promises,

- physical and verbal abuse,

- complex and unexpected emotional outbursts,

- irresponsible and unsuitable behavior in public and at home, and

- inability to give love in return for love received.

Most addicts who abuse substances have good days when they can control themselves better, and family members constantly hope they will at last stop drinking and become loving, responsible people. With this hope in mind, and to adapt to the situation and survive emotionally, families adopt **dysfunctional rules** that help them get around the problems an addict introduces to the family, but that don't actually fix them:

- Don't talk about problems.

- Don't express your feelings openly.

- Don't speak directly about your problems, but rather gossip and complain.

- Don't be selfish—that is, don't take care of your needs or set boundaries.

- Don't be childish—that is, take on the responsibility of an adult.

- Don't rock the boat—that is, don't complain.

- Don't tell anybody on the "outside" about our family secrets.

- If an authority figure in the family breaks one of these rules or otherwise acts poorly, do as they say, not as they do.

- Conform to unrealistic expectations of strength, goodness, fairness, and perfection so the family can be proud of you.

These rules often limit communication, add further damage to the basic insecure attachment, and hinder the development of the children in the family. They certainly don't leave much room for healthy growth.

To comply with the family's rules, children can adopt **roles** that allow them to obtain some approval and apparent safety in this toxic environment. The typical roles in the addicted family are:

- The **Perpetrator**, typically the addict. The Perpetrator often interacts with the Rescuer and the Victim.

- The **Scapegoat**, the person who enables a dysfunctional family to stay together by acting as a convenient person to blame for everything that goes wrong. It's important to note that the Scapegoat often does not ask for this role, but other members of the family thrust it upon them.

- The **Invisible Child**, the "good guy," who stays in their bedroom all afternoon or at the playground until dusk to avoid the drama in the kitchen. Usually a Scapegoat's sibling, the Invisible Child might play aggressive video games to vent their feelings.

- The **Superman/Superwoman**, the family's star, an overachiever and workaholic who works hard to get away from the family as much as possible.

- The **Rescuer**, who takes sides with the seemingly weaker members of the family and becomes a codependent. The Rescuer often interacts with the Perpetrator and the Victim.

- The **Victim**, who is seemingly helpless and often attacked by the Perpetrator, but actually capable of manipulating everybody else with feelings of guilt. The Victim often interacts with the Rescuer.

Mark's Story

To get an idea of how the atmosphere in a person's family of origin can influence their marriage as many as twenty-five years later, read this testimony of an "Invisible Child"—Mark, 36, husband to Iris, the client whose story I shared earlier in this chapter. Their relationship is not a coincidence, but rather proof of the underlying forces that shape the lives of the victims of dysfunctional families.

> *My dad always came home from work at 5:00 p.m., and that's when we had dinner. Every day, without exception, my mom fixed dinner for him. But when my sister had leukemia, everything was turned upside down. Every day after school, Mom would go by bus to the hospital, and there*

she stayed all afternoon. When I came from school, the house was empty. There was no dinner. I had lunch at school, but I don't remember what Dad ate. They did take care of my basic needs, but what was missing was the feeling that there was somebody there for me, to take care of my other needs, to be responsible for me. I had an idea of how sick my sister was, but I couldn't have imagined what my parents must have been going through. I don't remember begrudging my mom then, but later the resentment emerged in my own relationships. It is so damn painful to be pushed away by the person you love the most. Mom must have suffered, but she hid her fear, and it appeared as if she had everything under control. I suppose this was also the case with Dad, but he seemed more like a robot on the outside.

Perhaps that's what made it easier for me. I didn't feel it was that difficult. Mom never cried or showed any weakness in my presence, and Dad never let himself show any vulnerability. We visited my sister at the hospital, and she looked happy to see us. From everything I was allowed to know, I must have concluded that my sister's illness wasn't that bad and would work out well. And it did! My sister recovered, but we all bore some consequences. Our parents' inability to show their emotions left an imprint on us. I can say that at that time, I was abandoned, even though my parents seemed to think I was getting everything I needed. I wasn't angry at Mom for abandoning me, but rather sort of disappointed. After that, I constantly tried to prove my existence. I craved the attention that was stolen from me and never returned. I felt left out, unimportant.

When Iris and I became a couple, I felt the same whenever we were out with friends. She went, was happy with them, had fun . . . and I felt like little Marky, cast away, unimportant. I didn't try to change the situation or say anything. I just withdrew and radiated that damned negative energy. It was always the same, and Iris and I were constantly arguing about it. At home, I acted like a robot, showing no feelings. I was stubborn; things had to be my way, and if they were, I felt accepted and loved. If Iris re-sisted my ideas of how things were supposed to be, I felt un-important and left out. And so, I started to withdraw more and more. I didn't hear her. I didn't listen. If she didn't want to listen to me, I didn't want to listen to her. I know that she was sometimes right, but I also thought I was right. There was a wall between us. But I still loved her, and never even thought that we might go our separate ways.

For a child, their family is their entire world. The child accepts their family's rules, roles, and games as they are dis-played, never questioning their validity—not even when the child grows up. Of course, growing up means taking respon-sibility for your decisions and your life—but when the source of the philosophy on which you base your choices is dysfunc-tional, you can get older without growing up emotionally. You behave like a child, dependent upon others, feeling worthless, and replaying old patterns, even when you have your own chil-dren. This is how dysfunctional behavior is passed to the next generation.

Traumatic events and their consequences

Trauma is a deeply distressing or disturbing experience that prompts emotions too powerful for a person to bear. This experi-ence need not involve tragic events caused by great catastrophes like war or natural disasters. For the children involved, domes-tic abuse and addiction are essentially a war perpetrated within the family. Growing up in a dysfunctional family is a source of **chronic** trauma—meaning it is repeated so often, family mem-bers' coping mechanisms fail to repair the damage it causes. In such a family, fear and dependence replace love and attachment. There is no safety; instead, there is a prevailing feeling that one is incompetent, vulnerable, unimportant, and simply not good enough. There is shame, and more shame. Relationships in such a family are shallow and unstable; betrayal and abandonment are expected. And worst of all, the perpetrators of the traumatic events are people the child is supposed to love.

Abuse in childhood can increase one's risk of developing an addiction, as it occurs during the most sensitive and critical stages of psychological development and has severe long-term effects. Remember Sara, the girl from the first chapter, who was sexually abused by her neighbor? *Sexual abuse in childhood* wreaks havoc on a child's developing psyche, crushing their ability to discern right from wrong and good from bad and convincing them they are worthless—especially if that abuse is perpetrated by a family member or trusted adult such as a teacher, priest, or nanny. Did you know one in five children endures such an experience?[24] I didn't—at least not until I started working as a psychotherapist. But once I did, I was appalled at the number of my clients who carried such terrible memories in their hearts. And in most cases, the addictions from which they were suffering began as coping mechanisms that helped them deal with their trauma when no one else wanted to know about it.

The connection between repetitive traumatic events in childhood—**chronic relational developmental trauma**—and the development of addiction is well known, and has been proven by extensive research. Understanding the consequences of childhood trauma is extremely important for recovery.

But first things first! To examine any childhood trauma fully, we must first understand not only its consequences, but its causes. However, one remarkable feature of trauma that can complicate this effort is the fact that victims often *don't remember* what caused their trauma. Their memories of traumatic events are hidden in their subconscious, seemingly forgotten. But when recovery begins in earnest, these memories start reemerging. Unfortunately, they are usually painful, adding more stress to the addict's already difficult situation. This stress can tempt a recovering addict to return to old habits to alleviate their pain, and can therefore jeopardize addicts' hard-won sobriety.

Though addicts cannot forever put off working through these memories, I recommend my clients do all they can to ensure a stable recovery by achieving and maintaining abstinence

---

[24] "Child Maltreatment," World Health Organization, WHO, September 19, 2022, https://www.who.int/news-room/fact-sheets/detail/child-maltreatment.

from the focus of their addictions before they allow themselves to delve deeper into their newly unearthed childhood traumas. In my experience, the best time to deal with childhood trauma is in the second year of sobriety.

11

Problems at the Level of Society

After having so closely examined the painful experiences of an abused child, it feels almost insensitive or disrespectful to pull back and discuss the problems society has with addiction. Nevertheless, it is important we do so. In this chapter, we'll discuss:

- Society's attitude toward addiction,

- The changes addiction causes in families,

- The influence of the media in the development of addiction, and

- The effect of the continuous struggle for perfection.

Society's blasé attitude toward addiction
Society's current attitude is that it is normal to drink or use drugs in moderation. Indeed, most adults do so, even in front of their children. Of course, not everyone who uses drugs or drinks alcohol will become an addict, but some will, and society's tolerance of that kind of behavior lends them to going too far.

Similarly, behavioral addictions are now so common, society seems to have accepted them as normal. We do not seem able to celebrate or mourn, to love or part, without the soothing effect of some substance or behavior. Everyone seems to be seeking pleasure, while efforts to avoid painful feelings and difficulties in general are considered normal. We seem to have forgotten that striving for something and overcoming obstacles is how we grow into better people. Is bettering oneself and the world around us even a goal for most anymore? Or have we replaced it with the goal of becoming popular, sexy, or rich? As a society, we seem to have abdicated personal responsibility for the world we live in, believing modern science or political change will solve all our problems—inequality of the sexes, climate change, or some war on the other side of the globe. We feel we have no power to influence these things anyway, so we may as well be satisfied in grabbing as much pleasure as possible and shutting everything else out of our awareness.

Addiction is one of those unpleasant things we do not want to think about—until it hits us so hard, we cannot ignore it anymore. As an example of how socially acceptable addiction seems to have become, and how its consequences are underestimated and even romanticized, I offer one of my own fairly recent movie theatre experiences. A few years ago, I went to see the Oscar- and Golden Globe-nominated movie *A Star Is Born* (2018), and was very disappointed—not at the movie itself, but at the effect it had on the audience. The film tells the story of a musician who helps a young singer find fame even as drug and alcohol addiction ruin his own career. Jealous of her success, he humiliates her by wetting himself and passing out on the stage while she is receiving the Grammy Award, ruining her celebration. She responds by marrying him. From their ecstatic reactions, I gathered most of the audience found this very romantic—but all I saw were the symptoms of advanced alcohol and drug addiction, an older and more powerful man's exploitation of a naïve young girl, and her full-blown codependency, from the first scene to the last.

Later, I discussed the movie with clients from my therapy group. Most of them had experienced firsthand the troubles of having an alcoholic family member—so I couldn't believe it when the majority of them told me they saw the movie as a very romantic love story. Contrary to what the movie's most famous song might claim, we're not beyond the "sha-ha-shala-la-la-llow!"

Lack of family time

Families, too, are no longer what they used to be as little as two or three generations ago. In the Western world, the "nuclear family," consisting of a couple and their children, has replaced the extended family as the primary domestic unit. No longer do grandparents and unmarried uncles and aunts all live under the same roof with the family—and for the first time in history, mothers and fathers are expected to take care of their children alone while also providing for the family. To support this self-sufficient lifestyle, most parents work all day, leaving their children in the care of professionals who may view this task as simply a job and may not try to establish a long-lasting loving connection with the children. The number of families with only one parent is also growing: many couples live separately, and children spend half their childhoods with just one parent, only visiting the other—if they visit at all.

These changes and pressures have led to chronic stress in parents and fear of abandonment in children—both of which can lead to addictive cravings. Life is becoming more and more of a struggle, leaving no room for moments of serenity and the contemplation of beauty in art or nature. We feel this lack and try to make up for it by buying new gadgets and clothes, or by overachieving—but while these little victories and material goods may provide moments of satisfaction, those feelings quickly fade, only to be replaced by new artificial "needs." What an insane perspective!

The influence of the media

Making our feelings of hopelessness even worse is the strong influence of the media—a pillar of life that has changed considerably in the space of only one generation. Much of today's most widespread media content is violent and sexual, with everything from entertainment to commercials featuring shocking imagery. Advertisers know the intense emotions generated by such images draw our attention, and therefore make us more likely to remember and buy products associated with those images. And since most productions are now made with, or at least augmented by, computer-generated graphics, there are no limits to what they can create. The fact that we know certain scenes are artificially generated does not help much, as the brain often does not distinguish between imagination and reality very well. We naturally believe what we see with our own eyes is real, and therefore react to violent and sexually explicit images as if they were real: with stress, fear, disgust, or sexual interest.

But the effect of the media doesn't stop there. In addition to artificially created entertainment, the media constantly shower us with reports of real-life catastrophes, violence, and wars. Every plane or ship that crashes anywhere in the world becomes headline news. Interest in "true" crime and violent sex is increasing. Several studies report half of Americans enjoy watching TV shows about true crime, and almost half of those people reported the experience worsened their view of humanity or made them feel less safe in their daily lives.[25] Many of us have even become suspicious and cynical of people who care for others, believing they have a hidden agenda.

Clinical experience has shown that bystanders and witnesses to violence are often traumatized along with its direct victims, and in some ways, suffer similar psychological consequences. It can be traumatic for a child to witness his brother being beaten up, even though he himself is spared physical violence. But by broadcasting daily news of the most horrible scenes of war, death, and suffering right into our living rooms, where our children play, mass media make us all witnesses to such violence. Indeed, it is our youngest children who are most mercilessly exposed to this intrusive media bombardment, as they spend much of their time fixated on screens of various kinds, while being too young to have established boundaries that would help them distance themselves from depictions of aggression.

---

[25] "True Crime Obsession: Exploring America's Love Affair with True Crime," SuperSummary, SuperSummary, September 13, 2023, https://www.supersummary.com/true-crime-obsession.

Most adults, on the other hand, have established these boundaries—but at a price. To listen to reports of such horrible disasters, we must deny the instinctive, fearful feeling that we are as vulnerable as the people on the other side of the camera or screen, and pretend that these terrible tragedies could only happen to somebody else. People's capacity for self-deception is truly enormous—but *what is the cost of shutting down the pain in our souls to be able to fool ourselves into thinking others' tragic circumstances are irrelevant to our lives?* We pay the price in the loss of our sense of the meaning of life, and of what is essentially good within us. Even new scientific achievements, which should improve our lives, instead add to the loss of these values: the hole in the ozone layer, climate change, new weapons . . . day after day. As a citizen of the former Yugoslavia who experienced war at my doorstep, I can no longer pretend I will be unaffected by the tragedies I see played out on screens every day. Can you?

The continuous struggle for perfection

The extreme opposite of such hopeless tragedy, which the media also presents and curates, is the struggle for beauty and perfection. In our everlasting competition and pursuit of the "faster, higher, stronger,"[26] we have come to ignore human limitations, pressuring the best athletes into using drugs to enhance their performance, lest they be left behind. The Olympic motto is an excellent motivational slogan, but it is unrealistic—for in most athletes, striving to overcome nature will result in exhaustion, injury, and confirmation of the primary addictive thought: "I am not good enough!"

Unfortunately, through the influence of the media, even ordinary people are fooled into believing the sky is the limit, and that they can achieve anything if only they try hard enough. If we experience disease, death, and suffering in our lives, we are told, it is because we have failed to take care of ourselves—the original sin of the average consumer, who is advised to buy this or that product to prevent this or that

---

[26] The Olympic motto.

malady. As a breast cancer survivor and advocate, I have spoken at many cancer conferences, and talked to survivors. They told me that the idea that a certain lifestyle can contribute to getting cancer made them feel as if their disease were their fault. As a medical doctor, I had been used to advising my patients to implement certain lifestyle changes as part of their treatment. When I found myself "on the other side," in the patient's role and struggling to understand why cancer had affected me, I felt offended by my doctors' supposition that the cancer might have been prevented if I had acted more "correctly." Their view was a typical effort at denial: "If someone is good enough, they will be fine." But cancer and other tragedies affect good people, too.

After my experience with cancer, I could no longer buy into the idea that being perfect and buying all kinds of products could save me from the challenges life brings. The illusion dissolved, leaving me to confront a chaotic, apathetic universe—and yes, it was scary! From this perspective, it was easy to see why many prefer the more comfortable illusion.

And society does its best to push that illusion—by encouraging everyone to put up a façade of perfection. In an attempt to ignore the unpleasant realities of life and sell us products from food to books to exercise programs to plastic surgery, our capitalist society imposes standards of beauty, youth, and fitness on men and women alike—standards that only models and athletes who work out their whole lives can actually maintain. In the unforgiving quest to have perfect bodies and perfect lives, many of us have lost our connection to our essences, our inner sparks, our true sources of love and connection, and our awareness of our purpose in life. This has left a painful void in our souls, which we try to fill with everything else under the sun—and often in a way that contributes to the development of addictions. But, as they say, *you can't get enough of what you don't need!*

I always recommend that instead of worrying and obsessing about what society demands and what others should do, people should focus on dealing with their own problems. In this way, they would take care of the only piece of the universe for which they are truly responsible, and over which they had any modicum of control—themselves. If everyone did that, I believe the world would truly be a better place.

How the levels work together

All the levels of human experience we have discussed thus far, from the personal to the societal, influence how we understand addiction. It's important to understand all these different viewpoints so as to form a coherent picture of the problem.

It's also important to understand how these levels contribute to the lies addicts tell themselves to make themselves believe their behavior isn't that bad. All too often, I hear statements like these:

- Everybody drinks, so it's okay!

- I've been smoking for ten years and have experienced no consequences.

- I *have to* work so much because that's what my job demands.

- My father drank around me while I was growing up, and it didn't harm me, so taking my son to the bar with me is no big deal.

- A boy should learn early that life is hard, so exposing my son to violent movies or video games is no big deal.

- A girl should learn to be seductive and submissive.

These justifications can soothe the conscience in the moment—but a lack of understanding of the potential long-term consequences of an action or belief can make it easier for people to fool themselves into believing their behaviors are not (yet!) harmful. As a result, they allow those behaviors and beliefs to persist for too long. When that happens, a habit is formed—and sometimes, if the circumstances are right, this can lead to full-blown addiction.

12

What Contributes to Addiction

If you were to ask addicts what they believe caused their addiction, you would receive many different answers, from "I was influenced by my peers on the street" to "I just wanted to have some fun" to "I had a difficult childhood." As we have just proven, however, addiction is a multidimensional condition that manifests on many different levels. Furthermore, the roots of addiction begin to grow in a person's early childhood, and can take decades to develop to the point that people recognize the person's behaviors as evidence of addiction and start doing something about it. A drop of water may not do much harm, but given enough time, water can carve out even the Grand Canyon!

Instead of causes, it is better to speak about the *factors that influence the development of addiction*. These are some of the best-researched:

- Genetic factors (addiction in the family)

- Environmental factors (mode of upbringing)

- Biological factors (comorbidities, trauma, being exposed to mind-altering substances at young age)

- Cultural factors (tolerance to addiction)

Genetic factors
For years, experts have argued over the influence of "nature

versus nurture" on a person's development, including the development of addiction. Which one has the most significant effect? Really, the answer is *both!*

People usually underestimate how large a part genetics plays in who they will become. When I give lectures, I often ask my audience to raise their hands if *none* of their immediate or second-degree relatives are alcoholics or addicts of any kind. (Before doing so, I instruct everyone to close their eyes so that nobody but me sees the raised hands; I don't want anyone to avoid acknowledging their family secrets due to potential shame.) For every one hundred people who attend my lectures, usually only three or four arms are raised, whether I am lecturing to medical doctors or a gathering of recovering alcoholics. Only 3 to 5 percent of the population are not burdened by genetic factors that might play a part in causing addiction!

Environmental factors

While genetic factors contribute to more than half the likelihood of developing addictions, a person's environment and biological makeup as a result of how they behave—how they live, work, and sleep, and even the foods they eat—play a role in how those hereditary factors influence them. In short, a person's upbringing and life experiences can make them vulnerable to addiction. We discussed this earlier when we talked about the role of the family in shaping a person's core beliefs and defense strategies. Unfortunately, if a person is born into a family of addicts, they get an upbringing *and* the genetics that make them vulnerable to developing an addiction themselves.

Biological factors

Since genetics strongly influence a person's susceptibility to addiction, if you have blood relatives who are addicts, you should think of yourself as vulnerable. Cooccurring psychiatric conditions can also make someone more vulnerable to developing an addiction. These conditions are typically treated with many drugs, most of which are mood-altering substances: dopamine, for example, is used to treat Parkinson's disease and low blood pressure while Adderall, which is often prescribed to children with attention deficit and hyperactivity disorder, contains amphetamines, which stimulate the nervous system. We have learned that the brain uses these substances to communicate, and administering them in large doses affects the way people think and feel. These drugs are usually advertised as safe for consumption, and since trained doctors prescribe them, you may feel they must indeed be safe. However, many people have developed addictions to prescription medication.

Traumatic life experiences and events can also make people vulnerable to addiction because *trauma permanently changes the brain*. Chronic trauma, including a traumatic upbringing, is even worse in this regard because constant stress knocks the body's stress management systems permanently out of balance. And of course, doing something to numb your feelings in an effort to recover from the problems caused by both short-term and chronic trauma makes sense. In short, trauma invites those behaviors that can lead to the development of addiction.

We have also mentioned that the brain is particularly vulnerable to addiction in adolescence, when most people first come into contact with mood-altering substances. Peer pressure is also an important factor in the development of addiction—and no group is more vulnerable to peer pressure than adolescents. The absence of a solid spiritual attitude can also increase their vulnerability. As such, you can see that for adolescents, many factors that invite the development of addictions converge, creating a potentially dangerous combination.

Cultural factors

The influence of a person's cultural environment on their potential to develop an addiction is significant—especially when it comes to their culture's attitude toward addiction and addicts. We have already discussed this in the chapters relating to problems in the family and society.

All the information from the previous chapters will now help us understand how addiction works—and specifically, how it works in your case.

13

How to Understand Addiction

In this section of the book, we have learned many new facts about addictions. You now know that addiction is not merely about doing bad things too much, but that there is a system beneath it all. This system causes cravings and unpleasant feelings of withdrawal that perpetuate the addiction cycle.

Recall that the addiction cycle starts with feelings of **toxic shame** and inadequacy. To reduce the discomfort of these feelings, you resort to your favorite **comforting behavior**. For a brief moment, you feel relief—but then you are confronted with *additional shame over the consequences of that behavior*, and find yourself in nearly the very place you started—only a little worse off, feeling more shame and needing more addictive comfort with each turn. This is how comforting behaviors turn into addictions.

With this knowledge in hand, we have moved from *recognizing* to *understanding* the problem. Now, let's wrap up what we have learned with a new set of exercises that will transform you from a passive observer of behavior to someone who is not only aware of the problems this behavior can present, but ready to take the first steps toward resolving it.

In completing the exercises in Part One, you may have concluded your repetitive harmful behaviors have addictive characteristics. But it's important to note that even if you accept that realization, as well as the scheme representing the addiction cycle, feeling that cycle in operation is quite different from comprehending it on an intellectual level. Each addict's addiction cycle is a very personal and emotional experience—a cocktail of feelings, beliefs, behaviors, and sometimes substances that form a cascade of actions, each more involuntary than the one before, until they completely lose control and the "tornado" of the cycle sucks them in.

To stop the addiction cycle in yourself, you must first understand how it works for you personally. The next set of exercises will reveal to you the elements that form your personal **addiction cycle** and help you construct a scheme that describes how it functions. You will also construct a **timeline of your life** that will allow you to understand how the most significant and most traumatic events in your life correlate with your addiction.

Exercise 4: What am I ashamed of?

We have said that **toxic shame**—belief one is not "good enough"—is the core feeling of most addicts. This belief makes them feel bad about themselves, prompting them to do almost anything to numb it: pretend, fantasize, or lie to themselves and others. When their illusions stop working, the addict turns to substances and behaviors that can temporarily change their mood—setting up a vicious circle and introducing the potential for addiction.

In this exercise, you should list the *events from your past* of which you are ashamed. Be thorough, as even events that happened in your childhood can be significant. What are the *beliefs about yourself* that resulted from these events? How did these beliefs later affect your behavior?

Example:

Event #1*: My parents divorced.*

Resulting Belief*: They divorced because I was not good enough.* (Although this logic is faulty, it helps the child by allowing them to believe they have some control over bad events. "If I were good enough," the child thinks, "my parents wouldn't have divorced.")

Consequences*: I built on the resulting belief, developing the following core belief: I am basically a bad and worthless person, unworthy of love. I must avoid getting close to people because they'll abandon me once they get to know me.*

Event #1:

....

....

Resulting Belief: ....

Consequences: ....

Event #2:

....

....

Resulting Belief: ....

Consequences: ....

Event #3:

....

....

Resulting Belief: ....

Consequences: ....

List your thoughts while working on this exercise:

....

....

....

Discuss your answers with a trusted friend, and take notes on your conversation:

....

....

....

Exercise 5: What are the consequences of my addictive behavior?

Actions have consequences—and avoiding action has consequences, too. This fundamental law of life shapes our behavior: everybody knows you can't eat all you want, have sex with everybody you like, or always have fun and never work. Consequences prevent us from engaging excessively in pleasurable behaviors—after all, we don't want to get fat, be involved with the wrong person, or be financially dependent on others.

Human existence comprises the following four major dimensions:

- Physical

- Psychological

- Social

- Spiritual

Addiction can have negative consequences in each of these dimensions. Let's list the potential consequences of addiction, grouping them according to the dimension of human existence under which they fall.

The **physical consequences** of addiction show up as physical conditions and diseases. Long-term stress, to which addiction often contributes, impairs the body and leads to the development of physical illnesses. Most "contemporary" diseases like high blood pressure, stomach ulcers, asthma, thyroid dysfunction, and some skin diseases are caused by chronic stress. In addition, some diseases can be brought on by repetition of a particular behavior characteristic of certain addictions: sex addicts are more likely to contract sexually transmitted infections; alcoholics may experience cirrhosis of the liver due to their excessive consumption of alcohol; and cigarette smokers may develop chronic bronchitis or cancer.

The **psychological consequences** of addiction can include low self-esteem, anxiety, depression, burnout, suicidal thoughts, or trauma due to the events an addict experiences or acts they commit while in the throes of addiction.

Social consequences of addiction can include broken relationships, dysfunctional family relationships, and loss of the ability to work.

Finally, the **spiritual consequences** of addiction can include the loss of feelings of connection with the universe, or even loss of the ability to love.

In completing the following exercise, you will identify the negative consequences of your addictive behaviors, in the hope that recognizing these consequences will motivate you to stop acting out. Check the boxes that match the consequences you have experienced as a result of your behaviors:

Physical consequences

- Exhaustion

- Sleep disorders

- Chronic fatigue

- Burnout and inability to work

- Extreme obesity or emaciation

- Bodily injury due to violent or reckless behavior related to your addiction

- Stress-related diseases (e.g., ulcers, high blood pressure)

- Diseases that are consequences of acting out (e.g., cirrhosis of the liver, pancreatitis, STDs, AIDS)

Psychological consequences
- Despair

- Loneliness

- Depression

- Paranoia

- Guilt and shame

- Suicidal thoughts

- Suicide attempts

- Fear of the future

- Fear of losing your mind

- Intrusive thoughts, including thoughts of violence

- The feeling of living two separate lives—one public, the other hidden

- Dysfunctional expressions of anger (e.g., rage, passive-aggressive behavior)

Social consequences

- Problems in your relationship
- Spousal abandonment or threats of abandonment
- Problems with children (e.g., conflict, diseases, harmful behaviors, addictions)
- Loss of your partner's or children's respect
- Endangering the interests of the family
- Alienation of parents and siblings
- Loss of friendships
- Lack of friends, except for drinking buddies
- Loss of efficiency at work
- Lack of promotion at work
- Loss of coworkers' respect
- Termination of employment
- Doing work below your abilities and educational level
- Lack of opportunities to do what you love
- Loss of interest in hobbies and activities you previously enjoyed
- Problems in school (e.g., bad grades)
- Lack of opportunities to study
- Poverty and financial irresponsibility
- Fraud and other civil or criminal offenses, especially to finance the addiction
- Legal suits

- Incarceration

- Fines

Spiritual consequences
- Anger at God or another higher power

- Complete loss of faith or spirituality

- Abandonment of life goals and expectations

- Acting contrary to your values and beliefs

- Feeling abandoned by God or another higher power

List your thoughts while working on this exercise:

....

....

....

Discuss your answers with a trusted friend, and take notes on your conversation:

....

....

Exercise 6: My Addiction Cycle

As we have previously noted, the addiction cycle starts with feeling shame for who you are and trying to do something to feel better. However, when these methods fail, the eventual addict feels additional shame for failing—which prompts them to try again, and again. At the end of each cycle, they feel a little worse than before.

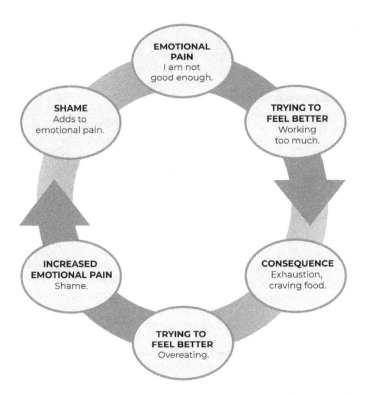

*Example: Let's look again at the example of Karen from the chapter about the consequences of addiction at the level of thinking (**page 65**). Her addiction cycle begins with the shame and humiliation she feels when she shows up late for work. She tries to make up for it by working extra hard, but is resentful that she works harder than her colleagues and afraid they are planning to terminate her employment. At this point, the **work addiction cycle** begins, and the thought that she is not good enough starts rolling around in her head. By skipping lunch, she fails to take care of herself, prompting the start of her **food addiction cycle**. Both cycles now drive one another, leaving her feeling like a victim, entitling her to compensate by going on a binge and engaging in emotional eating. In the end, she feels like a loser, and puts off the start of abstinence until the following day. . . .*

We will now arrange all we have learned so far into a comprehensive scheme to help you understand the forces driving you into your own addictive system.

A. Shame: Write down the addictive behaviors you are ashamed of. (For help identifying these behaviors, see Exercise 1.) If you have trouble deciding which behaviors to choose, select the three you consider the worst.

....

....

....

....

B. Belief: What negative belief do you hold about yourself as a result of these behaviors?

....

C. Stress: How do you feel when you cannot stop thinking about the object of your addiction?

....

D. Craving: What do you crave?

....

E. Using and acting out: What do you need to do to stop these cravings?

....

F. Consequences: What are the consequences of your addiction? (For help identifying these consequences, see Exercise 2.)

....

Back to A: Additional shame and remorse builds up to basic toxic shame under A. The cycle is complete—but you feel worse every time you go around, and need to engage in your comforting behavior more and more often.

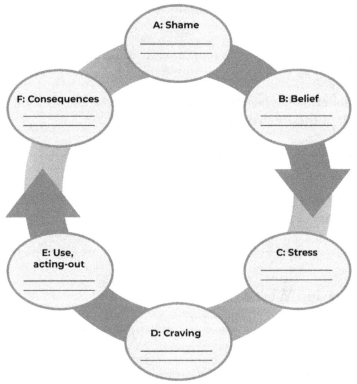

List your thoughts while working on this exercise:

....

....

....

Discuss your findings with a trusted friend, and take notes on your conversation:

....

....

....

Exercise 7: My Addiction Timeline

To overcome your feelings of toxic shame, you need to understand yourself and your decisions in the context of your life story. Creating an Addiction Timeline that chronicles your personal history can allow you to do just this. Placing certain events in the context of your life will help you understand why you made decisions that you may now regret, by helping you realize trauma or lack of understanding and resources contributed to your decision making at the time. *The Addiction Timeline is a tool you will need throughout your recovery, and you should update it continuously as you recall additional events from your past.*

To begin this exercise, take a large piece of blank paper and colored pens. Draw a long line across the middle of the paper. At the beginning of the line on the left-hand side, mark the date of your birth, leaving some room for the nine months before. Then extend the line, mark the current date on the rightmost side, and divide the line into equal parts. Depending on your age, you might use one-year, three-year, or even five-year increments.

Next, below the timeline, list the *important events* that occurred in your life and connect them to the appropriate date on the timeline with a line. You might include your siblings' birthdays; your parents' divorce; a move to another town; the start of kindergarten, middle school, or college; your marriage; separations or divorces; the beginning and end of meaningful relationships; and other significant events that shaped your life. Above the timeline, in another color, list the *traumatic events* you remember: hospitalizations, accidents, diseases, loss of friendships, loss of family members, loss of pets, and so on. If necessary, try to reconstruct the past from old photographs. You'll probably find what your parents remember will be less helpful here; you need to draw upon your own memories, which are likely to differ from those of other family members. Don't forget that a child's age and understanding decide what consequences an event will have on their life. You may notice periods full of events, as well as some almost empty spaces.

Next, use yet another color to mark the *beginning, the course,* and if applicable, *the moment you began to abstain from each of the addictions* you believe you might have *ever* had. Observe the interrelationship of trauma and acting out behaviors.

I suggest you keep this timeline and hang it up somewhere private but easily accessible, like inside your wardrobe or closet door. Every time you recall new events, add them to the timeline. Remember, everybody needs a logical and consistent story of their lives to understand and know themselves. Filling in the gaps in one's memory is the most fundamental part of in-depth psychotherapy. This work will change you completely!

IMAGE 4: Your addiction timeline

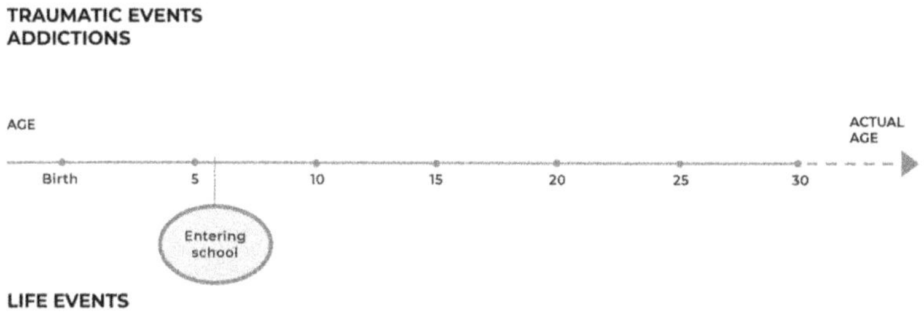

TRAUMATIC EVENTS
ADDICTIONS

AGE

ACTUAL
AGE

Birth | 5 | 10 | 15 | 20 | 25 | 30

Entering
school

LIFE EVENTS

List your thoughts while working on this exercise:

....

....

....

Discuss your findings with a trusted friend, and take notes on your conversation:

....

....

....

PART THREE:

BEHAVIORAL ADDICTIONS

Addiction is not about feeling good;
it's about feeling less.

14

From the General to the Specific

Learning about the brain is exciting and interesting—but how can it help you with your particular situation? You need the most up-to-date, fact-based, expert advice to help you find your way—not a heap of ideology. After all, you're facing problems and seeking answers to questions that seemingly have little to do with the theory of how addictions work.

As a start, you've figured out that your own behaviors, or the behaviors of someone you may care for, are out of control. Now, let's get down to the business of regaining control.

From here on, you can use this book in two different ways:

1. You can read it linearly and learn about most behavioral addictions; or

2. You can simply choose to read only the chapters about the behavioral addictions relevant to you (see Exercises 1–3), and then continue to Part Four: How to Recover from Addiction.

Putting theory into practice
Almost fifty years ago, when I started studying medicine, I was so excited. Finally, I was about to learn what was inside people, what drove their behaviors, and what made them human. For me, it was a great mystery: how can a bunch of jellylike cells like the brain generate something as sophisticated as a human soul?

To my great disappointment, all they taught us in medical school was the arrangement of the brain's white and gray matter and how some common reflexes worked. This was unable to explain all the sophisticated thoughts, feelings, and behaviors of which humans are capable.

But I kept learning. The following years brought with them some great scientific discoveries and advancements. By now, scientists have deciphered how the parts of the brain interact and what happens when they're off-balance. But we still don't know how the mind is connected to the brain. We don't have much of a clue where delicate emotions, thoughts, and decisions are generated. And we don't know what love means on a biological level, except that it's vital for our survival as infants that we attach to a nurturing adult. We have no idea where, much less *how*, all the delicate impulses we know from personal experience—fantasy, creativity, and compassion—are generated in the brain. In many ways, we're still wandering around in the dark.

But to recover from addiction, you need a map to show you how to get out of trouble. It's time to integrate all the theories we've learned about addiction with your personal life experience. Along the way, my clients' personal stories will help you understand how each addiction might look for them, and how their struggles with that addiction influence their lives. Perhaps you will even recognize yourself and your behavior in some of their experiences—for although people's personalities and experiences can be very different, they can also have much in common, especially if they are addicted to the same behavior.

In this part of the book, we will discuss what we know about the following specific behavioral addictions:[27]

1. **Addictions to Food**
    a. Bulimia Nervosa and Compulsive
       Overeating

---

[27] The official medical classifications like the *DSM-5* and *ICIDH* do not yet support listing all the behavioral addictions under the category of addictions, though their addictive characteristics are widely recognized by experts and laypersons alike. I decided to list them as such for greater clarity for the readers.

    b. Anorexia Nervosa and Orthorexia

2. **Addictions to Work, Money, and Risk**

    a. Work

    b. Money (Spending, Shopping, Debt) and Risk

    c. Gambling

3. **Addictions to Electronic Media (Cyber Addictions)**

    a. Video Games

    b. The Internet and Social Media

4. **Addictions to Relationships**

    a. Romance

    b. "Love"

    c. Codependence and Addiction to Destructive Relationships

5. **Addictions to Sex**

    a. Sex Addiction

    b. Co-Sex Addiction (Sexual Codependence)

    c. Sexual Anorexia

The structure of Part Three

1. **Definition and short overview** of the five broad categories of addiction listed above, along with a list of associated **behavior types**—that is, ways in which these addictions can be expressed.

2. **Introduction** including some information characteristic of the whole category.

3. **Chapters on each behavior type**, each including the following information:

a. The **name** of the specific addiction.

b. A **definition** and short explanation of the specific addiction discussed in the chapter.

c. List of **typical behaviors** (see Exercise 1), a reiteration of the part of Exercise 1 in which you were asked to list the behaviors that may be problematic for you. This will help you identify the chapters to which you need to pay special attention.

d. A **discussion** of some typical symptoms and behaviors associated with the addiction.

e. An examination of the **scope of the problem**, which offers statistics about the prevalence of the behavior.

f. An **example** featuring a true story from my rich treasury of client experiences.

g. **Advice** for the addict, and for family members and friends who may want to help.

We'll categorize the different addictions by the behaviors in which the addicts indulge because that's how they're typically described. But let's not forget that the brain does not discriminate between different sources of oblivion. Whether you are addicted to a substance or to a behavior—for example, computer games or gambling—does not make much difference when it comes to the way the brain functions while in the grip of addiction. *As long as the behavior is used to escape reality or block out pain, the same brain circuits are involved; and most people use many substances and behaviors for that purpose, anyway.* Each addict has their own individual cocktail of substances and behaviors—the magic potion they use when things get too painful to bear. And every day, new substances and behaviors can be added to replace old ones that have stopped working, or to induce an even greater escape from reality.

Still, personal experiences with addiction vary somewhat

based on each addict's "drug of choice." We're going to delve a little deeper into these experiences, in the hope that they may help you find a way out of your own addictions.

Finally, at the end of each chapter, you'll find some sound advice on how to help addicted relatives or friends. I hope it will help you take further steps toward your or another's recovery.

15. Addictions to Food

a. Bulimia Nervosa and
   Compulsive Overeating
b. Anorexia Nervosa and Orthorexia

15

Addictions to Food

Introduction

Addictions to food are actually a combination of substance and behavioral addictions. The concept of addiction to food is still controversial. Some authors describe food addictions as addictions to substances—for example, addictions to sugar, chocolate, or other "comfort foods." Others emphasize the abnormal eating habits common in food addictions—binge eating, dieting, or choosing only certain foods—and prefer to think of various presentations of food addictions as different types of eating disorders. Some have even suggested calling food addiction "eating addiction."

Regardless of what we call it, addiction to food is characterized by *a person's pattern of dysfunctional obsessive and compulsive thinking and behavior with regard to food*—almost a sort of love-hate relationship they have with it. Although their behavior toward food is initially voluntary, after some time, the addict experiences intense cravings and a loss of control surrounding food and eating. If they engage in specific behaviors involving food, like avoiding or excluding certain foods from their diet, starving themselves, purging, or eating to achieve a "sugar rush," they may experience significant changes in their modes of feeling, thinking, and behavior, and warrant a diagnosis of addiction.

Addictions to food can manifest in several behavior types. To an observer, these types may seem very different from each other, but those who have food addictions typically share the basic mindset that food and eating are both problems and the solutions to those problems, and that they should be rigorously controlled.

Behavior types of addictions to food

a. Bulimia nervosa and compulsive overeating

b. Anorexia nervosa and orthorexia

The behavior patterns found in food addiction vary from one type to another.

TABLE 3: Behavior types of food addiction

Behavior Type	Behaviors
Bulimia nervosa	Binge eating alternating with purging
Compulsive overeating	Periods of extreme overeating wherein one eats an enormous quantity of food in a short time without purging
Anorexia nervosa	Extreme dieting, with or without purging
Orthorexia	Obsession with eating foods one considers healthy, and systematically avoiding specific foods one believes to be harmful

As you can see, many different behaviors concerning food can escalate into addictive behavior. Some of these patterns of behavior and their physical effects on the body are so different that they may appear to indicate the presence of what doctors have classically defined as entirely separate diseases. For example, food addicts with behaviors associated with the bulimia and compulsive overeating behavior types will probably gain weight while those exhibiting behaviors associated with the anorexia and orthorexia behavior types may look malnourished or even "normal." Still, for a person experiencing food addiction, what starts as one pattern of behavior can sometimes transform into another over time—or, behaviors associated with different behavior types may present at the same time in the same person. Whatever behaviors the food addict exhibits, it's important to remember that a food addict's appearance and body weight are not specific signs that allow an observer to understand what is going on behind closed doors. Since people with these conditions are usually ashamed of their behavior around food and hide it from even their closest family members, it can sometimes be challenging to identify whether someone is experiencing food addiction at all.

Another important thing to remember is that despite the apparent differences in some of these presentations of food addiction, all of them cause or stem from the same *underlying thoughts and feelings* commonly found in those suffering from any type of food addiction:

- Extremely low self-esteem and negative self-image or self-hatred;

- Dissatisfaction with one's appearance;

- Distorted body image, wherein the person is convinced that their body weight is too high, while they may actually be seriously malnourished and skinny;

- Obsession with efforts to achieve the desired "look" (which can sometimes be very bizarre), including extreme dieting, purging, fasting, and exercise;

- Obsession with using tricks to rid one's body of ingested food so as not to gain weight, including purging, abuse of medications, induced vomiting, and forced excretion of urine and feces;

- Suppression of one's emotions;

- Self-induced isolation; and

- Rejection of emotional and physical intimacy, or a fear of sexuality.

So how does food addiction start? Based on what we have learned about addiction at the level of the brain, we can identify a simple answer. Feelings of satiety and hunger are generated in the brain, in the same neural pathways we mentioned when we explained what happens in addiction at the level of the brain (see Chapter 7). The ingestion of sweet foods is followed by the release of dopamine, which induces the person to want more of those foods.

IMAGE 5: The seesaw of addiction

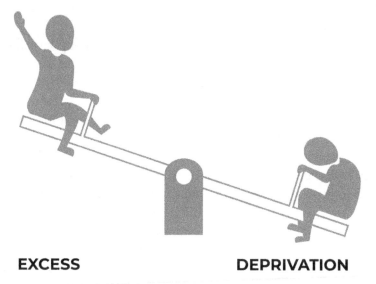

EXCESS　　　　　　　　**DEPRIVATION**

However, this answer doesn't account for those behavior types of food addiction that drive an addict to consume *less* food, such as anorexia and orthorexia. To account for these types of food addiction, we must note that although we are used to thinking that addictions are driven by **excesses** of a substance or behavior, **deprivation** can also start the addiction cycle. Like a seesaw, both extremes prompt the internal "mechanism" of the brain, and influence the levels of dopamine in the body. This is important, as it also accounts for the transformations from one behavior type to another in cases of food addiction, and reminds us that while *sometimes it may seem that someone is getting better, they may actually just be changing the pattern of their behavior, and getting worse.*

How body image, intimacy, and sexuality interact with food addictions

Girls usually become conscious of how others see their bodies around the onset of puberty, when they typically start to receive more attention for their looks. If they have low self-esteem—like so many of those children whose upbringings did not allow them to form secure attachments as infants—they may see their bodies as a means of obtaining validation. Suddenly, the "puppy fat" on their hips becomes their number one problem.

These girls may start dieting—but, after a couple of failures, their dieting can turn into an obsession, and into anorexia. After some months or years, they may give in to their cravings and find they can no longer follow the extreme rules they've set for themselves in an effort to lose weight. These girls start bingeing, then learn to purge, which can then turn into bulimia. When they binge and gain weight, they may find they become "invisible" to potential lovers who are put off by their looks. After a while, perhaps wanting to feel validated for their looks as they originally did, they may resume some control, lose a lot of weight, and become sexually provocative and seductive—until dieting once again becomes too complicated or difficult for them, and they retreat into becoming obese and nonsexual as they did before.

As these addicts go through life, their behavior may switch between the two extremes many times, often accompanied by other behavioral addictions like sex addiction. Since being fat is generally considered unattractive, and may lead to reduced interest from potential partners, some people who fear being preyed upon sexually and losing control during sex—especially victims of sexual abuse—unconsciously manipulate their bodies to avoid being seen as sexual, as a way to deter potential predators or even partners who may bring up bad memories they aren't ready to deal with. In some cases, the lives and bodies of these food addicts alternate between two extremes: they are either thin and seductive, desiring validation and love; or heavy and isolated, protecting themselves from potential pain.

Indeed, research has shown many food addicts, especially those suffering from binge eating and bulimia, also have issues with their sexuality.[28] Unfortunately, this is no surprise, since studies show that around 30 percent of this population are victims of childhood physical and sexual abuse—a slightly higher percentage than that found in other types of addictive populations and a full 50 percent higher than the percentage of child abuse victims found in the average population. Yes—terrible figures! When I first read the studies, I was sure they were exaggerated, and child sex abuse was just a fashionable topic of psychological research. But later, my own clinical experience confirmed the numbers. And it makes sense that young victims of abuse would become food addicts, as well—after all, what "drug" does a five-year-old have at her disposal with which to medicate the emotional pain and self-loathing resulting from such a traumatic experience? Food, of course. Children can usually obtain sugary, high-calorie foods long before they can get their hands on alcohol or other drugs, and stuffing themselves creates a comfortable feeling of satiety and oblivion that soothes the pain they may feel in other areas of their lives.

Emotional eating

As we have demonstrated above, *eating disorders and food addictions, like all addictions, are not about eating, but about controlling emotions.* Stuffing oneself with food can help suppress unpleasant emotions. So can depriving oneself of food. When certain types of food addicts don't want to feel emotion, they may drive it away by introducing a physical feeling that overpowers it: hunger. Many of these addicts also fear that, should these defense mechanisms fail, all their suppressed emotions would rise up and be vomited out of the body with no way

---

[28] Susan M. Mason et al. "Abuse victimization in childhood or adolescence and risk of food addiction in adult women," *Obesity* 21, no. 12 (2013): doi: 10.1002/oby.20500.

of stopping them. This explains some of the seemingly more confusing features of food addictions—like, for example, the fact that even emaciated anorexics can appear to be *afraid of eating*, or even of food. These addicts actually adore food, while appearing to fear it at the same time; but in fact, what they are really scared of are the emotions they would feel and the world they would experience without the protective cushion of their cherished friend and worst enemy—their addiction.

Of course, even food in significant quantities cannot satisfy emotional needs. As they say, *"You can't get enough of what you don't need!"* And in the words of Oprah Winfrey, who herself admitted having suffered from compulsive overeating, "For most of us who overeat, extra pounds correspond to unresolved anxieties, frustrations, and depressions, which all come down to fear we haven't worked through. We submerge the fear in food instead of feeling it and dealing with it. We repress it all with offerings from the fridge."[29]

For most healthy people, food is supposed to be the fuel we need to keep going, and hunger the physical signal that we need to refuel. Between meals, we ought not to think about food so much. This was one of the rules I wanted to follow in raising my children—but unfortunately, other influences in their lives seemed determined to contradict my efforts. Early on, their kindergarten teachers presented them with a different rule: "Be good, and you'll get candy!" And when we visited my relatives, I couldn't stop their doting grandparents from bringing all sorts of sweets to the table. Their grandmothers accused me of being too strict because all they wanted to do was show their grandchildren they loved them; and when my head was turned, lollipops or chocolates changed hands under the table.

This kind of thinking, common across many cultures, impresses upon young children that *food is a reward*, in the case of the classroom; and that *food symbolizes love*, in the case of the visits to my relatives. Both messages encourage us to associate food with emotion rather than hunger—which can lead to disordered eating later in life.

---

[29] Oprah Winfrey, *What I Know for Sure* (New York: Flatiron Books, 2014), 223.

I was especially frustrated by my children's grandmothers' accusations because I had my own share of problems with food. I was always on one diet or another, but my weight kept oscillating around the same (too-high) figure, and I couldn't hide it from the kids. Nor could I control the constant stream of comments and remarks they heard at the table—comments about who had taken too much and who should clean their plate; comments that a certain person should eat this or that, and *look at the girl next door! How good she looks now that she has lost weight!* Even though I was aware of the epidemics of obesity and eating disorders at the time, I wasn't able to protect my daughters from the damaging idea that food was love, nor from the idea that food was dangerous—*because if you eat too much, you may get fat, and then nobody will like you!*

When my daughters entered adolescence, they started to view their bodies critically, and even hatefully. They started comparing their looks to those of their classmates and started to think they ought to be different—thinner! At first, they just wanted it, and were disappointed at being compared to others, with no real idea of how to act on their feelings. But as they grew older, their willpower started to grow, too. They started their first diets, which at first only lasted until dinner. Nevertheless, their "failures" resulted in guilt and anger that they directed at themselves. These feelings worsened progressively into despondency and depression, and they took to lying on the couch all afternoon, angry at themselves. Sometimes they mustered enough energy to go running at night when nobody could see them. Other times, they comforted themselves with large bowls of ice cream.

Even though my daughters luckily never became food addicts, they exhibited some behaviors characteristic of food addiction—behaviors with which I'm sure most parents of adolescent daughters are familiar. Indeed, such behavior surrounding food and body image is a phase most girls, and many boys, go through in adolescence. However, the eating disorders that sometimes develop from these behaviors are much more severe than just a phase—they are deadly diseases.

Laura's Story

Laura, 32, told me her story of how she developed a food addiction as early as childhood:

> *When I was ten, I started dieting. My mother was overweight, divorced, and miserable, and I didn't want to end up like her. Most days over the next five years were spent thinking about what I wanted to eat but mustn't. I was living in a world where there were only two participants: food and myself. Other people could barely get through to me. As long as my sole focus was on food, the size of my wardrobe, the cellulite on my thighs, and the fantasies of my life when I would finally lose weight, nobody could really hurt me. My obsession with food was far more intimate than anything I had experienced with a boyfriend or a lover. When I felt rejected, I pretended the person was rejecting my body, not me, and that everything would be fine when I lost the weight. I got a lot of attention from the boys at high school. I went out with many of them but couldn't hold their attention for long. In my sophomore year at high school, I fell in love with Michael, who played on the football team. We dated for a while, and then he left me for a girl who was a lot heavier than me. I heard him commenting that he preferred her curves to my bones. I was devastated. I started skipping classes and staying at home, where I would binge eat. I stopped dieting. I could tolerate the pain of his betrayal only when my stomach was so full that I could hardly move. Of course, I gained a lot of weight in a short time. My mother started hiding food from me, my clothes no longer fit, and I was ashamed to go out. I thought everyone was talking about my body, as I'm sure they did! Every time I looked at myself in the mirror, I felt disgusted, like a pig, and was so full of shame that I hardly talked to anybody.*
>
> *During the school holidays, I shaped up and got back on my diet, and by the beginning of the next term, I was thin again. I started going out with boys again and discovered*

that the excitement and sexual pleasure of it all helped me stay on a rigorous diet. I was proud of my thin body and liked to dress in a way that showed it off, making me very popular with the boys. Everything in my life revolved around boys, sex, and food, or the lack of it.

When I started going to college, far away from home, I was really homesick and didn't have any friends. Everyone already seemed to be committed to some groups, so I stayed in my room and ate. The cycle was repeating itself...

15.a. *Bulimia Nervosa and Compulsive Overeating*

Bulimia nervosa is a behavior pattern characteristic of food addiction—an eating disorder characterized by repeated episodes of consuming large amounts of food in a relatively short time (binge eating). This bingeing is followed by a sense of loss of control over eating as well as feelings of guilt and shame, leading the person to engage in compensatory purging behaviors such as self-induced vomiting; fasting; excessive exercising; and the misuse of laxatives, enemas, or diuretics. Compulsive overeating is similar, only without purging. At their core, both disorders can be thought of as a type of behavioral addiction to food.

Typical Behaviors (see Exercise 1)

- Constantly thinking about or obsessing over food

- Devoting a lot of time and effort to maintaining a certain diet, and being extremely upset if you are unable to do so

- Obsessing over maintaining a certain body type

- Obsessing over your and others' body weight

- Constantly commenting on or controlling your own or others' eating habits

- Constantly comparing your body and eating habits to others'

- Planning meals well in advance, and becoming irritable if you are unable to stick to the plan

- Wolfing down food while alone, but eating little or nothing in public

- Eating enormous quantities of food in a short time, and even feeling unable to stop eating (**bingeing**)

- Purging by inducing vomiting after meals or abusing large quantities of laxatives

- Trying the latest "wonder diets" to lose weight or achieve some other goal, but abandoning them after a few weeks or months to start another diet

- Becoming ashamed and angry at yourself for overeating

- Losing control over your consumption of food (e.g., being unable to stop after only one piece of candy)

- Comforting yourself with food (**emotional eating**)

- Gaining and losing weight rapidly (e.g., fluctuating up to twenty pounds per month)

- Obsessing over exercise and becoming extremely restless if you are unable to work out

- Other: ....

Binge-purge syndrome

Binge eating is far from ordinary eating. It involves consuming enormous quantities of food—much more than a healthy person would feel comfortable eating. It also involves more than merely eating too much at a party because the food was so delicious and you just couldn't resist, or nibbling on snacks all day long. Instead, like alcoholics who drink to get drunk, food addicts binge eat to achieve the *feeling of fullness*, triggering the neurological pathways responsible for feeling satiation, dizziness, and numbness. Their normal feelings of being full are eclipsed; instead, they feel a terrible emptiness in their chests and stomachs, as if there were a hole there that is impossible to fill.

Often, these food addicts are ashamed of their behavior, so they binge alone. Before going out to a party, they may eat at home and only nibble a little while in the presence of others. Later, when they return home late at night, they empty the fridge, eating until they're so full it hurts. Sometimes, they empty their stomachs through self-induced vomiting, after which they may start eating again.

A food addict's binges are triggered by negative feelings, such as sadness, anxiety, relationship conflicts, or insecurity. As they say, "It's not what you're eating, but what's eating you!" While bingeing, the addict enters a sort of trance: an altered state of consciousness in which they find themselves numb to their bad feelings and unable to stop eating, even if they want to. When they awaken from the trance—either because they ran out of food or are simply too full to continue—they usually start to feel guilty, accusing and blaming themselves for breaking promises they've made to themselves and others, and despising their own helplessness and lack of control.

Between episodes of bingeing, food addicts who display this behavior type of food addiction usually choose low-calorie foods or skip meals in an effort to lose the weight they've gained as a result of bingeing. Paradoxically, the bad feelings this sort of deprivation creates can also prompt an addict's binges, putting them right back where they started.

Some addicts don't engage in any of the above behaviors between binges, and instead attempt to keep their weight down by **purging**, using laxatives or enemas or inducing vomiting in an attempt to get rid of the food they've recently ingested. Most addicts purge by sticking their fingers down their throats to trigger the vomiting reflex. This is physically stressful, but since the act of vomiting releases built-up stress hormones, a successful purge session often has a numbing effect on the addict's body, making them feel better as the body relaxes and the burden of food is no longer present.

Addicts who display this behavior type may also experience **cravings**. These cravings are more than just intense hunger—they are actually an altered state of consciousness in which the addicts can think of nothing but food and wolfing it down. Often, cravings concern a specific food and cannot be satisfied by other foods.

Of course, eating to excess prompts weight gain. Some of the addicts I've met who struggle with bulimia have told me they can gain more than twenty pounds in a couple of weeks if given the opportunity—such as during the holidays. Then, when the holidays end, nothing fits anymore, so they force themselves to lose weight as quickly as possible. Such rapid weight gain and loss is very harmful to the body, so, knowing they are unable to control their eating habits, some of them decide not to eat at all—which, of course, only harms their bodies in another way.

What bulimia does to the body

Whether the food addict suffering from bulimia overeats, binges and purges, or fasts in an attempt to lose the weight they've gained due to bingeing, symptoms of bulimia and binge eating affect their whole bodies. In some cases, although the addict may ingest plenty of food, they may be malnourished as a result of purging, which depletes the body of essential minerals called electrolytes. One of these electrolytes, potassium, plays a vital role in helping the heart and other muscles work, while other electrolytes such as sodium and chloride can become imbalanced by purging, leading to fatigue, muscle weakness, heart failure, and even death.

Food restriction and purging via vomiting also interfere with the normal process of digestion, and can lead to stomach pain, bloating, nausea, additional vomiting, blood sugar fluctuations, and other complications. Repeated vomiting can cause the salivary glands under the jaw and in front of the ears to swell. Often, the body tries to compensate for inadequate nourishment caused by purging by failing to process food at a regular pace, leading to constipation; and as a result, parts of the addict's digestive system may develop mechanical obstructions, or even rupture.

Symptoms of bulimia can affect the brain as well. Although this most vital organ weighs only three pounds, it utilizes up to one-fifth of the body's ingested calories. Dieting, fasting, deliberate starvation, and erratic eating prevent the brain from obtaining the energy it needs, leading to emotional and psychological consequences, such as an obsession with food or difficulty concentrating.

Of course, deprivation affects all of the body's systems, not just the digestive system, heart, and brain. For example, the body makes many of the hormones it needs from the fat and cholesterol we consume. Without enough fat and calories in the diet, hormone levels, including the levels of thyroid hormones and the sex hormones estrogen and testosterone, can drop—causing changes in girls' menstrual cycles and significantly decreasing their bone density, which increases the risk of fractures. Over time, binge eating can also cause the body to become resistant to insulin, leading to type 2 diabetes. Without enough energy to fuel metabolism, core body temperature drops, making addicts feel constantly cold. Starvation can also damage the immune system, resulting in frequent infections.

These symptoms should not be ignored—for addicts like this can die of starvation even when they live in abundance. In fact, people with eating disorders are six times more likely to die during any given year than a member of the general population, mainly due to causes like starvation, substance abuse, suicide, or, because their immune systems are typically compromised, cancer and infections.

The scope of the problem

Eating disorders are often enacted in private. Ashamed of their behavior—like many addicts of other kinds—these addicts are embarrassed that they cannot seem to control such a trivial thing as what goes into (and sometimes, out of) their mouths—so they lie about it. As a result, we can safely assume that this type of addiction is much more prevalent, and the problems much more significant, than official statistics tell us.

But even official figures are bad enough. According to statistics from the National Eating Disorder Association, up to thirty million people in the US suffer from eating disorders such as anorexia nervosa, bulimia nervosa, or binge eating disorder—almost 45 percent of the global figure. When it comes to binge eating specifically, 2.8 percent of American adults suffer from this disorder in their lifetime, and 1.5 percent of American women suffer from bulimia nervosa. In fact, this type of food addiction, which often first presents when the addicts are in their late teens, occurs most often in females—and only one in ten sufferers seeks and receives treatment. Considering the deadly complications, it's safe to say that bulimia and binge eating is a national health problem in America.

When considering these figures, it's important to remember that disordered eating and eating disorders are different. A person who worries about their looks and engages in disordered eating to change their body may not necessarily have an eating disorder.

Caren's Story

Caren, 26, described the powerlessness binge eaters feel as part of this grave disease in the following letter to me:

> When I wake up in the morning, I'm terribly hungry. But I have a plan: only one slice of whole wheat bread and some yogurt. I start eating, and as I do, I want to eat more and more. It's not enough. I have a feeling that I've had nothing to eat. I could eat two, three times more . . . and more and more. I can never feel satiety anymore, as though I never knew how it felt. No matter how full I am, I just don't think that I've had enough. It takes a lot of effort not to eat even more. I shudder, and I can't think of anything but food. My whole body craves food. I try to think of something else. I go out for a walk to get my mind off eating. Being outside makes it a little bit better. I can relax a little. I am starting

to question why I am only hungry at home. I'm alone in the house, and I can't stand the loneliness. When I'm alone, disturbing thoughts come to my mind. I feel guilty for having done nothing all these years. I hate myself for it. I see no brighter future ahead, just the same old dreaded emptiness. And when I think like that, I feel so hungry . . .

I go to the fridge, looking for something sweet. Chocolate, pudding, cookies. I have no sense of how much is enough. I just shovel food in my mouth. At first, it's a great relief. A feeling of calmness and happiness. Satisfaction washes over me. I think more positively; something is going to give, and everything will be all right . . . but these are just thoughts, just dreams to comfort me. Anyway, I never do anything to make them come true.

And suddenly . . . boom . . . I become aware of how much I have eaten. There's chaos inside me. What am I supposed to do now? I feel full, fat, and horrible. The tension is back. I feel like I'm as fat as a pig. Nobody will ever like me. Nobody should see me like this.

Of course, there's a solution. I go to the bathroom, drink a bottle of water, and put my fingers down my throat. I vomit. More! More! And more! Until I'm sure that all the food is gone. Then I feel better. I relax—but now I'm so tired, I have to take a nap.

I feel hunger when my mother comes home. Whenever she looks at me, I feel fat and worthless—especially when she looks down on me. In such situations, I wish I could make myself invisible. When she's around, I feel the tension all the time. And I'm hungry.

How does this feeling of hunger begin? It starts with anxiety and tension. I don't know where they come from. Then I start craving food. If I resist, I start shuddering, or become nauseous or dizzy. Nervous. Anxious. I feel that nobody likes me, and that everything is terribly wrong. I can see nothing good in the future. Everyone gets on my nerves. I just want to scream and lash out. Everyone has to leave me alone.

When I feel the craving, if I don't eat chocolate that very instant, my body starts trembling, and I would do anything to get some. I can think of nothing but chocolate. I cannot control my thoughts. Trying to escape them, I go running. The tension subsides. I get tired. My hunger subsides. I keep running, as if I want to run away from the pressure. And yes! Suddenly, I'm completely calm. I'm relieved. But for how long?

Advice for addicts

Like certain substance addictions, bulimia is very serious, in that it is one of the types of behavioral addictions that can most easily lead to death. If you are struggling with bulimia, you must seek professional help. The earlier you do so, the greater the likelihood you will recover physically and emotionally, without long-term consequences to your health. Please refer to the personalized recovery plan in Part Four of this book for sources of assistance.

Advice for the addict's family and friends

As a relative or friend of a food addict who exhibits behaviors typical of bulimia, you may witness the addict bingeing or purging—but you also might not, as addicts often practice their addiction in secret. Rapid changes in the addict's weight might be easier to notice. If you live with the addict, you might notice that food quickly disappears from the fridge, that the trash contains a lot of empty packaging, and that your friend or loved one is obsessed with their weight, or with dieting. You might also find empty packages of medication used for purging.

If you're concerned about a family member or friend whom you believe may be struggling with bulimia, you might be tempted to try to fix, control, or explain the addict's behavior. However, what the addict really needs is professional help. If you create shame in the addict by engaging in a long-term struggle with your addicted friend or family member, you could inadvertently perpetuate the negative feelings that are responsible for their addiction cycle—so, to help you cope with feelings of helplessness in the face of your loved one's addiction, I advise you also seek professional assistance.

15.b. *Anorexia Nervosa and Orthorexia*

Anorexia nervosa is a behavior pattern characteristic of food addiction—an eating disorder characterized by the avoidance of food and the resulting extreme weight loss (or lack of appropriate weight gain in growing children); difficulty maintaining a body weight appropriate to one's height, age, and stature; and a distorted body image. People with anorexia restrict the number of calories and types of food they eat, purge via induced vomiting and laxatives, and exercise compulsively. Some people with this disorder also binge eat.

Typical Behaviors (see Exercise 1)

- Rapidly losing weight or failing to gain weight when your weight drops below 15 percent of that expected for a person of your age and height, or when your BMI is less than 17.5

- Constantly thinking about or obsessing over food

- Experiencing extreme dread at the thought of gaining weight

- Devoting a lot of time and effort to maintaining a certain diet, and being extremely upset if you are unable to do so

- Bingeing and purging

- Sticking to an extremely restrictive diet, refusing to eat certain types of food (e.g., carbs or fats), or eating only certain foods

- Having an unrealistic perception of your body (e.g., viewing yourself as overweight even if you are dangerously underweight)

- Obsessing over maintaining a certain body type

- Obsessing over your and others' body weight

- Constantly commenting on or controlling your own or others' eating habits

- Constantly comparing your body and eating habits to others'

- Planning meals well in advance, and becoming irritable if you are unable to stick to the plan

- Fasting to the point of experiencing extreme fatigue, dizziness, or faintness

- Experiencing **amenorrhea**—the absence of a menstrual period in women, or failure to begin a menstrual cycle in girls—in combination with low body weight

- Constantly feeling cold

- Exercising to an extreme degree in order to "burn calories"

- Experiencing suicidal thoughts

- Undertaking extreme or unbalanced diets, or fasting to "cleanse" your body

- Being afraid of food

- Other:...

How anorexia begins

Like bulimia, anorexia usually begins in adolescence, around the time children's bodies start changing and young girls get their first periods. In my clinical experience, children who develop anorexia often come from well-to-do families that usually don't seem dysfunctional from the outside. Before the onset of the disease, they are usually "model" children, hardworking, well-adjusted, and doing well in school—in short, perfect girls and boys.

But though their families may seem perfectly normal, there may be an invisible elephant in the room. Maybe Dad is seeing another woman, and Mom is controlling, acting out her insecurity and rage toward her husband by obsessively cleaning the house. If these problems are never discussed—or worse yet, if they are actively ignored, with family members explicitly or implicitly forbidden from bringing them up—the children don't know how to resolve them; yet they feel unduly responsible. The family members are estranged, hiding behind work, problems, and TV; but they can feel the tension. Something is about to happen.

In a world they don't understand and can't control, children may discover dieting is all they can do to get their minds off the tension at home. Although boys can also engage in the disordered eating that leads to anorexia in pursuit of a specific body image, girls in particular are more likely to express an interest in becoming more like society's "ideal"—the skinny fashion model worked over in Photoshop. But when they force their organ systems out of balance through starvation, anorexics trigger an emergency response mechanism in their bodies.

Interestingly, in the beginning, parents sometimes praise their daughters for losing weight, and it takes time before they sound the alarm. A girl might hide the true effect of her addiction on her body by dressing in baggy clothes, claiming she is always cold; and act out secretly while behaving normally in public. She may even eat normally, but hurry to the bathroom to purge after lunch. As the disease progresses, the addicted child loses weight disproportionately, first losing her skeletal muscles, which are hidden beneath the layers of clothes she wears. Her face, however, often remains the same, thanks to the swelling of her salivary glands, which hides her protruding cheekbones. In this way, the most dangerous consequences are invisible, as the heart—which is also a muscle—grows weaker. The anorexic is often left with just enough power to maintain the illusion that nothing is wrong, dragging herself around as she attempts to get through each day. She might even insist on running for hours a day—to "burn calories"!

Extreme self-deprivation of this nature is very stressful on the body, which adapts to the lack of resources by shutting down all functions not essential to survival. To assist in this transformation and ease the body's stress, dopamine and cortisol are released into the brain, and the addict enters an altered state of consciousness: calm, detached, and prepared to shut down.

This is the physical draw of anorexia. More than the achievement these girls feel in becoming more physically similar to their favorite models and influencers, the dopamine they receive at this stage of the disease helps shut down painful feelings—which is the first, most basic step in the development of an addiction. Remember, dopamine is the main chemical involved in most addictions, and it is a hundred times more potent than heroin!

Unfortunately, while manipulating the body into extreme starvation alleviates psychological pain, it also produces other serious side effects: nonspecific gastrointestinal pain, dizziness, fainting, muscle weakness, difficulty concentrating, and impaired immune functioning and wound healing, which are also present in cases of bulimia. Depleted of important nutrients, the body is forced to slow all its processes to conserve energy, resulting in even more physical consequences: menstrual irregularities or even cessation; the emergence of fine hair on the body (**lanugo**); and increasingly thin, dry, or brittle hair on the head. Self-induced vomiting to maintain a low-calorie intake and achieve the altered state of consciousness and numbness caused by dopamine can also cause telltale consequences: cuts and calluses across the tops of the finger joints, dental problems, tooth sensitivity and discoloration, cavities, and swollen salivary glands. And finally, as the disease progresses and the addiction worsens, serious electrolyte imbalances caused by a lack of essential minerals can cause the addict's heart to beat irregularly, resulting in arrhythmia or even death.

I once saw a thirteen-year-old girl die of anorexia at the

pediatric clinic. She was lying in bed, unable even to sit up, with artificial liquids flowing through tubes leading into her veins. She lay there, emaciated, detached, and numb, with chocolates of every kind stuffed under her pillow and all around her—but she had crossed a line, and her body couldn't recover anymore. In the end, no one was able to help her.

Orthorexia

Perhaps more than any other addiction, orthorexia demonstrates how almost any behavior can become obsessive and even addictive if not practiced in moderation, and if it is used (and abused) to escape one's problems or numb one's feelings.

A behavior type of food addiction related to anorexia, **orthorexia**—a new name for an old condition that has only recently been described in the context of food addiction—is *an eating disorder characterized by an obsession with eating foods one considers healthy, and systematically avoiding specific foods they believe to be harmful.* Of course, eating healthy food is good for you—but some people can drive this idea into an obsession, taking the old saying, "You are what you eat!" deadly seriously. It is not necessarily as dangerous as anorexia in all cases, which may account for part of the reason it is not as widely recognized as an addiction. However, even if an addict's orthorexia is not extreme enough to result in the same deadly consequences as anorexia, this addiction can stem from similar maladaptive thinking, and cause unwanted disruption and shame in the addict's life. In this way (among others), orthorexia shares some common behaviors and basic beliefs with food addictions—which is why it is useful to include here.

Orthorexia seems to have become increasingly common in recent years. As a clinician, I have met quite a few clients who professed that certain bizarre food restrictions could save lives or even lead to instant enlightenment. According to Steve Bratman, the physician who coined the term "orthorexia," this disorder usually begins with a desire to overcome chronic illness or improve general health. Orthorexia nervosa develops when the victim becomes obsessed not with the *quantity* of food eaten, as in the case of anorexia or bulimia, but the *quality* of the food. What starts as a devotion to healthy eating can evolve into a pattern of incredibly strict diets, with addicts becoming so focused on eating a "pure" diet—usually of vegetables and grains—that the planning and preparation of food come to play the dominant role in their lives. Such people, who are often insecure, obsessed with food, or secretly struggling with anorexia, develop their own rules for eating, typically as a response to their fear of losing control in other areas of their life. Some stick to raw food, while others eliminate certain ingredients. And some even try to plan their meals according to strict dietary recommendations, to the gram and to the minute—for example, no protein until noon.

Restrictions of this nature often mimic fad diets, or are even prompted by them. These days, we are bombarded by commercials for these diets, which try to sell us everything from specific foods to a certain way of life, claiming they are all one needs to achieve absolute happiness. Every commercial or archaic (but recently rediscovered) diet has a fancy name—paleo, gluten-free. Behind each diet, an anecdote or a story, probably published in a bestselling book, explains in layman's terms what miracles readers can expect if they stick to the diet—or, conversely, warns readers of the risks of eating certain foods, or of the chemicals used in food production. They may claim you will get cancer or some other disease, or even die sooner if you continue eating certain foods, or if you use this or that additive. And people follow these tips by the thousands! One could easily spend days researching and attempting to comply with all these recommendations, musts, and must-nots—but if you do, obsessing over eating healthily and avoiding foods that may harm you can become more than just a healthy choice. It can turn into an obsession—and an addiction.

To stress the difference, the necessary ingredients for a "healthy" diet are not sold in ordinary supermarkets but in special sections or shops, and are considerably more expensive, increasing their emotional value. It's considered healthy and good for you if you make a special effort to go out and

get this particular food, prepare it according to the special recommendations, and measure it carefully. This can be feasible,
especially if you live alone—but addicts who conform to this
behavior type of food addiction often impose their strict rules
onto family members and even pets, offering them no choice
in the matter. Such behavior can easily fall under the umbrella
of psychological manipulation, or in some cases, even cause
physical harm; in fact, I know of some tragic cases of infants
dying of severe malnutrition as a result of having been fed
strictly vegan food.

Ultimately, it is this maladaptive thinking and the harm it
can cause that mark orthorexia as a type of addiction. The body
is a wonderful natural instrument that can metabolize almost
any organic substance into the basic building blocks it requires
to sustain and nurture itself. It needs no special essential ad-
ditives, provided the food we eat contains adequate nutrients.
It functions best if we know how to listen to what it tells us,
in the form of hunger and other feelings. But addictions and
other obsessions try to override these feelings with cravings or
habits. If we stop listening to the messages our bodies send us,
illnesses and tragedy can result.

The scope of the problem
Due to the effects of weight loss and starvation on the body
and brain, anorexia nervosa is a life-threatening disorder. According to available research, the lifetime prevalence of anorexia nervosa in the US may be as high as 0.3 percent among
males and 4 percent among females.[30] Other sources, including
the National Association of Anorexia Nervosa and Associated Disorders, maintain that eating disorders affect at least 9
percent of the population worldwide,[31] and a review of nearly fifty years of this research confirms anorexia nervosa has

[30] Annelies E. van Eeden, Daphne van Hoeken, and Hans W. Hoek. "Incidence,
Prevalence and Mortality of Anorexia Nervosa and Bulimia Nervosa," *Current
Opinion in Psychiatry* 34, no. 6 (2021): 515–24, doi: 10.1002/oby.20500.
[31] "Eating Disorder Statistics," ANAD, National Association of Anorexia Nervosa
and Associated Disorders, 2023, https://anad.org/eating-disorders-statistics.

the highest mortality rate of any psychiatric disorder.[32] A full 20 percent of people suffering from anorexia will prematurely die of complications related to their eating disorder, including suicide and heart problems. What's more, about half of the patients who suffer from anorexia also have other conditions such as anxiety and mood disorders, including obsessive-compulsive disorder and social phobia.

Jessica's Story

Jessica, a young girl in her late teens, describes her way of thinking while she was in the throes of anorexia in the following way:

> *I have always hated family meals. Well, not always. When I was very young, I loved them. My mother would cook my father's favorite soup all day to show him how much she loved him. I loved the feeling that they loved each other. My mom was always on a diet and only ate salads. I somehow believed that a woman had to always be on a diet—that it was normal.*
>
> *Then the divorce—a new husband, and a new baby. A new wonderful family for her, and now she could correct all the mistakes she made with us. Good for her! What's in it for my brother and me, I don't quite know! Neither does she, I guess! But we still have to come to family dinners and sit there and pretend we're a happy family. I hate it when somebody munches at the table. It seems so dirty and disgusting, like having sex at the table. I don't know why. Probably because they enjoy it so much.*
>
> *Of course, these meals we have to sit down to always end up in a fight because my brother can't hold his tongue and says what I dare not. I always keep silent, stare at my plate with a lump in my throat till the end of dinner. Then I go to my room, clutching my knees like a baby in the*

---

[32] Daphne van Hoeken and Hans W. Hoek. "Review of the Burden of Eating Disorders: Mortality, Disability, Costs, Quality of Life, and Family Burden," *Current Opinion in Psychiatry* 33, no. 6 (2020): 521–27, doi: 10.1097/YCO.0000000000000641.

womb, and cry for hours. Nobody ever comes to comfort me; they've probably got no idea. No one seems to notice I never touch my food. I suppose my mother would be happier if my brother and I disappeared, and she could forget our father.

But every morning, it's time to "weigh the cattle." If I'm smart enough, she will let me be all day. It seems that the number on the scale tells me how much she loves me that day. I'm cornered. I want the number to be as small as possible, but she'll start to question me if it is too low. So I wake up at five and drink two large bottles of water and a large pot of tea. Since I'm awake, I do my exercises. I'm so full of water it hurts and makes me sick, but I can't use the bathroom before being weighed. Secretly, I attach weights to my feet and wear two pullovers. I'm disgusted at myself for being so weird, but if I succeed, we can pretend all day that everything's fine.

I only touch food in the evening. Daddy always taught me to save the best for the last.

I love food, and I'm afraid of loving it too much, so I'd rather not touch it. I've buried the pleasure I get from eating, and instead have charts and numbers. If anybody interferes with my habits, I'm overcome with feelings I can't describe: rage. Fear. Shame. Everything I want to suppress. I always eat at 10:00 p.m. on the dot. Then there's peace, and nobody's watching. I never eat anything that doesn't have a label showing the number of calories on the packaging. If I did, I would feel so dirty. I'm afraid of what would happen if I gave up control. I know I'm weird and am ashamed of it.

I think about food all day. When I'm really hungry, I sort out the yogurts by their expiration date or prepare a meal and flush it down the toilet. And when I do that, I get the same feeling as when I eat the food I allow myself to eat at the time I allow myself to eat it. I feel good and clean, knowing I have won the battle over food. The lump in my throat gets smaller. I feel like I'm in a peaceful, very comfortable trance, like I'm on a "high." This is the only pleasurable feeling I ever have. Everything else is just tears, pain, and shame.

Anya's Story

Anya, 17, told me how her father's obsession with eating raw food affected her family:

My father is an alcoholic. When I was ten, he went into treatment because my mother threatened to divorce him. He has been sober from then on, but I still fear him coming home at night, hearing his staggered footsteps and him yelling in the courtyard. When he was drinking, it was horrible, and every day we wished he would go into treatment, expecting that that would solve all our problems. But it didn't. It actually got worse. He would line up my brother, my mother, and me in the kitchen to listen to his drunken preaching of how he was doing everything for us and how ungrateful we were. After that, he would go to sleep, and the next day, he would avoid us.

But now, he's on our backs all day long. He's obsessed with eating raw food. He doesn't let my mother cook ordinary meals for us. We have to eat raw fruit and vegetables, just like him, and nothing else. Our basement is full of apples, and every day, I have to listen to how healthy they are. I crave the delicious soups my mother used to make. Whenever I can, I try to cheat, and a piece of bread is sooooo delicious, but if he catches me, I have to pay for it by listening to him preaching how my body will degenerate and become fat and bloated. Actually, I have lost some weight, but I always seem to be hungry and crave "real food." I feel sorry for my younger brother, who's bullied at elementary school for not eating meals with his classmates. He's still so young, and he believes everything our father tells him. He thinks he'll fall ill if he eats like the others and doesn't understand why they mock him.

My mother doesn't want to confront my father, so she seemingly sticks to his rules, but I have seen that she's started smoking. Whenever father sits us down to listen to his monologues of how the world is filthy and the dangers lurking outside, my mom says she needs to visit her friend across the street, and I see them smoking on the balcony. She often comes home smelling of alcohol, and that is a smell I will never forget. My father must have smelled it too, but he doesn't say anything. I can hardly wait for the day when I turn eighteen and will be able to leave home. If it weren't for my brother, I'd have already left. . . .

Advice for addicts

Like certain substance addictions, anorexia can be very serious, in that it is one of the types of behavioral addictions that can most easily lead to death. If you are struggling with anorexia, you must seek professional help. The earlier you do so, the greater the likelihood you will recover physically and emotionally, without long-term consequences to your health. Please refer to the personalized recovery plan in Part Four of this book for sources of assistance.

Advice for the addict's family and friends

Unfortunately, when it comes to anorexia, an ounce of prevention is worth a pound of cure. Given the high prevalence of anorexia, especially among young girls, parents are best served by trying to prevent their children from heading down a path that could lead to anorexia by offering positive affirmations and examples of what it means to have a healthy body image. They should be aware that commenting on their child's body weight could have serious consequences when it comes to their self-esteem, and be careful not to instill in them the belief that a person must be a certain weight in order to be attractive.

However, success in this area can be difficult to achieve, especially since parents are up against a media conglomerate that relentlessly depicts images of perfectly airbrushed bodies, both male and female. With all these messages being pushed constantly through television, the Internet, and print media, a child will learn soon enough that they will be judged by their looks. Add bullying at school and even doctors' or coaches' recommendations for losing weight, and they may decide to start dieting regardless of their parents' or guardians' positive messages on this subject. And while this happens more often in girls, boys are not exempt from this kind of thinking—especially if they practice a sport.

Ultimately, the best way to prevent a child from developing anorexia is for the whole family to commit to maintaining a healthy relationship to food. But what if you believe someone you love might already be sliding down the slippery slope that leads to this type of addiction? What are the signs?

In spite of all the possible indicators, it can be hard to identify an anorexic in trouble. I was made aware of this problem at a parent-teacher meeting when one of my daughters was in junior high school. At that time, my daughter told me six of her classmates always went to the bathroom after a meal, and became extremely nervous if they were unable to do so. All the girls in the class knew, but the teachers had noticed nothing. After talking to the girls and gaining their confidence, we discovered even more girls were involved. The participation of so many girls serves to emphasize the fact that once this type of addiction has taken root, it can very quickly escalate out of control.

In the beginning—as scared as they are of losing that control—young anorexics may take pride in being so thin. Wanting to engage in their new weight loss habits without interference, they learn to cheat and lie to their parents, guardians, and other authority figures, telling them they have already eaten. Relatives of a child—or adult—in this position may notice the addict is fussy about food, doesn't eat certain foods, or chews food for an unusually long time. At family meals, they may eat normally, or even claim they have already eaten. After meals, they might rush to the bathroom or toilet to purge, becoming nervous or aggressive if unable to do so. One day, you may notice the chocolates that have been kept for Christmas are missing, or find some empty boxes. You may also notice that they drink a large amount of water, to try to fool their empty stomachs into believing they are full. If you stand in line at the cashier behind them at lunchtime, notice whether they only buy chewing gum and Diet Coke. No calories—calories are their enemy!

Usually, friends and family also notice that these addicts don't see their bodies as they actually are. They may think they're too fat, even when they're actually starving. Their actual body weight may be average, or they may be slightly overweight, or their weight might fluctuate. They may also complain of various symptoms, such as stomach cramps, and gastrointestinal issues like constipation or acid reflux. They may have difficulty concentrating, feel dizzy, or even faint when getting up quickly. They may feel cold even when the weather is hot, or be unable to sleep. A visit to a doctor will reveal abnormal laboratory findings—anemia, low thyroid and hormone levels, low potassium, low blood cell counts, a slow heart rate, and so on.

Physical changes can be visible as well. You might notice the addict's face looks round due to the swelling of the salivary glands, that their teeth are yellowish or damaged, or that they have calluses and abrasions on their fingers from inducing vomiting. For adults and older teens who fell into this addiction earlier in childhood, their addictive behaviors may even have affected their body's release of growth hormones in adolescence, resulting in arrested physical development.

You may also notice changes in the addict's way of life. They may alternate between excessive exercise to "burn the calories" and depressively lying on the couch and bingeing TV series. They may go running even when the weather is terrible, or if they are tired, ill, pregnant, or injured.

If you are the parent or guardian of a young child or teen and all or even some of the above indicators feel familiar to you, please get them professional help. You may be confused by your child's behavior, and secretly wish that somebody would solve the problem for them, or make it disappear. All too often, people see what they want to see—and parents who are insecure in their parenting abilities may choose not to see a problem if they feel they cannot handle it. But a child in such a state is seriously ill, and often needs to be taken to the hospital to help return these processes to normal. What's more, if all the hospital staff do is feed the patient back to their normal weight, the improvement will only be temporary. What an anorexic really needs is psychotherapy. You are your child's most important ally; if you can't handle the situation, how can they? They need you to take action on their behalf. As an adult, you need to take on the mindset that if you cannot deal with a problem, you should get help from someone who can. *Please don't underestimate the problem. Find expert help!*

16. Addictions to Work, Money, and Risk

a. Addiction to Work

b. Addictions to Money (Spending, Shopping, Debt) and Risk

c. Addiction to Gambling

16

Addictions to Work, Money, and Risk

Introduction

Addictions to work, money, and risk are behavioral addictions whereby a person achieves an altered state of consciousness through extreme manipulation of resources—money, energy, and time—all with the intent of numbing and escaping pain. These types of addiction are similar to food addiction in that excess (in these cases, overworking, overachieving, and earning) and deprivation (burnout, procrastinating, spending, and acquiring debts) with regard to the subjects of the addiction both serve as sources of stress, and have numbing effects on the addict's brain.

Manipulating resources to boost one's self-image

At first glance, money, energy, and time have little in common; but in fact, they all have to do with resources. We need them to survive—as we need food, or even relationships.

In all these cases, *the way we handle our resources reveals how we position ourselves in relation to the world*. Some people, for instance, feel entitled to all the good that life has to offer, and therefore gravitate toward hoarding goods. On the other hand, some pride themselves on being able to live deprived of what most of us would consider certain basic essentials, and deny themselves the right to be well off, balance work with rest, or relax.

Often, whether an addict gravitates toward excess or deprivation in their addiction is mainly the result of their upbringing. When we discussed the effects of addiction on families in Part Two of this book (see Chapter 10), we explained that people who are insecurely attached to their caregivers carry this dysfunctional attachment style into their adult relationships—and this includes not only their relationships with people, but also their relationship to resources such as money, work, and time. When such people try to compensate for their insecurities and feelings of uncertainty or a lack of safety, they may do so in two distinct ways: either they cling to the soothing relationship, object, or in this case, resource, and try to hoard it; or they trick themselves into believing they don't need it at all. Usually, one of two extreme "solutions" will result, as depicted in the table below:

TABLE 4: Excess and deprivation in handling resources compared to other behavioral addictions

	EXCESS	DEPRIVATION
MONEY	Hoarding money, excessive borrowing or earning	Debts, shopping, gambling
ENERGY	Overworking, overachieving	Burnout, inability to work due to psychological reasons
TIME	Procrastination, being chronically late	Constantly feeling you are running out of time
RISK	Gambling, dangerous sports, cryptocurrencies, stock market	Burnout, social phobia
FOOD	Bulimia, compulsive overeating	Anorexia, orthorexia
RELATIONSHIPS (LOVE)	Codependence, "love" addiction	Relationship anorexia (social phobia)

Remember the seesaw from page 119, when we discussed how both excess and deprivation drive the addictive system? As the table shows, this type of interaction applies to all behavioral addictions involving basic resources.

People who have low self-esteem, as addicts do, can abuse the social power that lots of money and a prestigious career can bring them to improve their low self-esteem. Money is the most concrete and obvious of these resources, as well as an unavoidable fact of life. It offers social power—and if we don't feel good about ourselves, we can use the power of money to make us feel better. Meanwhile, incurring a debt means you're entering into a relationship with a creditor—a relationship in which you are not likely to be abandoned. Someone's worth can be measured by how much others are willing to loan them. Spending money can also make you feel good—at least, this is what all the advertisements try to tell you.

Devoting one's energy to working excessively can also bring an addict social power and prestige—and of course, money. And finally, as we all know, "time is money," as well. How do you handle your time?

How our beliefs shape our destinies

When we try to understand and react to what happens around us or within us, we are seldom aware that we are actually not responding to the events themselves, but rather to the meanings we have automatically assigned to them based on all the experiences we had so far. The memories of these experiences and the meanings we derive from them are organized in our minds as "mental world maps," which serve as the basis for assigning meaning to everything we encounter. Different people have different experiences, and therefore different mental world maps, which unfortunately causes many misunderstandings between people. These "mental world maps" are particularly prevalent when it comes to the mental images of what you want and expect in a relationship, which then guide the way your actual relationships unfold. (We call this type of mental world map a "love map," and will return to these in our chapters on relationship addiction.)

The unconscious assessment of whether the world is either benevolent or hostile is the core element of a person's mental world map.[33] It is the lens through which we "see" everything, influencing the meaning we assign to everything later in life. This belief is too deep to be easily changed through learning or persuasion, but it can be changed, usually through a therapeutic process that takes a couple of years and a secure relationship with a therapist or similar professional.

The "rules of safety" we learn in our families of origin are essential parts of our mental world maps. The rules established by our families of origin[34] influence what we feel is safe. We either blindly adhere to them or rebel and do just the opposite, but we are bound by them in both cases. This was best explained by Eric Berne,[35] who introduced the idea that our destinies are bound by **life scripts**: the *"early decisions, made unconsciously, as to how life shall be lived."* He proposed that from the early interactions between mother, father, and child, the child's life plan unconsciously evolves, limiting their freedom of choice to only a few possibilities by means of injunctions and counterinjunctions. The idea was further developed by Claude Steiner[36] who described some of the most common scripts and explained that some life scripts, typically those leading to addictions, are self-destructive. People bound by them derive unconscious "payoffs" from situations where they are hurt, betrayed, abandoned, deprived, or in danger, thus proving their "core belief" that the world is dangerous, people are evil, and themselves powerless. As problematic as it is, confirming one's core beliefs can actually make people believe in the illusion

---

[33] See the chapter on addiction as an attachment disorder, wherein we discuss secure and insecure attachment styles (pg. 73).

[34] See Chapter 10: Problems at the Level of the Family, on pg. 72.

[35] "Eric Berne (May 10, 1910 – July 15, 1970) was a Canadian-born psychiatrist who [in the mid-twentieth century] created the theory of transactional analysis as a way of explaining human behavior." In addition to life scripts, he also evolved the theory of games, which we discussed earlier. "Eric Berne," Wikipedia, Wikipedia Foundation, Inc., September 2, 2023, https://en.wikipedia.org/wiki/Eric_Berne.

[36] Claude M. Steiner, *Scripts People Live: Transactional Analysis of Life Scripts* (New York: Grove Press, Inc., 1990).

that they have some control, so they feel safer.

Let's look at an example of a life script of a "workaholic."

Life script of a "workaholic"

A child is brought up in a home where he sees his mother struggling hard to make ends meet. His alcoholic father abandons them. He learns that you have to struggle and give up on things you enjoy in order to survive. The mother's **injunction**—*Don't exist!*—is communicated indirectly through her words: "If I weren't pregnant with you, I wouldn't have married your alcoholic father! My life would have been so much better without you!" As a result, the child's **belief** becomes: "The world would be better without me. I'm worthless and unimportant. Nobody loves me as I am." The mother's **counterinjunctions**—*Please me! Work hard! Be perfect!*—now come through: "Now that your father has left us, I'm counting on you to be the man of the house, regardless of what you're capable of doing." From these interactions, the child develops a **life decision**: "Only if I work hard, am perfect, and please others am I permitted to exist."

The child now believes they are not allowed to exist unless they work harder than everybody else and are perfect in their performance. Indeed, for them, doing so is no longer a choice—as the injunction "don't exist" is activated if they stop obeying the counterinjunction (*Work hard; please me; be perfect!*), resulting in terrible anxiety and possible burnout. As a result, adult workaholics feel as if something terrible may happen unless they continually control their workplace and accept more and more work. Their feelings are exaggerated to the point of endangering their health and family relationships.

On the other hand, other people with different scripts may attempt to comfort themselves and quiet the anxiety created by their life scripts by shopping and incurring debts disproportionate to their financial means. Some may behave as if money has no value for them. Still others adore money and believe having it will make all their problems go away—so they hoard it, becoming excessively frugal. Or they may become money-anorexic, feeling superior if they can get by with as little as possible. Others may subconsciously sabotage their chances of financial success because they believe being rich means being dishonest. Everyone is different, and so there are numerous possibilities of getting hooked into this "if this, then that" game—which is another example of people continuing to engage in certain behaviors despite knowing those behaviors will cause harm, a feature so typical of addiction. And as you can see, this circle of injunctions and counterinjunctions looks dangerously similar to the addiction cycle we already know!

The way we handle *money in relationships* reveals the meanings we assign to it. Misunderstandings and manipulations are often the reason for irreconcilable troubles between partners. Money is power, and our relationship to it affects how we distribute power in our marriages. It allows for all sorts of psychological "games" of revenge and manipulation: if your spouse is financially irresponsible, you may have to cover their debts, which influences your relationship. If you fear your spouse is thinking of leaving, you may be tempted to exploit their fear of poverty to keep them in the relationship. If your spouse is losing interest in you, you can get revenge by using their credit cards to go on a shopping spree.

Money and *work*. How much of our daily personal and family lives revolve around these? Let's dig a little deeper into each of these behaviors to understand the different behavior types of this addiction.

The behavior types are:

1. Addiction to work

2. Addiction to money (spending, shopping, debt) and risk

3. Addiction to gambling

16.a. *Addiction to Work*

Addiction to work is a behavioral addiction whereby a person works compulsively and excessively, to the detriment of their health and other pursuits such as family or free time. It can appear in anyone, not only among high earners or those who have a career society views as very important; a workaholic can get caught up in obsessively doing charity work, or even mundane housework. Workaholics have a strong work ethic, are constantly working, and take little time for personal enjoyment. Although they may claim their job demands they work long hours, they actually do so to escape their problems in other areas of their lives. When unable to work, they are apprehensive and restless. Eventually, their extreme and exaggerated behavior can lead to exhaustion and burnout, leaving them unable to work at all—sometimes for months.

If you accuse your spouse of being a workaholic, you probably don't mean to accuse them of being an addict—but rather to tell them they need to be more engaged with the family and take on more family obligations. However, by now, you have probably realized I don't speak lightly about behavioral addictions, but in terms of obsession, loss of control, preoccupation, and continuing despite adverse consequences. Engaging in too much work *can* be a sign of addiction—and we will discuss that addiction in more detail below.

Typical Behaviors (see Exercise 1):

- Constantly working overtime despite health problems, conflicts in the family, and signs that your children are being neglected

- Feeling anxious if you cannot control what is going on at work (e.g., during your vacation time)

- Losing your sense of time while working

- Working even when you are sick out of the belief something terrible might happen if you stay at home and rest (e.g., that you'll be laid off or demoted)

- Experiencing rage-fueled outbursts, irritation, sleeplessness, tension, impatience, forgetfulness, problems with concentration, and changing moods if you are unable to work

- Feeling extremely anxious if you cannot achieve perfection at work

- Constantly thinking about what else needs to be done at work

- Burning out and being unable to do any professional work for a long period

- Alternating between working too much and being unable to work at all

- Believing you are irreplaceable in your work role

- Believing work is the most important thing in life

- Other: ....

Losing oneself in working too much

Society values work—and as a result, it respects and appreciates those who work a lot. But some people choose work over themselves, their family, and their friends—not because they have to or want to please an unsupportive boss, but to escape everything they consider wrong with their lives. These aspects of their lives are usually connected to the trauma and abuse they experienced during childhood, and driving themselves to work to exhaustion may be a kind of trauma repetition (discussed in my next book, *Courage*). They hide their feelings of inadequacy behind the smokescreen of their "busy-busy" persona, but their chaotic and hysterical preoccupation with work reveals their belief that the world requires their superhuman efforts and self-sacrifice. In reality, their belief that the world would stop turning if they didn't toil from dawn to dusk is an indicator of their low self-esteem. Although they assign themselves the super-important role of a savior, they actually feel they are not allowed to breathe unless they work twice as much as others (see the example of a life script in the previous chapter). At the same time, they may actually cause drama with their unrealistic planning—for instance, by promising to finish a task in half the necessary time, and then becoming exhausted or making so many mistakes that the job actually takes even longer to be finished.

Workaholism has to do with avoiding emotional closeness, which may trigger painful feelings for the addict. As devoted as they are to resolving problems at work, workaholics are usually passive when it comes to personal relationships—often ignoring them entirely, or at least wishing them away. They're also ignorant of the potential physical consequences of an imbalance between work and rest. They don't feel their bodies, and they're numb to their relationship problems. When they cannot control what is happening at work, they feel lost, disconnected, or in danger. Even on holidays, they need a plan; spontaneity threatens them.

Employers may think a workaholic is a model employee, working until the wee hours of the morning and enjoying it, too. But no! Remember that addicts lose the ability to enjoy things. Instead, workaholics are driven to work by their inner demons. Lack of sleep and chronic stress impair their ability to concentrate. More often than not, they abuse chemical stimulants, starting with coffee and progressing to cocaine and other drugs.

Workaholics experience a number of different symptoms as a result of their addiction. **Physical symptoms** are the result of chronic stress and exhaustion. They can start with headaches, fatigue that doesn't go away with rest, chest pain, shortness of breath, facial muscle spasms, or dizziness. If the stress continues, thyroid dysfunction may occur as a result of overloading the stress system. They can also experience **emotional and behavioral symptoms**, which can be outbursts of rage, restlessness, irritability, impatience, boredom, forgetfulness, inability to sleep or relax, inability to concentrate, and mood swings. In an attempt to hide their failures, the workaholic may start lying about how much they work, and about their success.

Workaholism destroys families! Even when they are at home, workaholics are emotionally absent and obsess about their work. Compared to the cosmic dimensions and extreme importance of their work, their children's school problems, athletic victories, and first loves can wait. The family gets used to not being able to count on them. The initiative to start therapy usually comes from their spouses, who are angry to the moon and back! My clients' spouses often tell me they feel they are living with a zombie. They miss someone to share all those little but important things that make up a partnership, and they feel exploited because they have to do their spouse's share of the parenting and household chores. They're angry when they see how the children try in vain to arouse their parent's attention. Forty percent of such marriages end in divorce.

Putting all your eggs in one basket is risky. A disease or a work crisis may result in sudden unemployment—and for a workaholic, this is the end of the world. They may become seriously depressed or suffer so-called **burnout**[37] a severe condition characterized by emotional exhaustion, reduced feelings of work-related personal accomplishment, physical fatigue, and cognitive weariness.

The scope of the problem

Studies that consider workaholism a behavioral addiction don't just measure working hours but include the obsessive quality and inability to stop despite serious consequences. These studies estimate that around 8 percent of people—mainly those in the upper middle class—suffer from the condition. This is in line with findings that 5 to 10 percent of the general pop-

---

[37] "Burnout is a syndrome conceptualized as resulting from chronic workplace stress that has not been successfully managed. It is characterized by . . . feelings of energy depletion or exhaustion; increased mental distance from one's job, or feelings of negativism or cynicism related to one's job; and reduced professional efficacy." "Burn-out an 'occupational phenomenon': International Classification of Diseases," World Health Organization, WHO, May 28, 2019, https://www.who.int/news/item/28-05-2019-burn-out-an-occupational-phenomenon-international-classification-of-diseases.

ulation suffers from some form of addiction.[38] In Japan, they even have a word for workaholism: *karoshi*, or simply "working to death." Technological advances such as smartphones and company-supplied laptops have allowed employees potentially unlimited access to their work, and changes in where work occurs (e.g., telecommuting) may further blur the lines between work and home. Recent adaptations to work from home due to the COVID-19 pandemic further blur the boundaries between work and leisure or family time. Some find this potentially positive, at least initially; but the common opinion of most researchers nowadays is that the negative psychological consequences seriously outweigh the positive ones.

Frank's Story

You may still think addiction to work is not as serious as, for example, drinking or gambling. You may even be proud of your ability to put so much effort and concentration into your work. But read about how Frank, 30, a successful entrepreneur, struggled with its consequences:

> *I started working and earning money already when I was in high school. Every day, I fought my fear that I would be left alone, without anything. My grandmother, who took care of me, was quite old, and I had no other family to look after me. I took any work I could get, from physically exhausting construction work to fixing computers. I knew they took advantage of me, but the money I saved made me feel a bit better. The more money I had, the safer I felt—and most important of all, I had proof that I was good. I got a lot of praise when I succeeded in something difficult, and it made me feel I needed to work even more.*
>
> *Despite all this working and striving, I somehow found the time to get married. After a couple of years of marriage, my wife started complaining that we needed to work on*

---

[38] Mark D. Griffiths, "Work Addiction and 'Workaholism': Are These Two Constructs the Same?," *Psychology Today*, Sussex Publishers, February 12, 2018, https://www.psychologytoday.com/us/blog/in-excess/201802/work-addiction-and-workaholism.

our relationship. I had no idea what she meant. I had built everything in my life—my education, reputation, business, and house. But our worlds kept drifting apart. We made a deal that one day a week would be devoted to just us. I kept my promise and stayed at home—behind the computer and with a telephone in my hands. I didn't understand her complaining that I "wasn't present." She often complained that I would be a lousy father if we ever had kids. Those words hurt me a lot. Am I really becoming like my father, who—despite my successes—never knocked on my door to tell me how proud he was of me? I kept looking for praise and money. I worked two, three jobs simultaneously, traveling worldwide, meeting business people from abroad, and enjoyed meeting important people. After a while, my wife threatened to divorce me. I had nowhere to hide, so I agreed to look for help. I was sure that the therapist would understand my way of life and help open my wife's eyes, telling her that she should support my efforts. But instead of that, she gave us some homework which was difficult for me— one hour of closeness a day.

No telephone, no computer, just us, on the sofa, talking about us and our feelings.

The first hour felt like a hundred years! I remember I sat in such a way that I could watch the clock over my wife's shoulder. The clock hands just wouldn't move! What should I talk about? Ask me about the stock market, or the latest nanotechnological achievements . . . anything but how I was feeling. I sat there feeling anxious, looking into my wife's eyes, full of expectations. And I couldn't stop thinking about work, the current projects I was working on, and the things I needed to do. . . . For a long time, that hour was the most stressful part of the day. Worse than complex business negotiations I was so good at.

Advice for addicts

On the surface, work addiction seems quite innocent when compared to other substance or behavioral addictions. Still, it brings with it grave consequences: burnout, depression, poor physical health, career and life dissatisfaction, conflicts between one's work and family, and relationship and marital conflict. If you have found that a couple days off can no longer alleviate your stress, or if your doctor has warned you about developing stress-related diseases, something needs to change. Please refer to the related sections in Part Four of this book.

Advice for the addict's family and friends

Many workaholics hide behind the social, societal, and organizational culture that surrounds us, which glorifies excessive work and competition in the workplace. And as many times as you may tell your workaholic loved one that they should "work to live, not live to work," they will not hear you. Their "life scripts" have their own logic. If a workaholic stops working, unless they are totally exhausted, their inner injunction "Don't exist!" is activated—and their profound anxiety with it. Workaholics have to work to get their inner demons' permission to live! This is why, as much as you may plead, argue, persuade, or even threaten divorce, none of these efforts will work long-term. In cases of workaholism, individual and family therapy is recommended. Please refer to the later sections of this book to develop a comprehensive plan of action for your workaholic loved ones.

16.b. *Addictions to Money (Spending, Shopping, Debt) and Risk*

Many obsessive behaviors involving risky decisions and the irrational acquisition and spending of money often occur together. When they do, they often indicate a certain lifestyle in the addict—so it makes sense to explain them within the same chapter. In addition, addictions to money and risk are often found together with other behavioral addictions—and when they are, they form **addiction interaction**.

Money

Addictions to money are behavioral addictions characterized by obsessive and out-of-control behavior involving hoarding, spending, shopping, incurring debts, and even avoiding money. In acting out these behaviors, the addict uses money and their relationship to money to escape, improve, or otherwise manipulate their own negative emotions, especially their feelings of low self-worth. For people with insecure attachment styles, as addicts are, the whole world feels dangerous, and they may find that certain behaviors like hoarding money help them feel less anxious—thus affecting the pleasure and reward pathways in the brain. On the other hand, addicts can even act out a negative sense of self-worth by self-sabotage in acquiring or spending money. In this way, these addictions bear some similarities to gambling addiction, in that they also involve irrational behavior relating to money and may get the person into trouble or dependent relationships (in this case, between a creditor and a debtor) that may mirror the addict's traumatic childhood relationships.

Risk

Addictions to risk are behavioral addictions characterized by obsessive and out-of-control behavior involving excessive risk-taking. Risk-taking in itself can be a component of many behavioral addictions, such as gambling, gaming, playing the stock market, using cryptocurrencies, procrastinating, and engaging in extreme sports and immoral or forbidden sexual practices. The amount of risk one can handle depends upon their secure or insecure attachment. Adrenaline, the hormone released when we are stressed or in danger, is one of the essential neurotransmitters and a powerful accelerator of pleasure pathways. Adrenaline addicts are sensation-seekers; they need the rush of excitement to sweep those things that may be wrong with their lives "under the mat." Adrenaline is closely related to dopamine, the pleasure-seeking drug. Danger also triggers the pituitary gland and hypothalamus to secrete endorphins, the pain-suppressing and pleasure-inducing compounds that opiates mimic. By intentionally putting themselves in danger, people activate their fight-or-flight response. Firefighters, police, Wall Street brokers, and individuals who participate in extreme sports may fall into this group. Like workaholics, when on vacation, they become nervous and have to constantly check in on their work.

Addiction interaction

As you can see, *one addiction can turn into another*, like gambling turns into debt addiction. *One addiction can replace another*, or *many behaviors can complement one another* to reach the desired effect of numbing painful feelings and escaping harsh reality. Sorting behavioral addictions by the behaviors that are abused complicates things. It's not just about the name. I know of a successful playwright who was an alcoholic, chain-smoker, and relationship addict. Then he went to a casino and developed a gambling problem. He stopped drinking because it interfered with his gambling and soon became obsessed with gambling and work. However, to the people who knew him as an alcoholic, he appeared to be miraculously cured. But the addictive energy flowing through his body was more or less the same, as well as his out-of-control lifestyle.

Replacing one addiction with another and keeping a dangerous, out-of-control obsessive lifestyle is not recovery. That is why people in recovery must understand how addicts can swing their addiction cycles. Behavioral addictions are made up of behaviors we all sometimes do, and that's why we underestimate the threat. For addicts, they should be avoided or controlled.

Typical Behaviors (see Exercise 1):

- Believing your happiness depends on how much money you have

- Obsessing over earning money

- Hoarding money or luxury items

- Obtaining money in unfair or illegal ways (e.g., fraud, scams, selling useless or stolen objects)

- Shopping to improve your mood

- Being "in the red" most of the time

- Taking out loans to cover loans

- Investing in risky businesses, lending money to unreliable people or gamblers, or investing in money chains or cryptocurrencies

- Refusing to spend money you have saved for important things, like buying or renting a place to stay; or preferring to remain living in poor conditions so you can save

- Spending your partner's money as revenge when they neglect you (**financial infidelity**)

- Being constantly in debt to people who are emotionally important to you as a means of maintaining a connection to them, or using money as a measure of how important you are to loved ones (**financial dependence**)

- Taking responsibility for paying off the debts of addicted family members (e.g., gamblers or drug addicts) so they do not leave you (**financial enabling**)

- Taking excessive financial risks

- Borrowing from dangerous or unreliable people

- Making risky business decisions

- Ignoring and violating financial regulations

- Driving dangerously, engaging in high-risk sports, or otherwise living "on the edge"

- Other: ....

Obsessive lifestyles

Risk-taking and danger are addictive in themselves, and though most people find the feeling of high stress unpleasant, for some, it's a way of life. These people drive dangerously, always arrive late, invest in risky or illegal businesses, gamble, live on the edge, or spend money they don't have yet. They fear boredom, and feel fully alive when they manage to escape danger in the last second.

Fear, threats, expectations, shame, guilt, and fantasy drive their bodies' and brains' stress mechanisms into high gear, and the chemicals released during these moments are highly addictive.

People typically handle money, debt and risk based on the injunctions, counterinjunctions, and decisions dictated by their personal life scripts. Their behaviors around spending, saving, hoarding, worshiping, and even fearing money and poverty can become compulsive or obsessive. If they are not stopped despite the severe consequences they encounter, the diagnosis of an addiction is warranted. Typically, this kind of addiction presents itself as shopping and spending addiction, debt addiction, or even money avoidance.

An addict who engages in **compulsive spending** spends far beyond what is necessary to feel better and avoid negative feelings like anxiety and depression. Shopaholics spend more than they can afford to in reaction to feeling angry or depressed. Afterward, they feel guilty for spending so much and may even try to return the goods—but they may also go shopping again as a way to feel less guilty about a previous shopping spree. Their relationships suffer because of their compulsive spending. What sets shopping addiction apart from other harmless types of shopping is that the behavior becomes *the person's primary way of coping with stress*, to the point where they continue to shop excessively, even when it clearly harms other areas of their life. And while some studies have found shopping addiction is more commonly found in women, others have shown an equal propensity for developing this addiction in both genders.

Addiction to excessive financial risk-taking—or a lack of such risk-taking altogether—may be a part of the addict's money and work management, or a lifestyle. Again, compulsive and obsessive habits can turn into addictions. Habits form in childhood, and parents and families alike have a significant role in teaching their children how to manage risk in their lives. Life scripts play an important role in narrowing the choices one has in life.

Debt addiction is more complicated than compulsive shopping or spending. It has to do with risk-taking and gambling. Debt is not just about money—it comes with a relationship to the creditor. How much debt you can get away with shows how much they care for you. Someone we owe money to will not likely forget about us or abandon us; they're interested in what we're doing. If our family supports us financially, they show they care; but on the other hand, they earn the right to interfere with our financial decisions. Harmful life scripts about money and debt are not rational—rather they hide the unconscious life decision that one is powerless, unimportant, or simply bad, and the "payoff" is shame and having to work hard (a counterinjunction). One of my clients grew up on a farm where her parents had all the latest equipment and machinery, but she was only allowed to wear secondhand clothes. Later in life, she was always in debt, but she didn't spend the money on herself. She took out a bank loan to finance her boyfriend's business and another one for her friend at work. Both were financially much better off than her, and both soon left her in the lurch after they had collected the money. She paid off both debts, despite being a single mother with two kids, living hand to mouth.

Someone addicted to debt uses it as a crutch for solving their financial and personal problems, despite not having any plan whatsoever for living differently or getting out of debt. Other signs include living from paycheck to paycheck, never planning for the future, constantly being in a financial crisis, or being unwilling to take care of oneself to repay creditors. Running up debt to avoid having to acknowledge you don't have the money to provide for yourself or your desired lifestyle is a dangerous thing to do.

Addiction to debt is a large part of a gambler's story; the addict may gamble for some hours or days, but paying off the incurred debt can take years.[39] They may have to juggle paying off debts to different creditors, banks, family members, and sometimes loan sharks, which leaves them in constant fear that their elaborate repayment plans may collapse, exposing them to the world as losers.

---

[39] Interestingly, Eric Berne claims that the "payoff" in the Alcoholic Script is not the pleasure of drinking, but the hangover and shame the next day. Ibid.

The scope of the problem

Addictions to behaviors surrounding money and risk are typically combined with or secondary to other addictive behaviors and substance addictions, appearing as an **addiction interaction**. As a result, the picture of these behaviors is blurred by the many other behaviors addicts use to achieve the desired addictive effect. Unfortunately, this makes obtaining reliable information about these behaviors as addictions all but impossible. However, we can get an idea about the scope of the problem if we consider that the overall national average credit card debt in the US—exclusive of student loans or mortgages—was $6,569 in 2021.[40] Actual data about the number of addicts hoarding, spending money, incurring debts, and taking risks are hidden within this average. But for an addict who is trying to sober up, it is simply important to be aware that these behaviors may be part of the addictive "cocktail" they abuse, and should be taken seriously during recovery.

Maya's Story

After Maya, 46, was forced into bankruptcy by her own reckless business decisions, she entered treatment to change her relationship with money. Here's her story:

> *Money! In our family, it was the greatest of all evils. This is how it was when I was born, when I was growing up, and still is nowadays. My parents didn't like money, although they both wanted it. Money always triggered fights, although the real reasons were elsewhere. My father feared debt and wanted to control everything, but my mother was absolutely nonchalant about money and always spent beyond our means. I craved financial security and paid a high price for it. The power of money should be as strong as the power of love, but in our family, both were lacking.*
>
> *I became a successful musician, but halfway into my career, I decided to change the direction I was heading in*

---

[40] Matt Schulz, "2023 Credit Card Debt Statistics," LendingTree, LendingTree, LLC, September 18, 2023, https://www.lendingtree.com/credit-cards/credit-card-debt-statistics.

life and became a businesswoman, driven by the desire to learn how to handle money. And yes, I did—but I paid the price! I let myself be exploited, shamed, even mobbed at work. Then I tried to overindulge my financial pride and opened my own company, which was the last slap in my face on my business journey. I was burnt out and left with nothing but debts that I still have to pay. I ignored reality, denying everything I felt, for I was driven by an obsessive craving for security. My work was always done correctly, but unfortunately, I didn't know how to appreciate myself.

I was angry at my mother. As a child, I had never learned how to save money, and neither did my brother. Living in constant fear of poverty led to unhealthy boundaries, and I let them be crossed. I never considered the person I was signing a contract with, the one on the other side, who was to pay for my hard work. I was so happy that I had a job at all. Many a time, I spent hours sitting behind my desk, working for next to nothing. The fear of poverty occupied my mind. Now that I'm writing this, I'm well aware of my poor self-image. Merry on the outside, I was constantly struggling inside. To think how well I fooled myself into being able to manage it all was the worst. I never saw the accurate picture. To personal bankruptcy and beyond, until my health turned against me. And all this is because of my addiction to risk-taking and craving financial security.

Advice for addicts

The life scripts that lead a person to develop the addictions discussed in this chapter are not something someone can change by themselves. If you have found that your problems with money, debt, or risk-taking are obsessive and compulsive, you need professional help. Hopefully, you still have a family member whom you can trust to take care of your money matters temporarily, so that you can avoid triggers while you are in treatment. You should also work together with a financial advisor and therapist to construct a payment plan and stick to it. However, at the same time, to truly address your addiction, you'll need to deal with the traumas that have affected your relationships to money, risk, and power.

Advice for the addict's family and friends

If one of your family members has this kind of addiction, their behavior may affect you in many ways. You may suffer from poverty or a lack of money, or feel a lack of attention and emotional presence on the part of your addicted family member.

My advice to you is similar to the advice I give to family members of gamblers. These addicts need a rational perspective to point out the differences between what they imagine is real and what is actually real. They cannot rely on their own perceptions, because their denial distorts reality. Instead, someone aware of their addiction has to be there to stop them from fooling themselves. This is why I believe money and work addicts cannot fully recover without the initial help of relatives or friends, or at least someone who oversees their financial matters—and my experience as a therapist supports this view. Specific advice how to overcome the family members' emotional betrayal and loss of trust is further discussed in the chapter about gambling addiction, as the consequences of both addictions are very similar.

16.c. *Addiction to Gambling*

Gambling addiction, or gambling disorder,[41] is a condition characterized by a person's inability to stop gambling, even when consecutive losses begin to take a toll on their relationships, finances, and career. Despite negative consequences to their physical and mental health, as well as to their familial, social, and work relationships, gambling addicts continue to gamble, and even cross moral and legal boundaries to do so.

Typical Behaviors (see Exercise 1):

---

[41] "Gambling disorder" is the diagnostic term the *Diagnostic and Statistical Manual of Mental Disorders, Fifth Edition,* or *DSM-5,* uses to refer to gambling addiction. The *DSM-5* is the reference manual for the American Psychiatric Association, widely used by North American psychiatrists to diagnose mental health problems.

- Gambling with the purpose of "earning" money

- Experiencing conflicts with family members due to gambling

- Being absent from work or school because of gambling

- Spending more money gambling than you can afford

- Gambling or "staying in the game" longer than you originally intended

- Going into debt as a result of gambling

- Committing fraud or theft to obtain money you can use to gamble

- Attempting to recoup your losses by doubling down and increasing your bets (**chasing losses**)

- Alternating between periods of obsessive gambling and periods of compulsively working to try to cover your debts

- Being convinced there exists a method for overcoming "the machine" or "the house"

- Believing fortune or luck is on your side and the big win is just around the corner

- Being convinced fortune will come your way if you always play your favorite machine, and feeling that if someone else plays "your" machine, they may get away with "your" money

- Other: ....

The attraction of games of chance

Games are supposed to be fun, exciting ways to spend one's leisure time—and initially, they may seem harmless. Games of chance, however, involve risk and betting, offering a plethora of opportunities to win or lose money; and this can be dangerous if you lose control.

Many people think of winning games like these, and thereby obtaining lots of money, as the way to ultimate happiness. Advertisements reinforce this perception: TV ads tout what you could do if you won the lottery, and billboards promote the excitement of casinos, sports betting, track and off-track betting, online gambling, and more. In the face of such opportunities, why go to the trouble of working and training hard when all you need is that special moment? Just buy a lottery ticket and let God or destiny do the rest. Let them shove enormous amount of money your way and show everybody that you are Fortune's chosen one.

Problem gamblers and pathological gamblers

For most people, gambling is fun—a way to make a dull day a little more interesting, or a way to spend your free time with friends. But some people get so hooked on gambling, they have problems stopping or controlling themselves. They may become problem gamblers or pathological gamblers. The difference is how deep they are in trouble, and whether they can will themselves to give up their habits or not. **Problem gambling** *is an urge to gamble despite harmful negative consequences or a desire to stop.* It is a progressive disorder characterized by a *continuous or periodic loss of control* over gambling, a preoccupation with gambling and obtaining money to gamble, irrational thinking, and continued engagement in the behavior despite adverse consequences. **Pathological gambling,** however, crosses the line from a temporary disorder to a *chronic and progressive mental illness, defined as persistent and recurrent maladaptive gambling behavior meeting at least four or more of the following criteria in twelve months.*[42] As you can see, most of the criteria for behavioral addictions are met in both categories:

1. **Tolerance**: needing to gamble with increasing amounts

---

[42] American Psychiatric Association, *Diagnostic and Statistical Manual of Mental Disorders*, 5th ed. (Arlington, TX: American Psychiatric Association Publishing, 2013).

of money to achieve the desired level of excitement.

2. **Withdrawal**: being restless or irritable when attempting to stop or cut down on gambling.

3. **Loss of control**: having made repeated unsuccessful efforts to control, cut back, or stop gambling.

4. **Preoccupation**: having persistent thoughts of reliving past gambling experiences, handicapping, or planning the next venture, and thinking of ways to get money with which to gamble.

5. **Escape**: gambling to improve mood or escape emotional problems (e.g., helplessness, guilt, anxiety, depression).

6. **Chasing losses**: returning to gamble on another day after losing money gambling, in an attempt to break even.

7. **Lying**: trying to hide the extent of their gambling by lying to family, friends, or therapists.

8. **Illegal acts**: breaking the law to obtain gambling money or recover gambling losses.

9. **Bailout**: relying on others to provide money to relieve desperate financial situations caused by gambling.

These are the *official criteria that must be met to warrant the diagnosis of pathological gambling*. Notice that we have used these same criteria in Exercise 3 on page 45 to help define if any of your repetitive adverse behaviors added to the addiction.

How do you know if the boundaries of addiction have been crossed?

The signs that a person's gambling has become problematic are similar to those of other addictions:

- Pathological gamblers *spend money they cannot afford.*

- They *spend too much time gambling,* and as a result, fail to fulfill their responsibilities.

- Pathological gamblers *think of gambling as a legitimate way of earning money,* rather than as a fun activity or pastime. They fantasize that they have insight into how the game works, and imagine they can use that insight to beat the system. Even when everyone around them sees they have been burned, they stick to that fantasy, believing they'll recover everything in the next round. When they lose, it's because they ran out of money just short of the final stroke of luck. They misjudge reality to a dangerous degree, and act accordingly, following their fantasy. But their ideas are nothing more than naïve delusion. No casino in existence was ever created to enrich its patrons—only its owners.

- A gambler's main problem often becomes their effort to *"chase losses."* When they start realizing how severe their losses have become, they begin trying to win the money back, only to end up sliding deeper and deeper into trouble. Anyone else would stop playing when they had lost the money they set aside to gamble. But not the pathological gambler! They won't quit—not even if they *win* big. Instead, they'll simply keep pushing their luck, until they are left penniless.

- Pathological gamblers *prefer to indulge in their habit alone* so that they can concentrate solely on the game. They're not interested in playing for fun with friends.

- When their money is gone, pathological gamblers *start borrowing money from friends, family, and the bank so they can continue playing.* Sometimes, they return a part of the loan when they strike it lucky; but in the end, they'll be left in severe debt. They are unbelievably good at making up stories of the misfortunes that have befallen them, and often lie so convincingly, they actually believe their own falsehoods. It's as if there were two people inside their bodies: one a loving father and charming neighbor; the other a cold-hearted gambler who uses his daughter's college money to "double up" on his bet.

- To finance their gambling habits, pathological gamblers *sell material goods, including personal and family assets,* at a loss; try to get others to take loans for them; get money from loan sharks; or even refinance their mortgages, insurance, or inheritance. Their spouses may not know how serious their problem is, and nothing will be able to bail the gambler out of trouble when the debt collectors come. What's more, it's as if there is a special "code of honor" in gambling: gambling debts are sacred, and obligations toward the family come second! This can be rationalized on the gambler's part by the fact that some people who lend money at high interest rates may become violent when they don't see that money returned.

- Gamblers may also *engage in criminal activity* to finance their habits. They may pretend it's alright to surreptitiously spend their wife's savings chasing losses—but in reality, it is theft. They may convince themselves it's okay to temporarily borrow their company's daily profits, which were supposed to go to the bank, but were "lost" at the casino along the way— in an effort to "double their earnings." After all, who will notice? And when their backs are up against the wall, they may be "forced" to engage in further illegal or criminal acts to compensate for unpaid loans.

- When there's nowhere else to hide from the debt collectors, as many as 20 percent of gamblers *attempt suicide,* leaving the rest of the family to deal with their debts. As a result, any thoughts or talk of suicide on the part of the gambler must be taken seriously, and they should be urged to seek help.

How I learned about pathological gambling

Thirty years ago, my family became victims of my then-husband's pathological gambling. One fateful day, I was bitterly surprised to discover he had taken our family savings and blown it all on slot machines. In fact, he had been doing so for months without my knowledge, and only revealed the truth because he needed my consent to sell the family car to pay his debts. He talked me into agreeing, explaining that it was the only way out of trouble.

But that was just the beginning—the tip of the iceberg. In a couple of months, angry creditors began appearing from every corner, and I became terrified. I tried to reason with my husband, telling him he was destroying our family, but I was dismayed to learn I was speaking not to the man I thought I'd known, but to a stranger who had thoughtlessly destroyed everything I thought was sacred to both of us. With a strange glare in his eyes, he kept arguing that he was only gambling for our benefit, for he had found a foolproof system for how to get money from the slot machine.

That was when I realized he had lost touch with reality. For me, it was obvious—money doesn't appear out of thin air, and the longer you keep playing just one machine, the likelier it is you will be left with only a fraction of money you have wagered, if any. But for him, it was only a question of time; as soon he got ahold of "his" money, it would justify all the lies, and he would pay back all the debts, lavish me with extravagant gifts, and prove his superiority to everyone. He could no longer be trusted—not with the money for the electric bill, not even when he said he was just going to pop down to the neighbors for a moment. Did I really totally misjudge the man I'd married and had two kids with, or did that damned disease change him so much? I felt helpless in the face of these changes.

I learned the hard way that pathological gambling is classic addiction driven by fantasy, risk, and excitement. Expecting a big win, "almost" winning, and even winning are highly stressful experiences, as is losing money. Stress hormones like adrenaline and cortisol flow through the veins of gamblers, blurring their sense of time and perspective and making them feel like invincible heroes. They imagine the big win they are anticipating in the next game will resolve everything their behavior has caused.

But sooner or later, there comes the day when all the money is gone, and the consequences must be faced. Reality slowly creeps in—and it's terrifying. This, too, causes a burst of adrenaline, as well as guilt, shame, and disgust. The gambler becomes preoccupied with making unrealistic plans of how to win back the money. They might borrow from friends, from the bank—from whoever wants to lend, and at any price. Some fall into what looks like workaholism. They make unrealistic plans to pay their debts by working incessantly and never calling out sick, sometimes working three jobs at a time. But all the money goes into that bottomless pit.

My own story with a pathological gambler did not have a happy ending. My husband chose his addiction over our family, and I gave up on our future together. But I devoted the rest of my life to learning about behavioral addictions like his, trying to understand the force that seemed *stronger than love*.[43]

How gambling addicts think

When a gambler plays, hormones that create feelings of pleasure, like oxytocin, are released in the brain. When the reward the gambler receives is better than he expected, dopamine, which contributes so much to addiction pathways, is released. Excitement and risk propel adrenaline and cortisol into the body. Together, these chemicals make up the magic potion that makes the gambler feel in control—but for the addict, this same potion is a poison!

A pathological gambler cannot stop gambling. The main difference between so-called "recreational" gamblers and pathological gamblers is how they react when they've spent the money they had put aside for playing. The former will stop gambling and go home, reminiscing on the fun day they've had. But not the pathological gambler! They'll spend the money they've put aside, and then feverishly start looking for

---

[43] My memoir, *Stronger Than Love*, details my experience.

new sources, taking out bank or credit card loans, pawning a watch or jewelry, and going to loan sharks. They aren't merely greedy for money—for them, cash is important simply because it allows them to stay in the game longer. When such addicts gamble, the processes in their brains change. They feel elated and ecstatic, and their feelings of low self-esteem are soothed. Gambling allows them to escape into a different world where they feel like epic heroes of a heroic drama or a tragedy. This is the principal reason they cannot stop—especially since the remorse and guilt they feel after losing more money spins their addiction cycle even faster.

Gamblers, as portrayed in the media, are often seen as charismatic, special people who are typically loners. Because they seem to risk so much, many consider them brave and cool. Instead of being chastised, they are often respected for behaving recklessly and taking dangerous risks with money, as the very wealthy do. When we watch them on TV, we want them to beat the casino, the impersonal fortress of wealth.

Take the case of Nicola Tesla—one of the greatest minds of the twentieth century, a man who was so good with numbers and who had seemingly supernatural insights into nature's workings. But did you know that he was, even from his school days, a pathological gambler—a mysterious, charismatic, misunderstood genius who dared challenge Lady Luck and grab her fortune from under her nose? Although he held many patents now worth billions of dollars, he died penniless and alone while others profited from his work. Bad luck—or bad decisions?

Gambling used to be a pastime for the rich, who could afford to lose money. But over the last century, this has changed. Casinos and similar venues now target the middle class, including some, like seniors, who may be very vulnerable because they may not handle money well.

The scope of the problem

According to reliable sources,[44] gambling disorders affect 0.2

---

[44] National Research Council (US) Committee on the Social and Economic Impact of Pathological Gambling, *Pathological Gambling: A Critical Review*

to 5.3 percent of adults worldwide. Gambling tends to run in families, but environmental factors, like accessibility to gaming venues, may also contribute. Symptoms can begin as early as adolescence. Men are more likely to start gambling at a younger age, while women are more likely to begin later in life. The advent of the Internet has made gambling more accessible through online betting platforms and games of chance. As gambling becomes more easily accessed by more people, the number of lives negatively affected by gambling has also increased.

Suppose 5 percent of the entire adult population of a country is addicted to gambling. In that case, a lot of money flows away from impoverished families, and the tragedies hidden behind those numbers can be severe. The sad truth is, gamblers don't just take risks with their own money, but usually gamble with the assets and destinies of those closest to them. This kind of major risk-taking has little in common with how a real game positively stimulates its player, and more in common with perilous activities like skydiving, bungee jumping, and other extreme sports, which send enormous amounts of adrenaline through the body. But when you're dissatisfied and disappointed in the direction your life is taking, surging adrenaline and the fantasy of all the good things waiting for you just around the corner can serve as powerful antidepressants!

Nick's Story

Let's look into the mind of a gambler, as described by my client Nick, 32:

> *I have no idea how this wish to start playing entered my mind. It may have happened while I was driving and saw, for example, the road I once took on my way to a local casino or the place where we used to play poker. The memories of evenings spent playing on my computer at work or at the poker table trigger the "Gambler" in me. The wish*

(Washington, DC: National Academic Press, 1999), https://www.ncbi.nlm.nih.gov/books/NBK230631.

starts growing and becomes a craving, so I hurry to the first ATM or go to the Internet page. I'm well aware of how many times I have repeated the same mistake and how I've jeopardized my family's interests. I try to resist, but . . . I've already exchanged two hundred dollars for chips. I decide to start wisely, playing for small sums, and yes, I'm lucky! I'm winning! Suddenly I've got two thousand dollars in credit, and I know I should call it quits and go. But I'm already hooked. I need to up the ante because I've got a powerful feeling that finally, this is my lucky day. This is the day that I'll finally show them who Nick is! Whenever I win and lose significant amounts of money, the adrenaline that flows through my veins blurs my sense of time. I feel on top of things. Nothing's going to stop me! If I encounter a slight loss, it doesn't stop me but drags me down even deeper.

It may go on for days until I lose it all—the money I put in and the money I had won. Finally, I blow it all. There's no more cash. Reality hits. I'm so mad at myself! I throw things around the apartment and bang my head against the wall. But when my wife comes home, I pretend that everything's okay. Nobody knows what's going on inside of me. The world of poker is mine alone; there, I'm the master. I take a day away from it to calm down and then return because I want to win back the money I lost. I'm in agony. I try to play it cool, but I can't. Hoping to win back my losses, I put in a larger sum. I take out a loan and borrow from friends, telling them that I need the money for a medical emergency. But sooner or later, I find myself at the bottom again. I've failed my wife and my child, whom I sincerely love. I feel like a failure.

Advice for addicts

As with all addictions, recovery from a gambling addiction requires that you avoid situations and substances that might trigger you to engage in addictive behaviors. But money is everywhere, and is necessary for almost everything. How can you avoid using it?

For the first months to a year of recovery, you should not have anything more than a little daily pocket money at your disposal. The risk of relapse is simply too great. Someone of sound mind, such as your spouse, should take over your financial responsibilities and see that the debts are modified and paid off. This puts your spouse in a challenging position because money is power, and those who control the money in relationships have more power than those who do not. In this way, the balance of the relationship is disturbed, which can lead to resentment on the part of you and your spouse, even as your spouse helps you recover. But this resentment causes less harm than the alternative! In the case of gambling addiction, if you relapse, you run the risk of ruining not only your own recovery, but your and others' lives, returning to the very state of financial despondence in which you found yourself in the worst throes of your addiction, causing you to restart recovery completely, and likely with more debt.

Advice for the addict's family and friends

When you're trying to help a relative with their gambling problem, it can be hard to distinguish whether bailing them out is a helpful act, or a codependent one. Indeed, it can be either—or both! Since gamblers usually begin to realize they have an addiction thanks to the pressure of being unable to settle their acquired debts, paying those debts for them can prolong their acting out. Therefore, *one condition of any such bailout should include their agreeing to obtain treatment.* If cornered, they may surrender and acquiesce to obtaining therapy. It's not ideal because their own personal willingness to surrender typically is a precondition of any treatment, and will make said treatment much easier and more successful for everyone involved. But sometimes, all one can do to help an addict become willing is refuse to enable their disease.

But as much as I'm aware that bailing a problem gambler out of their troubles may be a sign of their partner's codependency, I also believe gamblers need help. Without that initial help from relatives or friends, gamblers have a tough time recovering. Their minds are deeply affected by defense mechanisms, and they tend to live fantasy lives which are—to them—indistinguishable from reality, seeing things only from their perspective. Due to their denial and distortions of reality, they can no longer rely on their own perceptions of themselves and the world. Someone who knows about their addiction must be present to stop them from fooling themselves. Even a therapist may not be able to help in this regard, for all therapists may not be familiar with the disease and, manipulated by an intelligent and outspoken gambler, may underestimate the depth of their compulsions and blame marital problems on the spouse. Only a peer group of recovering gamblers and their partners, led by a specialized therapist, may see through their delusions and help them build solid foundations for a new life.

While control is a sad surrogate for trust, restoring trust after a betrayal like this is a tough job, and it takes time. But if the addict successfully recovers, the control you must take from the addict will ultimately benefit both parties—and if the addict does not manage to recover, the financial control you assume will ultimately allow any relapses to cause much less damage than they otherwise might.

Finally, because their lives and finances are often inextricably linked, *spouses, partners, and children of gamblers also often need help themselves to be able to recover from the gambler's betrayal and the addiction's effect on their lives.* Counseling can help you see your family's strengths and realize your situation can change. It can also help you decide what actions to take, and help you manage any stress, anxiety, and depression that may have arisen due to the gambler's actions. We'll speak further on these topics in the section on codependence.

17. Addictions to Electronic Media (Cyber Addictions)

a. Addiction to Video Games
b. Addictions to the Internet and Social Media

17

Addictions to Electronic Media (Cyber Addictions)

Introduction

Addictions to modern electronic media are behavioral addictions characterized by a person's excessive and compulsive use of modern communication technologies like the Internet, social media, and apps, to the extent that they interfere with that person's everyday life. They may present as obsessions with these activities or as excessive time spent online, to the detriment of family, work, and leisure activities. In both cases, the addiction causes problems in the cyber addict's everyday life.

This disorder has many striking similarities to gaming and gambling addictions, which have recently been recognized by the *DSM-5*. However, even though both parents and members of the medical community have expressed growing concern about the increasing amount of time our youth are spending online, and signs that some online activities can be addictive, the lack of a proper definition makes it difficult to grasp the severity of this problem. Some studies on the prevalence of cyber addiction from as early as 2014 claim anywhere from 6 to 10 percent of Internet users exhibit this addiction.[45] After all,

---

[45] Cecilia Cheng and Angel Yee-lam Li. "Internet addiction prevalence and quality of (real) life: a meta-analysis of 31 nations across seven world regions," *Cyberpsychology, Behavior, and Social Networking* 17, no.12 (2014): doi: 10.1089/cyber.2014.0317.

when did you last see people in a train, subway, waiting room, park, or restaurant who weren't staring at and typing busily on their smartphones, utterly absorbed in online content and isolated from the real world? Your own observations are probably enough to let you know the problem must be widespread.

Addiction to the Internet, addiction to technology, cyber addiction . . . the fact that experts cannot agree on a name for this addiction says a lot about the confusion still present in this area. Of course, no one is addicted to the Internet itself, or even to a computer or smartphone, just as alcoholics are not addicted to the bottles in which their alcohol comes. Rather, it is the content these devices allow one to access that is addictive. Some online content may be very useful, entertaining, and even educational; but it can also be abused for the purpose of escaping negative feelings and numbing oneself to emotional pain. Online communication apps give people ways to escape real-life conflicts, but using them excessively for this purpose can turn into an addiction.

Again, to judge the extent to which modern electronic media use might be safe or unsafe, we can consult the general criteria for addictions listed in Exercise 3 on page 45: engaging in the behavior for longer than you originally intended; not managing to cut down on the behavior when you want to; experiencing cravings and urges related to the behavior; experiencing problems at work, at home, at school, and in relationships due to the behavior; giving up important social, occupational, or recreational activities to engage in the behavior; developing physical or psychological problems due to the behavior; developing a tolerance for the behavior; and experiencing withdrawal symptoms if you cease the behavior.

Behavior types of addictions to electronic media

It can be difficult to distinguish between addictive and nonaddictive content in media. We only have general criteria to tell us the differences. To better understand the problems, we can describe some distinct behavior types of cyber addiction. But note that as far as the addictive processes in the brain, body, and psyche are concerned, *there are more similarities between the various behavior types than there are differences.*

The behavior types of cyber addiction are:

a. Addiction to video games
b. Addictions to the Internet and social media
c. Addiction to online gambling (covered in the chapter on addiction to gambling)
d. Addiction to online pornography (covered in the chapter on addiction to sex)

The Internet is a medium that can bring users' fantasies to life with only a few clicks, and do so in such a powerful way as to make those fantasies seem almost real. Compared to the vividness of online content, real life may seem dull and real problems less important. Users' interaction with the Internet resembles a genuine relationship in many ways: the Internet learns about them, offers suggestions of what might interest them, and satisfies their every wish. It can actually determine their wishes based on their search histories; soon, with the help of eye movement tracking technology, it will be able to learn our preferences from the words on which we focus. It can give a person sitting alone in their room the illusion of connection to a large circle of people, as well as the illusion of importance. It can offer answers to whatever question you might have, whether clever or stupid, and serve as an infinite database of knowledge that prevents us from needing to recall information ourselves. And already, the Internet is almost everywhere, affordable, easily accessible, and allows its users apparent anonymity. People behave differently in online forums, as they never would in a public place, because they remain unaware that being online means being in public.

Recently, I traveled to China and found I had no Internet connection. I confess I missed it. We are all *dependent* on the Internet, and a sudden collapse of the system would cause an infinite number of problems. But not everybody is *addicted* to it!

Worldwide, playing video games and surfing the Internet is one of the most common sources of fun for tens of millions of kids and adults—and the more people who use the Internet as a source of entertainment, the greater the number of potential addicts. The Internet has brought not only many advantages, but also new dangers—the breadth of which we are not yet aware—as well as a cultural shift in recreation and entertainment. For five years now, I've been involved in creating content for educational TV programs for middle and high schoolers, supported by the Ministry of Education in Slovenia. Young adolescents, their teachers, and their parents meet with me on a videoconference and discuss their views and problems with cyber addictions. The resulting discussion helps all of us better understand each other and hopefully find working solutions to their problems. Here's what I learned: in the pre-Internet era, parents used to send their children out to the playground to play with their friends and explain to them that they had to stay away from strangers. Today, in my experience, parents prefer their children safe in the living room under their watchful eye, forgetting *they cannot keep an eye on them in the virtual world.* The older generation has little idea what adolescents are doing, which games they play, and with whom they are hanging out in virtual spaces. Even younger parents may underestimate the potential dangers of the Internet, being so used to spending time on computers themselves that they overlook the warning signs.

17.a. *Addiction to Video Games*

Video game addiction, or gaming disorder,[46] is a behavioral addiction characterized by a person's excessive and compulsive use of computer or video games—so much so that it interferes with everyday life. The condition presents itself as compulsive gaming, inability to stop gaming despite harmful consequences, social isolation, mood swings, diminished imagination, and hyperfocus on in-game achievements, to the exclusion of real-life events.

Typical Behaviors (see Exercise 1):

- Obsessively playing video games at the expense of other important activities (e.g., school, work, dating, friends, family, etc.)

- Losing track of time while playing video games, or playing longer than you originally intended

- Spending a lot of time thinking about video games, even when you are not playing them (e.g., reliving past experiences or planning your next game session)

- Needing to play longer to achieve your original level of satisfaction

- Seeking ever more stimulating (i.e., exciting, new, or more challenging) video games, or using more powerful equipment, to achieve the same level of satisfaction

- Feeling restless, moody, angry, anxious, bored, sad, or irritable when you are unable to play video games, or attempt (or are forced) to stop or cut down on the time you spend playing video games

- Playing video games as a way to escape or forget about personal problems or reduce negative feelings (e.g., boredom, frustration, anxiety, anger, shame, depression, etc.)

---

[46] **Gaming disorder** is the diagnostic term the *Diagnostic and Statistical Manual of Mental Disorders*, 5th ed. *(DSM-5)* uses to refer to video game addiction.

- Lying to family members, therapists, or others to hide the extent of your gaming

- Committing illegal or maladaptive acts related to the use of video games

- Losing work, educational opportunities, and relationships as a direct or indirect result of playing video games

- Performing poorly in school as a direct or indirect result of playing video games

- Experiencing health problems as a direct or indirect result of playing video games, and continuing to game despite these problems

- Feeling intense anger if parents or friends take away your computer, tablet, smartphone, or gaming console

- Neglecting sleep or recreational activities, such as hobbies you previously enjoyed, to play video games

- Getting angry at and insulting players who play poorly or make mistakes while playing a video game

- Other: ....

What makes video games so attractive?

Today, many people cannot imagine life without a computer. Many fall for the attraction of video games then become obsessed and preoccupied with them. Gradually, they begin to isolate themselves; neglect their families and friends; sit at the computer late into the night despite health, psychological, or spiritual problems; and even see their academic and work achievements fall behind their peers'. At some point, their unhealthy obsession with the game becomes a dangerous addiction. Nobody knows exactly when this occurs, but it always happens well before the addicts are aware of it. They are convinced their behavior is harmless, even as they slide deeper and deeper into addiction. Promises to hit the books after "just fifteen more minutes" turn into an all-nighter that ends in exhaustion. Parents become angry and worried, and accuse, bribe, and threaten—without any effect. Many of them don't understand the complexity and attraction of the virtual worlds present in games. Ultimately, the only way they'll be able to help their kids is by learning how video game addiction works.

The most addictive games often imitate the real world in many ways. However, in games, everything takes place more quickly and attractively, while offering many more rewards. These games place the player in the role of a hero who fights epic battles between good and evil, sucking them in. In the beginning, the games offer rewards in the form of additional equipment or advancement to a higher level until the player gets hooked. When players advance, they are rewarded with more power and a greater reputation, and the best players may even receive real-world benefits obtained through competitions. Games can also offer apparent social acceptance as players are encouraged to form groups and clans whose members value solidarity, hierarchy, and respect. This is just what a socially awkward teenager needs, but cannot seem to achieve in the real world. However, in the virtual world, he rules!

These days, increasing global connectivity has made the world seem small, but at the same time terrifyingly large, as the Internet opens up possibilities from far beyond one's neighborhood—and to position oneself and find a group of friends can be awfully difficult. Games offer an escape into a virtual world where individuals can achieve social acceptance with greater ease. Teenagers or socially inept adults have opportunities to control their progress and achievements in games that they don't have in the real world. If they don't value themselves, they may take on a role in the game, pretending to be who they would like to be instead of who they are; their fellow players will accept them as they portray themselves.

Games also offer an outlet for releasing aggression, as many games are based on some kind of warfare. Players can learn how to win these games, and gain social skills at the same time. Some computer companies are already discovering that players of online games acquire good leadership skills.

Children, who can be very clever, are often attracted to video games if the outside world does not offer them enough engaging stimulation. In games, they can explore new worlds and civilizations. These days, almost half the action films we watch in the cinema or on television are made, or at least highly modified, with technology that offers more and more realistic on-screen images. Sliding into virtual worlds as if they were real can present relief of anxiety for players, but "virtual reality" is no exchange for the real reality. Abandoning real-life chores and experiences will have consequences. People say that younger generations are *digital natives* (those have grown up in the information age), and *digital immigrants* are those of us who were born before Internet was invented. Let's hope our young ones don't become strangers in the real world.

Types of video games

Today, there are thousands of video games on the market, each with its own logic and jargon. However, "all games are not created equal," says Kevin Roberts,[47] who wrote a book about his own addiction to computer games as part of his recovery. He used his own experience to rate computer games according to their potential to become addictive. His system, which parents may find useful, takes into account a game's capacity to captivate the player's attention for multiple hours in one sitting, as well as its ability to sustain the player's interest over more extended periods—weeks, months, or even years. It also evaluates the reward potential of a game, which induces players to spend ever-increasing amounts of time playing.

The scale begins with video games that have a *low to moderate potential for excessive or addictive play:* puzzles; guessing games; word games; computer versions of card games; and games that require physical activity, such as dance games

---

[47] Kevin Roberts, *Cyber Junkie: Escape the Gaming and Internet Trap* (Center City, MN: Hazelden, 2010), 29-46.

and games that ask players to learn a musical instrument or a sport—*Guitar Hero, Madden,* or the *PBA Pro Bowling* series, to name a few. This tier also includes old-school console games for the Nintendo 64 or PS One. Games that have *a moderate potential to cause addiction* include the so-called **educational games,** which require knowledge of history (*The Cost of Life, TheorySpark, Rome: Total War,* or *Age of Empires*—the last of which can sometimes present a higher risk of addiction, if played in a certain way); and **games of control** or "God games," in which the gamer is given complete control over the creation of a virtual world. Such games include *The Sims; RollerCoaster Tycoon; Black & White;* and *Civilization,* which, like *Age of Empires,* can sometimes present an even greater risk of addiction. Parents should be aware that games of this kind can be addictive, and should be watchful for signs of addiction in their children.

In the next tier, we find *incredibly dangerous games that pose a high risk of addiction*—games in which a lot of players play simultaneously, each playing a different role. These games include:

- First-person shooter (FPS) games: games in which players typically engage in a great deal of target-shooting in the first-person perspective, like *Counter-Strike, Halo,* and *Call of Duty.*

- Real-time strategy (RTS) games: games that involve building a civilization and amassing technology to advance to higher levels of development, like *Age of Empires, Empire Earth,* and *Command & Conquer.* As "gateway games" that rapidly lead to addiction, RTS games carry an enormous risk.

- Adventure and role-playing games (RPGs): games in which players take on the roles of fantasy characters and embark on quests, like *The Legend of Zelda, Final Fantasy,* and *Warhammer.*

Finally, the "narcotics of the game world" allow many players to play together in real-time. In these so-called **massive**

multiplayer online role-playing games (MMORPGs), tens of millions of people across the world play simultaneously, organizing themselves online. They create avatars, fight together, and resolve problems in an ongoing virtual world, which operates on a server twenty-four hours a day. They join clans and guilds, unite to go on quests and adventures, chat with each other, and often bond. These games are so attractive, they have *the power to shift perceptions*. A strongly addicted player may relate to this online world as powerfully as real world, and consider their life outside the game as simply a necessary evil.

Among the most popular MMORPGs are *RuneScape, World of Warcraft, Civilization,* and *Heroes of Might and Magic.* Extreme caution is advised in approaching and playing these games, and confronting an MMORPG addict often requires professional intervention. To make matters worse, many players of these games use marijuana or massive doses of caffeine to enhance their ability to lose themselves in these games, risking addiction to these substances as well.

The scope of the problem
Since the 1980s, video gaming has become a popular part of the modern entertainment culture in most countries worldwide. At first, it looked like an innocent pastime. It has taken several years for the public to become aware that gaming could become a behavioral addiction, and even a national health issue.

Awareness of video game addiction is brand new: As of June 2018, the World Health Organization included **gaming disorders** in the eleventh revision of its International Statistical Classification of Diseases and Related Health Problems.[48] Just five years before, the American Psychiatric Association (APA) had concluded there was insufficient evidence to classify video game addiction as an official mental disorder, and declared further studies were needed. Some Asian countries appear aware of the danger gaming addiction can pose to their youth: China has recently barred underage online gamers from

---

[48] The **International Classification of Diseases** (ICD) is the international standard diagnostic tool for epidemiology, health problems, and clinical purposes.

playing on weekdays, and limited their play to just three hours each weekend. The Chinese authorities justified the restrictions by stating that they will help prevent young people from becoming addicted to video games.

While most people who play video games do not exhibit issues as a result of their gaming, some experts suggest that around 10 to 12 percent of gamers can be considered addicts, spending ten hours a day on the hobby. Statistics from a study that appeared in the medical journal *Pediatrics*[49] revealed Americans spend an average of twenty hours per week playing video games, and members of an estimated 72 percent of all American households play video games. Of these people, 9 percent show signs of video game addiction, and 4 percent were extreme users who played video games an average of fifty hours per week. But are these games innocent—or a dangerous trap?

Robert's Story

The story of my former client Robert, 29 is a good illustration of the effect video game addiction can have on a family:

> In elementary school, I liked sports, especially ball games. I enjoyed competing, and I wanted to win. Then, when I was in the seventh grade, we moved to town. Because I was injured at the time and wasn't able to train, I put on weight. At my new school, I didn't fit in so well. I didn't make any new friends. I began to stay at home in the afternoons and kill time playing computer games. I discovered a whole new world that drew me in, in which I was the hero, fighting evil creatures and conquering them. My mother thought I was studying, so she didn't get on my case about it.
>
> During the holidays, one of my school friends invited me to his birthday party. I got bored. They were playing one of those shooting games, and soon it was my turn to play. I started playing the game, advanced, and overcame obstacles as if they were nothing. After some time, I realized quite

---

[49] Douglas A. Gentile et al. "Pathological video game use among youths: A two-year longitudinal study," *Pediatrics* 127, no. 2 (2011): doi: 10.1542/peds.2010-1353.

some time had passed, and I should have let someone else play. I became aware that the partygoers were all standing around and admiring my skills. From that time onward, I was always invited to such parties, and I got a reputation for being really good at those things. I felt I had gotten my old life back again. Also, all my friends had computers, and instead of playing outside, we got together in the virtual world.

Then came high school, and my friends and I each went our separate ways. School was all the more demanding. I didn't have the time or desire to maintain contact with my elementary school friends, and those at my new school were like strangers to me. I just wanted to stay in my room. At first I spent time reading—more often than not fantasy stories like The Lord of the Rings and the like, in which the hero in the imaginary world overcomes evil. In time, I discovered games through which I could feel like a hero—only I didn't need to do anything with my imagination, as the game always offered me new challenges. I discovered games in which you could build entire civilizations. After completing certain tasks, you gradually become more important, advancing from an ordinary soldier to a commander-in-chief and then Caesar. It completely drew me in. My imagination was stirred up, and even when I wasn't playing, I spent more and more time thinking about strategies and future wins. Compared to my everyday life, my new life in the virtual world became more exciting, full of challenges, and satisfaction. Here, I was a pimply, awkward teenager without friends and no special recognition; while there, I was a skillful commander-in-chief or a prince who commanded his own army with a firm and righteous hand.

Whenever I was "in" the game and someone disturbed me, I would flinch and become aggressive. My mother tried to pull me away from the computer, first in a gentle way and then as a punishment, but it was easy to fool her. I began playing at night, and so I was tired at school and wasn't able to keep up in class. By the end of the second year, I had a whole heap of make-up tests to do, and I didn't manage to pass them all, which meant I had to repeat the year. I felt somewhat annoyed. I stayed at home. At school, they thought I was sick. After two months, my mother found out that I hadn't been attending school.

At the time, I discovered games you can play on the Internet so that many players can play at the same time from all over the world, where each has his own character, and they work together in real time. It completely drew me in. I became a member of a group of players from all over the world who meant more to me than my real friends, if I still had any. If we arranged to get together online at a specific time, I did everything to make that happen. If my mother tried to stop me, I would push her away. Slowly, she discovered that I wasn't going to school anymore and was livid. She took me to see some psychologist and wanted me to open up to her, but I resisted. At that time, I hadn't set foot outdoors for practically five months, and I ate in front of the computer because I was afraid of missing out on something important in the game. I didn't even want to go to the bathroom and held on as long as possible. I even thought how great it would be to have a diaper to avoid wasting any time away from the screen. My back hurt from constantly sitting down, and my eyes were always inflamed.

My room was a disgusting mess so that my mother didn't even want to enter it anymore. Then I began to lock my door to have peace and quiet, so I could get caught up in the game, undisturbed.

My mother organized a family meeting, and they all put pressure on me. At the time, I hadn't been attending school for almost a year. I didn't do anything and rarely left my room. I committed to playing only three hours a day and to reenroll in school. When I thought about my life, I didn't see any way out: I had fallen behind my classmates, I almost didn't know how to talk about anything other than computer games, and everything connected with school seemed so far away and foreign.

Nevertheless, I knew I couldn't play computer games my

entire life. I tried to limit myself but could do it only for two or three days before falling back into the old routine. When I took some kind of step in the right direction, a new game appeared, or the challenges of the game I was playing at the time rose to a higher level, and I was once again caught up in it all. The outside world became more and more of a drag until I transformed myself into the game's character, experienced many virtual world challenges, and achieved much success. In reality, it was all pretty pathetic.

Advice for addicts

Denying the problems brought up by gaming is the greatest issue you must overcome. It is very rare to find video game addicts who seriously want to cut down their playing. The only thing that can change their minds is the dire consequences of what they fail to do in the real world. Roberts[50] described the consequences: "Excessive playing and Internet usage have given me carpal tunnel syndrome and persistent back pain. They are the primary factor in missed appointments and have even cost me jobs, not to mention a whole lot of money. They have been a significant barrier that has gotten in the way of friendships and relationships. I have chosen video games over virtually everything and everyone close to me. I would chat all night online with 'friends' all over the world instead of going out with friends in the here and now. For much of my adult life, video games, and then later the Internet, assumed a place in the forefront, inexplicably drawing me away from social outings, dinners with friends, and even time with my family." But while in recovery, he added: "Video games and the Internet are not the problem, however. I am the problem. I do not blame these industries. I blame myself. I loathed myself in those moments when I would finally emerge from a video game flurry. In those times of reflection, I would wonder how I could possibly have been so weak as to fall under the gaming spell once again. The disgust would rise up within me, and I would swear to myself that I had learned my lesson. I would

---

[50] Ibid.

rid the house of all games. I would resolve to quit chatting online. But eventually, the urge would resurface and overpower my best intentions."

Cyber junkies like Roberts need professional help. Unfortunately, there are more than enough codependents around you who might enable you out of "love" and an unrealistic hope that you'll change.

Advice for the addict's family and friends

How do you feel when you watch your children play video games for hours, wasting time that should be spent playing sports or doing homework? If you try to intervene, they loudly protest that you're behind the times and that you're making a big deal over nothing. "All kids play them!" they argue. You sat them down in front of the screen with their first game because you discovered that a computer is a cheapest and most effective babysitter. Now, all of a sudden, you want to complicate things.

Still, it doesn't feel right. When you were young, you spent your days on the football pitch and hung out with your friends, while today, kids hardly get up from the couch, even preferring to eat in front of the computer rather than at the kitchen table. Is it really harmless for a child or a teenager to sit in front of a screen the entire day, shooting at imaginary dragons and giants? But won't this also bring out aggressive tendencies in them, which will show up much later on—and won't it then be too late? What will be the long-term effect of shooting games on children who are too young to have all of their moral filters activated?

To some degree, parents are responsible for introducing video games to their children. To get a little peace and quiet for themselves, they set their children before the television or computer when they are still very young, and encourage them to play. However, most parents underestimate the trouble their children may encounter by playing video games.

Parents' behavior is likely to change once social awareness of the addictive potential of video games grows. Sadly, this change will likely happen when the first generation of "cyber addicts" reach the age when they will be expected to get a job and provide for themselves, and find themselves unable to do so. To stave off this result, you must educate yourself on the potential consequences of video games and set necessary boundaries while you still can. *We used to teach our children to be streetwise and not talk to strangers; nowadays, we must learn to guide them in being safe in the virtual world.*

Of course, safety in the virtual world encompasses more than just regulating video game use, and we'll cover that subject further in the chapter about the Internet and media addiction. For now, here are some good rules and limitations you can set for your children to prevent them from getting hooked on video games:

- Learn which games are suitable for your children, depending on their age. The Entertainment Software Rating Board (ESRB)[51] issues guidelines to help parents understand which games are suitable games for children of different ages.

- When considering which video games to buy for your children, don't depend on advertisements alone. Instead, talk to parents and older children to get a holistic view of the game you may wish to purchase.

- Be a friend to your child, and play their games with them. There is nothing like hands-on experience! Teach them gaming is not necessarily harmful if approached properly. Take time to interact with them and win their confidence so that they are open with you and share their fears and joys.

- Beware of online gaming, as online games often feature unrated components. Online gaming may also offer

---

[51] "**The Entertainment Software Rating Board (ESRB)** is a self-regulatory organization that assigns age and content ratings to consumer video games in the United States and Canada. [It] was established in response to criticism of controversial video games with excessively violent or sexual content." "Entertainment Software Rating Board," Wikipedia, Wikipedia Foundation, Inc., August 30, 2023, https://en.wikipedia.org/wiki/Entertainment_Software_Rating_Board.

chat features that allow players to exchange ideas and information—including information parents might not want their children to encounter. To mitigate this risk, parents must teach their children, especially very young ones, about the potential dangers lurking online, and monitor their use of the Internet during online gaming.

- Invest in video game consoles and handheld devices that offer parental controls. This will enable you to limit the gaming content your children can access and ensure children only play games you deem appropriate for their age.

- Familiarize yourself with the games your kids play by reading reviews online, joining gaming blogs and forums, and watching game trailers and demos.

- Limit playing time in accordance with your child's age. Very young children (ages seven and under) should have minimal screen time, because screen time discourages movement, which is necessary for the development of their brain and motor abilities. Even though in several studies, children ages six to fifteen who played video games for one to three hours a day displayed significantly faster motor response than those who did not, additional time spent gaming did not improve these reactions any further. In addition, no difference in attention or memory skills was found between gamers and non-gamers, and gamers displayed functional brain changes in the circuitry involved in involuntary movements that were not observed in non-gamers.

- Place computers in the living room to discourage solo playing and allow you to monitor your children's time spent gaming.[52]

---

[52] "Screen Time and Children," aacap.org, American Academy of Child & Adolescent Psychiatry, February 2020, https://www.aacap.org/AACAP/Families_and_Youth/Facts_for_Families/FFF-Guide/Children-And-Watching-TV-054.aspx.

- Ensure children have plenty of other activities to pursue in their free time besides playing video games.[53]

Children aren't the only ones who can fall victim to this addiction. Many young adults spend a great deal of their time playing video games—sometimes even when they should be doing difficult but important tasks that will allow them to become responsible for their own lives and decisions. Some young adults, especially those with low self-esteem, may feel so overwhelmed by this prospect that they retreat into video games to escape their worries and soothe themselves. With the coming of "metaverses," they may find it even easier to lose themselves in the virtual world. Trying to make addicts reduce the amount of time they spend gaming may be a difficult task. As a parent of an adult child, you have very little authority to demand they stop, but you should ensure you don't enable them.

I remember a mother who once came to me for help, saying that her twenty-eight-year-old son had dropped out of school at sixteen to play video games. The boy's father had left two years later due to the crises his son's addiction created, and since then, the boy had never worked, nor returned to school. All day long, and most nights too, he was immersed in video games. This had gone on for more than twelve years, and now, she wanted to know what to do! Yet when I suggested she stop enabling him and let the young man suffer the consequences of his addiction, she said she couldn't, fearing his violent outbursts. I offered her support in setting boundaries with her son, along with therapy for her own codependence, but she chose not to accept.

17.b. *Addictions to the Internet and Social Media*

Addictions to the Internet and social media are new behavioral addictions characterized by a person's obsessive, excessive, and compulsive overuse of social media and compulsive

---

[53] "Video Games and Children: Playing with Violence," aacap.org, American Academy of Child & Adolescent Psychiatry, June 2017, https://www.aacap.org/AACAP/Families_and_Youth/Facts_for_Families/FFF-Guide/Children-and-Video-Games-Playing-with-Violence-091.aspx.

scrolling through online news feeds—apparently in search of entertaining or educational content, but in fact, to procrastinate or enter a state of numb oblivion—to the extent that it interferes with their everyday life. Although a specific addiction, disease, or disorder related to social media has not yet been officially medically recognized, behaviors characteristic of addiction are common when it comes to this topic. The proposed addiction has many similarities to gaming addiction, and even some similarities to gambling addiction. The brain centers that control reward and satiation are intensely stimulated by rewards, excitement, variable-ratio reinforcement, and drama, as well as by amplifiers like adrenalin and cortisol—creating the potential for addiction.

Typical Behaviors (see Exercise 1)

- Spending time scrolling through social media and news at the expense of other important activities like performing at your job, completing schoolwork, visiting family, or going out with friends

- Feeling unable to stop scrolling through social media despite the problems it creates (lack of sleep, isolation, etc.)

- Obsessively thinking about social media even when you are not online

- Feeling the need to post every trivial detail of your life online in anticipation of receiving reactions in the form of "likes"

- Feeling pressure to compete with and compare yourself to other users

- Feeling depressed and envious if you believe your life and achievements are not as impressive as those of other social media users

- Feeling the urge to check your news feed regularly each

day, and feeling anxious if you are unable to do so

- Frequently arguing with others over your use of social media

- Hiding your use of social media—especially dating sites—from your partner or family

- Using the Internet, email, or social media to send intimidating or threatening messages (**cyberbullying**)

- Procrastinating or wasting time by checking your news feed instead of working

- Anticipating "likes" and notifications to the degree that it interferes with your normal functioning

- Experiencing fatigue and stress, including sleep disorders, due your use of social media

- Using social media despite the potential for severe consequences (e.g., checking your messages while driving or while logged into a work computer)

- Experiencing health issues such as headaches, blurry vision due to strained eyes as a result of long hours staring at a screen, back and neck pain due to consistent bending of the neck to look at your phone, or carpal tunnel syndrome[54] as a result of your use of electronics

- Other: ....

What makes the Internet and social media addictive?

Many features of online content can make it addictive, but these are the major ones:

- Infinite scrolling

---

[54] **Carpal tunnel syndrome** is a medical condition caused by compression of the median nerve as it travels through the wrist, which occurs due to long hours of repeating the same movement with one's hands and arms.

- Rewards

- Erotic or terrifying imagery

- Illusion of relationships or familiarity

- Viral nature

Infinite scrolling keeps you glued to the screen by creating the expectation that something extraordinary may appear. American psychologist B.F. Skinner[55] proposed a theory about the way human behavior is reinforced by its consequences: If a behavior has negative consequences, the person engaging in that behavior will likely stop doing so. On the other hand, if the result is positive, they will continue until satisfied. But if the results of a behavior are sometimes positive and sometimes negative—that is, if they follow a **variable schedule**—continuing to undertake that behavior will be almost irresistible. That's the effect of dopamine, the neurotransmitter that prompts humans to expect extraordinary rewards, being produced in the brain's reward centers. It's the same mechanism that captivates gamblers, incentivizing them to keep pulling the handle of the slot machine, expecting to hear the rattle of coins. But unlike with slot machines, where the behavior requires an aggressive motion that demands the use of the entire arm each time, all that's required to receive new digital content is a swipe of your thumb on a screen, or of two fingers across a trackpad. *This ease of continuing the behavior, paired with variable-ratio reinforcement, is why scrolling through online content can be so addictive.* Even passively scrolling through the news and social media feeds without actively posting any of your own content can be addictive since endless scrolling offers variable reinforcement—meaning that it makes you imagine you may miss something important if you stop engaging in that behavior. After all, something pleasurable may be just one swipe away. In this

---

[55] "Schedules of Reinforcement," Burrhus Frederic (B.F.) Skinner, September 14, 2023, https://burrhusfredericskinner.weebly.com/schedules-of-reinforcement.html.

way, our phones are like portable slot machines. When we swipe our finger to scroll through our Instagram feeds, we're playing to see what photo comes next. The possibility of reinforcement keeps us scrolling through our feeds.

Rewards in the form of icons, emojis, likes, and notifications tap into your dopamine and other pleasure pathways, too—mostly due to what they represent. Let's say you post an image or tweet that garners a lot of likes. These likes ultimately offer three of the most powerful reinforcers of human behavior: attention, approval, and affection from others. Posting about oneself on social media is rewarding mainly because it delivers social validation. When people talk and think about themselves, it makes them happy and gives them a buzz. Researchers have performed MRI scans on people's brains to see what happens when they talk about themselves, which is an essential part of what most people do via social media. The result showed that *self-disclosure creates pleasure in the brain*. Whenever people receive notifications from social media platforms like Facebook, Instagram, and Twitter, their brain releases a small amount of dopamine, which makes them feel good on a chemical level. Each time they see a notification, their brain is stimulated. As a result, they post more, each time trying to outdo their previous post's like count. In other words, the reinforcement they receive from likes strengthens their behavior of posting.

These days, many people, especially children, use social media platforms to improve their low self-esteem by collecting positive comments on their posts. They go to great lengths to attract more interest, deliberately distorting their photos with Photoshop and even posting nudes or pornographic content. But this can backfire if the response is not as expected. A child, or even an adult, may find themselves subject to relentless vitriol posted online in response to their content. Cyberbullying is a real problem nowadays, and the rate of child suicide as a response to it is increasing dangerously.[56]

---

[56] See the documentary *Childhood 2.0 Movie* on https://www.childhood2movie.com.

Erotic or terrifying images are another online danger that can reinforce addictive behaviors. We have already explained how our brains cannot distinguish the images from reality. In the case of news feeds that deliver information about the catastrophes and wars occurring around the world, the images of horrors we see may as well be real, and they stir our stress response, releasing adrenaline and other chemicals that direct our attention to them.

Terrifying images in particular are a motivating factor in **doomscrolling**[57]—compulsively scrolling through social media or news feeds that share bad news. This relatively new phenomenon has become widely common in recent years, especially since the COVID-19 pandemic changed our social behaviors. At the beginning of the pandemic, when we experienced new dangers and learned of new preventive measures every day, it was truly necessary to know what advice we needed to follow in order to participate safely in society. The numbers of infected, hospitalized, and dead, and later the rates of the vaccinated, influenced how safe we felt and what we could and couldn't do that day. But for some, keeping abreast of this news turned into a habit, which may have grown into an addiction.

The **illusion of relationships** in the virtual world may replace sometimes more complex real ones. People are social beings, and have a natural tendency to seek the support of their communities. But for some, connecting with other people is difficult, mainly because they feel they're not up to the task. For them, becoming popular in the virtual world may be a surrogate form of acceptance, and may even have some advantages. But real friends are important. Not only can you have a lot of fun with them, but they will also let you know when you might be misbehaving or point out your weaknesses in an acceptable way. Virtual "friends," on the other hand, don't really know you. You can pretend to act as if you are already what you want to be, and they will shower you with praise. *Why work hard to achieve excellence when you can get as much—or even more—credit*

---

[57] The *Oxford English Dictionary* even counted doomscrolling among its "words of the year" for 2020.

204

by posting a funny video of a dance or a viral challenge? But this abundance of praise can just as easily be reversed. In a split second, you may find yourself a target of toxic criticism and name-calling from anonymous people worldwide—enough to destroy a person's self-respect and start the ball rolling toward a crisis and depression.

Finally, the **viral nature** of most content—and the idea that just one funny picture of your cat or a goofy trick you perform may elevate you to the "star of the day"—attracts many people, influencing them to perform extraordinarily foolish or dangerous acts to get just the right selfie, and the immediate short-term fame it brings. As we already explained, bad news, catastrophes, accidents, and wars capture our attention by releasing adrenaline and other chemicals and eliciting our stress response. Witnesses of an accident or violence may post images and videos of it on social media in the hope that their posts will be widely distributed. Pornography is also ripe for widespread distribution via the Internet, which makes it easily accessible from every device. More than any other content, sex, violence, the threat of danger, disgust, and hatred produce an explosive and addictive upheaval in our brains, gluing us to our screens.

Warning signs of Internet and social media addiction

Receiving messages or "likes" on social media is addictive, as is infinite scrolling. The more information or likes you get, the more you crave them. Their receipt releases dopamine, which creates a craving so that the person will want and search for more of the reward. People start checking their statuses and responding to their social media activities more often, and become anxious if they cannot do so. I once spoke to a college girl who told me she responded to approximately fifty messages during classes. How could she do this and follow along with her lectures? She couldn't! The same goes for playing video games during classes. Both have negative consequences, but this doesn't make the addicts stop. Remember, this is an essential criterion for addiction.

The typical signs of addiction to social media are those with which we are already familiar: checking your smartphone first thing in the morning, wasting time looking at silly and un-important posts, procrastinating, constantly monitoring "likes" and "shares," photographing and posting almost anything to receive "likes," becoming restless if unable to check social media. . . . Over the long term, this behavior becomes a habit, and then an addiction.

What about the dark side of the net?

The perceived anonymity afforded by the Internet gives some people the "courage" to speak in ways they would never dare—or get away with—face-to-face. Hatred, rage, contempt, humiliation, and name-calling are rife in online spaces, and can do actual harm to those whose self-respect is based on praise from others. Posting disgraceful comments and pictures to hurt one's ex-partner is becoming a common way to obtain revenge for abandonment. Once a lie or a photo you wouldn't want others to see is posted online, there is no getting rid of it—ever! The Internet does not know how to forget, and people rarely take responsibility for what they have said online.

Social media is an almost unavoidable part of our society now—but can it be a trusted news source? While the Internet is a great source of information, websites rarely employ authorities to be responsible for filtering the fake from the real. People used to think, "It was on TV, so it must be true!" Many people now apply this same line of thinking to content they find on the Internet—but this trust is not always warranted. We are witnessing the growing phenomenon of "fake news": false or misleading content including hoaxes, conspiracy theories, fabricated reports, clickbait headlines, and even satire. Such news can be posted just to get attention or change public opinion on a given topic—but it can also be deliberately created to deceive. Regardless of the authors' competence, anything can be widely distributed online based on algorithms and view counts. And of course, one can pay for views, and even make an advertisement look as good as hard-earned research.

Online dating, where most people present themselves as they want to be, not as they are, offers another example of the unwarranted faith people can have in social media. Online, people lie about their age, weight, and marital status; they post old or doctored photos to make themselves appear younger. They also sometimes act out their trauma surrounding abandonment by "ghosting"—ending an online conversation with someone interested in them by withdrawing from all communication suddenly and without explanation. They use intimate language and promise affection to many people simultaneously, but don't intend to live up to their promises. After all, words are easy, but actions are hard.

I read about a girl who left her family and job and traveled across the country to marry a man she'd met in a chat room—only to find "he" was actually a woman! Such naïve faith can be abused to lure young girls from their families and prepare them for sex trafficking. In another case of mine, a seventeen-year-old college girl was literally caught at the last minute before disappearing to a third-world country. Promised a job as an au pair, she'd stolen her grandmother's savings and gone to the airport because she believed in the sweet words of an Internet "friend"—whose addresses and all other data disappeared from her mailbox the minute the scam was exposed.

The scope of the problem

While social media helps keep the world connected, addiction to social media is becoming a global problem, and it only keeps growing. As of 2018, 3.1 billion people—roughly one-third of the global population—used social media. And this number is still rising—the number of social media users has grown by 13 percent (362 million) globally in the past year. In 2020, over 223 million Americans used social networks to post pictures, like and comment on content, or send private messages, and the average US resident spent 65 minutes on social media daily.[58] These services have become some of the most popular online activities of the past decades—the number of social network users in the US is forecast to increase to approximately

58 Stacy Jo Dixon, "Average daily time spent on social networks by users in the United States from 2018 to 2022 *(in minutes)*," Statista.com, Statista, June 2, 2022, https://www.statista.com/statistics/1018324/us-users-daily-social-media-minutes/.

243 million by 2025.

With numbers like these, it's no wonder scientists estimate over 210 million people suffer from Internet and social media addictions worldwide[59]—especially given the fact that the world's best marketing, neurobiology, and addiction experts deliberately design social media and online apps to be as addictive as possible, so as to keep users engaged as long as possible. The providers of the service are paid for the time users spend on their pages and look at intrusive, unwanted advertisements. It has been proven that when users later choose between similar products, they are more likely to buy those they have frequently seen before.

Anne's Story

Anne, 36, found out the hard way that her virtual relationships were not a match for real ones:

> I used to be very satisfied with my life until recently. I had everything: a loving family, lots of friends, a good job, a nice flat. I was writing a blog about my life and had thousands of followers. They made me feel important and gave me a sense that I belong to a group of like-minded people. It's true, that there were some people at work who tried to suggest to my boss that I should put more effort into my work and less into my selfies, but were just envious of my popularity.
>
> Then, everything crashed overnight. I got COVID, and was rushed to the hospital in an ambulance. I stayed there for three weeks, half unconscious, no visitors. I was recovering very slowly. The moment when I realized that nobody had wondered where I had disappeared, nobody missed me or asked how I was, was the moment when I started seeing the world in a different light, and it was scary. Everything I had thought I was had lost all meaning. I could not

---

[59] Phil Longstreet and Stoney Brooks. "Life satisfaction: A key to managing internet & social media addiction," *Technology in Society* 50, (2017): 73-77, https://doi.org/10.1016/j.techsoc.2017.05.003.

relate to people anymore, even to my family. I felt totally abandoned. The people who were my virtual "friends" and followers had moved on, and left me behind. For them, I was just an image passing by, a click on the screen, a fleeting moment. They never knew me. They didn't care. I felt as if I was invisible. If I disappear overnight, would anybody notice at all? I could not get back to work and face the pitying glances of my coworkers, so I just quit my job. I stayed in bed for days on end. I couldn't find the strength to get up.

I am better now and have started rebuilding my life. But nothing is the same. I chose a different job, and I feel better now. I choose my friends differently. I wish I could find someone to whom I would really matter. Not how I look, or how I can present myself online. Me, as a person.

Advice for addicts

Social media can be a great way to connect with people, but actual contact with others is vital as well. Technology exists to help us move forward, not so we can waste our time and be less productive. The time you may be wasting is your own precious life. Make the most of it. If you think your Internet and social media usage has signs of addiction (see Exercise 3 on page 45), follow the advice for making the personal recovery plan as suggested in Part Four, and stick to it.

Advice for the addict's family and friends

When trying to *prevent* social media addiction with your children and other family members, the same rules apply as with online gaming: limit the time the person spends on social media and the frequency with which they are allowed to check their news feeds, and encourage them to nurture real-life relationships and engage in physical activity. This sort of prevention is not easy. When *actual addiction* exists, trying to control social media exposure will not work—at least not permanently. Only if the addict decides to stop can they find a twelve-step group or a therapist to help them deal with the problem.

18. Relationship Addictions

a. Addiction to Romance

b. Addiction to "Love"

c. Codependence and Addiction to Destructive Relationships

18

Relationship Addictions

Introduction

Relationship addiction is an umbrella term for the many behavior types of chronic, compulsive, emotionally destructive, and unhealthy attachment patterns.

Relationship addicts obsessively pursue one-sided, unfair, and traumatic relationships. Their obsession, and the drama within the relationship that often results, help them escape their feelings of worthlessness and reduce their insecurity, regardless of any negative consequences those relationships may create.

The relationship addict's adverse childhood experiences typically prompt them to seek relationships that will bring them the "true love" they were not shown in childhood, when they were neglected, abandoned, or abused. However, they often end up subconsciously replaying the relationship traumas of their childhood in their love relationships. They are willing to take on extraordinary sacrifices; bear the greatest share of responsibility in the relationship; trust, even against their better judgment; and—somewhat paradoxically—endure abandonment, betrayal, abuse, and exploitation within the relationship—all the while believing that doing these things shows they are worthy of divine, everlasting love. *When my lover sees the depth of my unconditional devotion,* they think, *they will never abandon me!*

Much confusion surrounds the way different authors refer to relationship addictions of various kinds. Relationships consist of different aspects of love and attachment, such as sex, love, dependence, romance, caring and assisting, pleasing, or rescuing, and so the umbrella term for all behavior types is "relationship addiction." The difference between them lies in the degree of their most obvious dysfunctional aspect or behavior: either romance, "love," or codependence, which is reflected in the behavior type name.

In this introduction to relationship addictions, we will discuss the general traits most relationship addicts have in common. Then, in the next three subchapters, we will thoroughly explain each of the three most important behavior types and their differences.

The table below lists the behaviors typical of people who exhibit different types of relationship addiction:

TABLE 5: Behavior types of relationship addiction and the typical behavior patterns

BEHAVIOR TYPE	BEHAVIOR PATTERN
Addiction to romance	Obsession with being in love and the processes associated with being in love, rather than the person one loves
Addiction to "love"	Obsessive expectation that a specific romantic relationship will fulfill unmet developmental needs
Codependence and addiction to destructive relationships	Consistent selection of abusive or irresponsible people (e.g., alcoholics, drug addicts, or narcissists) as love partners; inability or unwillingness to leave bad relationships in spite of serious problems

Patterns of attachment and relationship addiction

Addictive love is an attempt to satisfy a fundamental, instinctive hunger for security, power, belonging, and meaning that everyone feels in early childhood. Relationship addiction develops in people who have experienced emotional abandonment by their caregivers in their childhood, and who try to heal (or at least hide) that pain by daydreaming about an ideal relationship with an imaginary person, in which they will eventually be repaid for the suffering they endured. They fantasize that their chosen partner will notice and recognize the depth of their pain and will understand that their love is sacred and special—after all, they have experienced the pain caused by an absence of love, so they believe they understand its true value better than others can. As a result, they believe no one else could love their chosen partner as well and deeply as they can, and that no matter how many obstacles come their way or how many times they are abandoned, someday, they will make their partner realize how precious their love is, making them want to stay with them forever. Waiting for that "someday," they ignore the warning signs in their relationship today, and subconsciously look to their love partners to "fix" the innate fear and discomfort left over from their painful childhoods—often tolerating abuse in the process, or even inflicting it themselves. In many cases, they even use and abuse the partners they claim to love.

But what exactly sets the stage for addiction such as this? Growing up in a dysfunctional family in which a parent is addicted to drugs or alcohol or is emotionally distant forces a child to adapt to survive. When their parents don't meet their needs, children may take on some of the adult's responsibilities, like caretaking, rescuing, and nurturing. They behave as "little adults," and often receive some praise for it from family members. But as children, they have not developed enough to understand the tasks they take on—so they often fail, and experience feelings of powerlessness and incompetence, or receive criticism instead of praise. Under these conditions, they fail to develop self-esteem. When they grow up, they lack confidence in themselves, and remain dependent on the praise of others. In adolescence, the instinctive expectation that someone will take care of them and satisfy their need for intimacy is maintained; but in the mind of a potential relationship addict, the responsibility for fulfilling those expectations is transferred from the mother or father to an imaginary Mr. or Mrs. Right. The potential addict starts daydreaming about the "right" partner, with whom they will form a romantic relationship so perfect, it will be worth the pain they suffered and the sacrifices they made in childhood. They expect that their chosen partner will not only offer them love, intimacy, and sex, *but also compensate them for their lost childhood*. This is why the relationship addict's ideas about love often don't fit the model of a love relationship between equals, but rather a parent-child relationship. However, while it's normal for a child to be dependent on their parents, this same dependent behavior in a thirty-year-old woman, for example, becomes a problem.

As a result of their painful childhoods, *relationship addicts obsess about other people, crave intimate relationships, and have unrealistic expectations about their own unconditional affection, believing it should provide a solution to all their problems by attracting people who will fulfill their every need*. This influences their love relationships and even their friendships, which often become complicated because nobody could ever completely satisfy their deep addictive cravings. By the same token, whenever these addicts are not in a relationship, they feel inadequate and unworthy. Their greatest fear is that they will be abandoned; to prevent this, they rescue, control, or try to change other people. However, that very tendency toward clinging and obsessive control often makes their relationships so unbearable that their partners finally decide to leave—making the relationship addict's fear of abandonment a self-fulfilling prophecy.

The neurochemistry of love and development of relationship addiction

Love and relationships are essential for everyone, and the mysteries of the romance involved in the process of falling in love can be a wonderful thing. But beneath this process is a complicated network of neurons communicating by way of various neurochemical substances that affect how we think and feel. Neuroscientists whose job it is to explain how underlying chemical processes manifest as human behavior have found that love consists of three different elements:

- Romance (infatuation, limerence)

- Relationships (partnered love, friendship)

- Sexual drive

Helen Fisher,[60] a researcher who has spent her academic life trying to figure out what goes on in the brains of those who are passionately in love, found that the brain areas associated with the production of dopamine and adrenaline are stimulated in those who are freshly in love. Remember dopamine and adrenaline? In the course of our discussion of the brain and addiction, we keep bumping into these two, and they are also present in our experience of romantic love.

However, when the first rush of romantic infatuation wears off, another mechanism takes over. We start to see our new partners as they really are, and feel friendlier toward, rather than infatuated with, them. During this stage of a love relationship, oxytocin, sometimes called the "love hormone," is released in the brain, stimulating the formation of a real, lasting attachment between partners. However, while this hormone prompts trust and bonding, the attachment formed can also have negative aspects, inciting feelings of jealousy, envy, and suspicion.

The third process involved in love relationships is—no surprise—sexual drive. Pleasant, sensual stimulation and orgasms increase dopamine and oxytocin levels in the brain, engendering both the sense of a romantic love connection and the deep attachment so critical in maintaining long-term partnerships.

For the relationship addict, the first process is typically what starts the addictive cycle in a new relationship. *Falling in love is an experience of altered consciousness.* If you've ever had a

---

[60] Helen Fisher, *Why We Love: The Nature and Chemistry of Romantic Love* (New York: Henry Holt, 2004).

crush, you probably remember how it was to be head over heels in love—when passion and intense erotic or romantic fantasies cause the brain to experience a pleasurable rush that would be addictive for almost anyone! Infatuation rids the brain of all negative emotions. Suddenly, the pain the addict feels is gone—all thanks to this new relationship.

However, while numbing the pain initially looks like a solution to the addict's problems, it does nothing to change their causes—so it needs to be repeated over and over. Meanwhile, the problems may grow out of proportion. A vicious circle arises, pushing the addict to engage in relationships that soothe them further and further. When this happens, some ability to stop engaging in the behavior that numbs the pain is lost—even if it later turns out their chosen partner isn't right for them.

If the addict's partner—the chosen "target" of their addiction, or at least the object that allows the addict to numb their painful feelings through a love relationship—leaves the addict, the addict will experience addictive cravings and withdrawal symptoms. In the final developmental stage of addiction—the formation of an addiction cycle and system—only one possible answer to every challenge will be left: acting out by performing the behavior to which they are addicted. In this stage, against their better judgment, they strive to get more of their "drug," compulsively seeking contact with past lovers and stalking them, trying to persuade them back into a relationship through blackmail or various other means, or attempting to get revenge on them for the pain they caused the addict. This is why, like all other addictions, relationship addiction is a disease—it changes the function of the brain and results in a loss of control and choice, obsession, compulsive, repetitive harmful behavior, and increased tolerance.

Should I stay, or should I go?

Many relationship addicts wonder whether leaving their partners—as painful as it may be—will allow them to recover from their addiction, like an alcoholic quitting cold turkey. Of course, they would prefer to let go of the problem and keep their partner—but often, their relationships are so rocky by the time they enter therapy, they are willing to consider the possibility that they must leave their partner to stop the negative consequences their addiction is introducing to theirs and their partner's lives.

While in therapy, most relationship-addicted clients of mine obsess over whether they should "stay or go," and cannot decide either way. As a result, they experience a lot of pain and confusion. To them, I often say, "If only breaking the cycle of relationship addiction were as simple as letting one person go, and your problems with them!" Unfortunately, it isn't. What if you let your partner go, and the problem remains? What if your obsessive feelings and problematic, addictive behaviors fade, only to reemerge in the next, even more troubled relationship?

Relationship addictions are not actually about one partner. Rather, they concern the "love maps"[61] and life scripts addicts learned as children, long before they first met their partners. I first try to redirect my clients to these underlying problems, the ones hidden beneath the "relationship problem." Staying or leaving is neither the problem nor the solution. What's more, "nothing major the first year" is a well-known and wise slogan in twelve-step groups, warning recovering addicts not to make premature choices they will later regret. And I couldn't agree more!

Most often, what relationship addicts need is therapy and a solid plan on how to move forward—not a change of partner.[62] Well into recovery, they may figure out a manageable way to communicate with their partner, thereby keeping the family intact. Or, if it's what they want, they may find it easier to leave their partner, as they won't fear abandonment quite as much

---

[61] A **love map** is a person's internal blueprint for their ideal erotic situations, depicting the idealized lover and the idealized program of sexual and erotic activity.

[62] There is one exception to this rule, however: if a relationship addict is suffering abuse, I do advise them to leave, even before they have begun to work through their addiction. I have zero tolerance for physical violence, and I never supported staying with abusive partners unless they, too, decide to come to treatment and change.

anymore. In either case, they win.

This leads us to another question, however: if leaving one's partner is not the answer, *what can one do to improve an unhealthy relationship corrupted by relationship addiction?* Different behavior types of relationship addiction demand different treatment approaches—so we will answer that question in the chapters related to each of those different behavior types. That being said, these differences are only superficial; to improve the relationship between a recovering relationship addict and their partner—who might also be a relationship addict—each partner must understand the problems they bring to their relationship and abstain from that harmful, addictive behavior. After that, once the addict has successfully maintained abstinence from their harmful behaviors for some time, ongoing recovery looks similar for most types of behavioral addictions, including all types of relationship addictions. We will learn a lot about that in Part Four of this book.

Now, let's look at the different behavior types of relationship addiction one by one, and explain what is to be done if you have found yourself in the throes of one of these addictions.

18.a. *Addiction to Romance*

Romance addiction is a pattern of preoccupation with being in love with ever new lovers, as well as with romantic intrigue, romantic rapture, and the magic of endless new infatuation. Romance addicts rely on romantic and sometimes sexual intensity as a way to escape emotional discomfort. When the passion of a relationship wanes, they seek a new one. Often, a new relationship is started before the old one has ended, just so the addict can feel the neurochemical rush of fresh romance. They nearly always have multiple online dating profiles, and they check these profiles constantly, focusing more on potential romance than on building a stable partnership.

Typical Behaviors (see Exercise 1):
- Constantly thinking about your romantic relationship

- Feeling desperate and alone when not in a relationship

- Using sex, seduction, or manipulation to attract or hold onto a partner

- Feigning interest in activities you don't enjoy as a way of meeting someone new or holding onto an existing partner

- Being unable to enjoy close relationships, even if you want to

- Constantly being in love, but changing partners, immediately entering a new relationship after a breakup, or even having several partners at once

- Using multiple dating sites to hook up with new lovers, or just to feel the rush of excitement when someone chooses you—even when you are already in a committed relationship

- Obsessively considering every person of your preferred sex as a potential love partner, regardless of their personal attributes

- Feeling worthless without a partner

- Missing out on important commitments (to family, your job, etc.) to search for a new partner or fix an existing relationship

- Repeatedly swearing to give up hunting for new relationships, but not following through

- Other: ....

Falling in love

Romance addicts, or **romance junkies**, are literally addicted to romance. They love it. They're good at it. They constantly look for new opportunities to fall head over heels in love. They come on strong, and don't hesitate to tell new partners what they long to hear. Unfortunately, next week, they may be saying these words to someone else.

For romance addicts, partnering up has more to do with the hunt and "scoring" than getting to know a person and developing relationships. They crave the excitement of the first phase of a love relationship—the so-called **limerence phase**—which they pursue to lose themselves in its romantic fantasy. Remember how the previous chapter explained that the areas of the brain associated with the production of dopamine and adrenaline are stimulated in those who have recently fallen in love? The experience is intense and often compared to inebriation with alcohol, and there is no doubt that it affects the way we think, feel, and reason, often against our common sense. To stimulate those feel-good hormones, romance addicts constantly seek out new romantic targets. The identity of their "target" matters less to them than being in love does—the people they choose can be their real partners or just crushes, whom they never approach and enjoy only in their own fantasies.

Romance addicts also daydream about the perfect romantic relationship. In their imaginations, they develop an elaborate script for a perfect romance, and get "high" on the feelings of rapture that belong to the early stages of infatuation.

Limerence, or infatuation, and the emotional pain that goes with it are probably known to everybody. You may find it hard to find a novel, a popular song, or a movie that does not feed on the limerence of unrequited love, proving that it's an important feature of our culture. A large amount of literature and popular music is based on stirring up these emotions, which seem to last longer whenever the lovers have to overcome countless obstacles to finally come together. Young girls in my therapy groups have explained how they love watching films and TV series in which many couples' fates intertwine, but the couples cannot be together for various reasons. "When, all eight couples finally come together at the end of the film, it's so, so romantic!" they say. For the spell to work, infatuation must exist at the beginning of the relationship.

If the lovers cannot be together for geographical or other reasons, the limerence phase can last longer than a couple of months. Still, eventually, it will either evolve into real love or fade altogether. *But not for the romance junkies!* When the rush of infatuation fades, they either go looking for a new target or spice up their current relationship with some adrenaline—by engaging in cheating, stalking, fiery breakups and romantic makeups, gossiping, victim and persecutor melodrama, or sadomasochism.

Interestingly, it's also possible to fall in romantic love with someone even if you haven't met them. Don't underestimate the power of fantasy! The growth of social media and chat rooms presents a new problem: people with partners falling in love with new friends they found online and have never met in person. Quite often they live on the other side of the world, and the addict spends enormous amounts of time and emotional energy writing to them, sharing their most intimate thoughts—all while living with their own partner, who is denied the knowledge of that which is so generously shared with total strangers.

The scope of the problem

We do not have reliable data on the prevalence of romance addiction alone.[63] A comprehensive review by Sussman et al. in 2011 estimated that the prevalence of relationship addiction in the general adult population ranged from 3 to 6 percent, while different studies reported widely different percentages—from 3 to 26 percent. The difference in the results of these studies can be explained by the fact that different researchers used different definitions of the addiction, defining the problem in different ways.

As we have said, human love consists of romance, a relationship, and sexual components. While people often seek therapy for the problems they encounter in relationships, they don't usually identify their problem as addiction to romance. Different therapists then try to help them in different ways, by,

---

[63] Sebastiano Costa et al. "The Love Addiction Inventory: Preliminary Findings of the Development Process and Psychometric Characteristics," *International Journal of Mental Health and Addiction* 19, (2021): 651-668, https://doi.org/10.1007/s11469-019-00097-y.

for example, teaching them how to communicate better, how to deal with trauma, how to interpret and work within family systems, and so on. Only if the same problems repeat, persist, or reappear in subsequent relationships—and if the client displays obsession, cravings, and an inability to stop performing certain behaviors in spite of adverse circumstances—are they diagnosed with an addiction—and often, not even then. Ultimately, the number of undiagnosed romance addicts out there might surprise everyone!

Tina's Story

There is no better illustration of this effect than this letter from Tina, 45, who realized how and why she resisted intimacy, yet craved it at the same time:

> This week, something happened that . . . suddenly enabled me to understand some of my behaviors. Peter! . . . I had hardly noticed him before. He was always so withdrawn, distant, and reserved. And then, suddenly, there he was. I couldn't stop thinking about him. How he corrects a lock of hair from his forehead. The way he walks, the way he smiles, the way he screws up his face. . . . I couldn't sleep. I couldn't eat. . . . He was constantly on my mind. It was obsessive! I kept looking his way, gazing toward him. Yes, I imagined sweet scenarios, daydreaming without having any realistic chance at all. But I couldn't make myself walk over to him and ask him out, although I was definitely obsessed with him. It was a huge crush. I was madly in love.
>
> Really? I don't even know him at all. And I've done nothing to get to know him. Crazy! To be honest, I don't want to get to know him. It's easier to dream. I can paint myself a picture of him whichever way I want to. I can make it a perfect relationship. I can imagine that he likes me, too, that he wants to be my partner, that there is no problem, and oh, he wants to spend his life with me. And all this with no risk, no vulnerability . . . and yes, I can change the object of my desire in a second! Only two weeks ago, it

was Rick. And Kevin before him . . . drama in my head. Different men. No real relationship. Crazy! Most of them are married, anyway, so they're safe.

Thinking back, I've been doing this since preschool. I thought it was just the way I was. Only now do I realize it's about escaping the reality I didn't like. I craved being seen, being noticed. Oh, my God! I'm still dreaming. At forty-five years of age! I had no idea! So many images, so many scenes on my inner screen. So powerful and uncontrollable internal dialogue. I keep talking to my imaginary lovers in my mind all the time. I'm everywhere but in reality. And I never open my mouth. Thinking about it, I remembered something from my childhood. My family ignored me. I was invisible. My mother criticized me, saying I was demanding and complicated. She sent me away to play in the courtyard because she had work to do. . . . I was overlooked . . . utterly alone in the middle of our yard. Just me and my kitten, the only living creature who was there for me at the time.

I think this is the source of my romance addiction. Longing and craving for someone to notice me, listen to me, and see me . . . to make me real. I didn't exist! Not at all. I could never have developed my sense of self. I was living through other people. That was my defense mechanism. Taking care of others, being preoccupied with them, daydreaming, never crossing the line to risk intimacy. Some emotional eating to go along with it . . . yes, the truth hurts, and I cannot ignore it anymore.

Advice for addicts

To recover, you have to stop chasing the elusive perfect romance and learn to live in reality. You need to understand love is not a constant fluttering of butterflies in the stomach, but has more to do with making a choice and sticking to it, even when times get tough. Then you have to address your underlying issues of abandonment and low self-esteem and resume your responsibilities in your existing relationships. Finally, you need to learn how to stay true to your promises, be vulnerable in your partnerships, and hold onto the friendly aspect of love. This change is best facilitated by a therapist, but there are also very high quality twelve-step-based self-help groups available, which call themselves S.L.A.A.[64]

Advice for the addict's family and friends

In this case, there is no advice for friends and family, for you have no power at all to interfere with or change the addict's affection. Believing that you can or trying to do so would make you codependent, as we will explain a little later. The power to decide whether to act either on their feelings or promises lies in the hands of the addicts themselves.

18.b. *Addiction to "Love"*

"Love" addiction is characterized by an obsession with select people, and by the fantastic, unrealistic expectations of those people's unconditional love, which would forever solve the addict's problems. Romance addiction focuses on the addict's experience of having the crush, while "love" addiction focuses on the actual person—the target of the addict's crush. To the "love" addict, this person is the "one-and-only magic person," who must be controlled and kept at any cost.

Partnerships with "love" addicts are very complicated and full of pain and betrayal, for no partner could forever satisfy the "love" addict's cravings and longings. In fact, "love" addicts are compulsively driven to control and change their partners. If they don't have a partnership to obsess over, they feel inadequate and worthless.

I have left the word "love" in quotation marks in this section to stress the difference between true love and this, its dark sister, which would be better described as obsession. I have nevertheless decided to use that expression, as it is well recognized and used in many excellent books, and—last but not

---

[64] "Sex and Love Addicts Anonymous is a Twelve Step, Twelve Tradition oriented fellowship based on the model pioneered by Alcoholics Anonymous. The only qualification for S.L.A.A. membership is a desire to stop living out a pattern of sex and love addiction." "What is S.L.A.A.?," Sex and Love Addicts Anonymous (S.L.A.A.) Fellowship-Wide Services (F.W.S.), The Augustine Fellowship, S.L.A.A., Fellowship-Wide Services, Inc., 2022, https://slaafws.org.

least—also makes sense from the point of view of "love" addicts themselves, who authentically believe what they feel is real love.

The behavioral characteristics of "love" addicts can be summarized as follows: "love" addicts assign a disproportionate amount of time, attention, and value to the person to whom they are addicted, and this focus often has an obsessive quality about it; they have unrealistic expectations that the other will love them unconditionally, and neglect to care for or value themselves while they're in a relationship. [65]

Typical Behaviors (see Exercise 1):

- Constantly thinking about your love relationship

- Expecting your partner to change or make your life perfect

- Feeling a loss of identity if a partner leaves you

- Feeling desperate and alone when you are not in a relationship

- Staying in destructive relationships out of a fear of abandonment

- Trying to control or change your partner to improve the relationship

- Giving up important hobbies, friendships, or activities you don't share with your partner

- Missing out on important commitments (to family, your job, etc.) to fix an existing relationship

- Stalking or blackmailing an ex-partner to convince them to return to you

---

[65] Pia Mellody, Andrea Wells Miller, and J. Keith Miller, *Facing Love Addiction: Giving Yourself the Power to Change the Way You Love* (San Francisco: HarperSanFrancisco, 2003), 10.

- Constantly struggling to maintain the sexual or romantic intensity in your relationship

- Using sex, seduction, or manipulation to attract or hold onto a partner

- Repeatedly swearing to end the relationship and focus on yourself, but not following through

- Other: ....

Partners or parents

Some of the most important characteristics of addiction to "love" are relying on others to satisfy the need for safety, power, identity, belonging, and meaning; expecting others to resolve all problems and deal with your anxiety, fear, and emotional pain; and insisting that others take responsibility for decision-making and helping to find your true place in the world. Children have every right to expect all of this from their parents. But suppose a grown woman expects such things from her partner, promising in exchange to be "good" and subordinate, turn a blind eye to mistreatment, and see her partner as her ideal, possessing magical capabilities—the "man of her dreams." This destroys the balance in the relationship. Such a relationship looks more like one between a parent and a child, rather than two equal partners. When someone gives up their personal strength in exchange for safety, you can bet that some kind of manipulation is going on. *"Love" addicts will not try to directly resolve their problems or ask for help, but rather expect their partners to take care of them.* And in exchange, they offer to please them! Only those with low self-esteem, who don't believe in their abilities to take care of themselves, would accept such a deal.

"I'll take care of you so that you'll be able to take care of me later!" The bargain recalls **covert** or **emotional incest**,[66]

---

[66] **Covert incest** is an emotionally abusive relationship between a parent (or stepparent) and a child that does not involve incest or sexual intercourse, though it involves similar interpersonal dynamics as a relationship between sexual partners. The parent expects the child to fulfill adult **emotional roles** while the

a situation in dysfunctional families wherein children try to take care of their helpless parents so their parents will later take care of them. The difference, of course, is that in "love" addiction, both participants are adults. However, at least one of them feels and behaves like a child, expecting fulfillment of their needs in exchange for admiration and subordination to the other. They feel safer in relationships with partners who seem powerful but are actually insecure. They promise to keep their embarrassing secrets, forgive them for their adulterous acts, do more than their share of housework; and in exchange, they expect their partner to be dependent, tolerant, and loyal.

Boundaries and enmeshment

It's wonderful for partners in a relationship to take care of one another. But in the case of "love" addiction, something manipulative and unfair lurks in the background. When a "love" addict's expectations are not fulfilled, the hidden negative side suddenly emerges. Then they feel entitled to cross their partner's boundaries. They stalk them, blackmail them with outbursts of rage, check their computer and phone contacts, and manipulate them into obedience by inducing feelings of guilt, manipulating their visitation rights, or withdrawing alimony.

"Love" addicts have problems with boundaries. They strive for unhealthy enmeshment: "You'll be strong for me, and I'll be emotional for you!" It's all about an unhealthy blurring of boundaries and a gradual loss of identity. Their repetitive attempts at control and dramatic outbursts of anger and jealousy may make the relationship so unbearable that their partners give up and start looking for a way out. If the relationship ends, not only is the addict faced with grief because of the breakup of the important relationship, but with it, they *lose a sense*

---

child's legitimate emotional needs are not met, thus hampering their healthy emotional development and creating reservoirs of repressed anger to be acted out in other relationships. Covert incest is a very common source of developmental trauma that may be misinterpreted as "real" love and loyalty, when it is in fact harmful to a child. Kenneth M. Adams, *Silently Seduced: When Parents Make Their Children Partners*, Rev. ed. (Deerfield Beach, FL: Health Communications, 2011).

of identity. Personal boundaries and identity are inextricably connected. "Love" addicts tend to mistake their roles for their identity, saying, "I am the wife of him, and the mother of them." Stripped of their roles, they become confused. So, if a partner threatens to leave them, how will they know who they are?

The underlying fear driving "love" addiction is the fear of abandonment. When relationships get complicated, "love" addicts come to the logical conclusion that their relationships are not working because there is something wrong with their partners. They have a definite idea of how their partners should change themselves to make the relationship work. After all, they have already sacrificed their own personality long ago, believing that doing so was vital to keeping the relationship alive. *Therefore, they are entitled to change their partner as well!* In a friendly or not-so-friendly way, they keep trying to save what they value over everything else: their idea of unconditional love. They never ask themselves what becomes of love in a relationship in which both sides are convinced they are victims and that their partner has to change.

Gradually, the stakes get higher and the battles rougher, starting with, at first, some everyday whining and complaining, then denying sex—which changes the relationship into a nonsexual relationship—then weeks and months of silence. Emotional blackmail is followed by a direct threat to end the relationship, after which follows a battle for alimony and visitation rights to the children.

The everyday dramas faced by "love" addicts are sources of daily stress that slowly eat away at their physical health. They fall victim to diseases resulting from chronic stress: high blood pressure, thyroid gland disease, obesity, asthma, and skin allergies. They are frequently exhausted and burnt out, and so resort to other types of behavioral or substance addictions to feel better. They try to lose weight obsessively to conform to an ideal body image, spend well beyond their financial capabilities to keep up appearances, and in relationships and sex, settle for things they don't even like in an attempt to hold onto their partner. They remain in destructive relationships and in situations from which they should distance themselves.

Intimacy and vulnerability

Another name for "love" addicts is "women who love too much," after a bestseller from the eighties.[67] Of course, not only women can be "love" addicts! However, in our patriarchal society, it seems that a relationship between a beautiful, helpless, and dependent woman and a strong, independent, and dominant man still passes for a "match made in heaven." It's expected that in such a relationship, a strong reciprocal love will prevail, as both partners are enmeshed and dependent on one another. There is no shortage of dramatic emotions, and it seems that fear of breakup and jealousy are signs of deep love, while in reality, there is only a mutual dependency. What is missing is the intimacy between them!

Intimacy comes from knowing somebody and letting oneself be known in a manner that creates a connection and safety. But being known also means that you risk vulnerability because you may be rejected and abandoned. Instead of showing their authentic self by expressing expectations and emotions, and risking rejection, "love" addicts *resort to the roles* of a perfect mother, wife, daughter, employee, and so on. With infallible sensors, they detect the partner's fantasies of an ideal mate and play that role impeccably. But every time they hold back the truth in a relationship, they lose a part of themselves, and sooner or later, the addict and their partner are nothing more than two strangers, standing opposite each other, perfectly adjusted in complementary roles, but incapable of feeling close. Overnight, one or the other could be replaced by a new partner, but the balance of the relationship would not change. The illusion that it is possible to have close relationships without risk and vulnerability is like a dangerous offshore reef, onto which the initial mutual attraction of partners can get shipwrecked and break apart into pieces. Yet, the addict might still choose not to end the relationship but instead stay with their partner and quietly suffer in their empty and formal relationship "because of the kids."

---

[67] Robin Norwood, *Women Who Love Too Much: When You Keep Wishing and Hoping He'll Change* (New York: Pocket Books, 2008).

The scope of the problem

As we have said, human love consists of romance, relationship, and sexuality, and different relationship problems are the result of all of these processes blended into a person's unique style or "script" of love. There are no reliable data about the prevalence of the different behavior types of relationship addiction. Rather, these behavior types appear together in different relationship addictions within the wide scope of the already cited 3 to 26 percent of adults reported to have relationship addictions.[68] However, it's useful to be aware of the different behavior types, as they seem very different in practice. Being in love with the process of love itself is romance addiction. But in "love" addiction, the obsession is focused on the special person, regardless if "love" has already turned into stalking, obsession, and jealousy. And a special type of "love," codependence, is the need to be needed, enabling dysfunctional behavior disguised as care. Things can go wrong in love relationships when romantic partners try to meet unmet relationship and development needs in adult partnerships.

Nina's Story

In a letter to me, Nina, 50, described her insight into how the events of her childhood repeated in the "love"-addicted relationship she had with her husband:

> My husband is a delicate seashell who—despite my efforts—has never opened to me in the twenty-six years we have been married. I never felt the flow of love between us. He always behaved like a little boy, incapable of adult problem-solving. Most times, he throws fits of rage, or sulks and holds grudges. In the beginning, I was totally blind to his weakness, but when I realized he withdrew every time I reached out or needed him, I couldn't fool myself anymore. So I started trying to change and rescue him, believing there

---

[68] Sebastiano Costa et al. "The Love Addiction Inventory: Preliminary Findings of the Development Process and Psychometric Characteristics," *International Journal of Mental Health and Addiction* 19, (2021): 651–668, https://doi.org/10.1007/s11469-019-00097-y.

was power in him that needed to be awakened.

A battle began that has lasted twenty-plus years. I was uplifting, supportive, and encouraged him, then ended up desperate . . . and after a while, I would start all over again. Failure, again and again, then going back to the starting point, where I, once again, tried to "make Daddy strong." I took it upon myself to constantly criticize and nag, but he wouldn't budge. I didn't accept him for who he was.

Now I know. On a subconscious level, I set about to repeat the game, not to succeed, but to bring me back to the starting point, where I could feel my father letting me down again. To be the victim. To re-experience him being a coward every time I fail to change my husband.

My father was a coward. To get away from my mother's whining, he retreated to his workshop. He abandoned me. He wasn't there for me when I was traumatized by my mother's ignorance and guilt-inducing maneuvers. I couldn't rely on him. He didn't fulfill his role. He didn't take me by the hand and take me to a world far away from my mother. He didn't show me the freedom that existed there. I never felt his presence. I was left in a deep, enmeshed, and entrenched relationship with my mother. Neither of them helped me to stand on my own two feet.

My father was a puppet to my mother. He never stood up for himself, he never had his own opinion, and he would rather retreat than fight. He left the upbringing to my mother. He never backed me up, even if he disagreed with her. His weakness left in me an empty space. A crack in my self-confidence. I lacked a strong arm to guide me into the world. The gap needed to be filled, the mission needed to be finished. The task I started with my father: to turn him into a powerful man. I found a husband who needed rescuing and nurturing. In essence, I was using him to keep the fantasy of my childhood going, changing my father so that his limp hand would finally become strong and take me out into the beautiful, safe world.

Advice for addicts

Recovery from "love" addiction is difficult. To break these patterns and learn new "love maps," you, like all addicts, must understand and admit you have problems. Most "love"-addicted relationships come to the point where arguing and emotional blackmail are at play most of the time, and eventually one partner or the other chooses to leave. The withdrawal "love" addicts experience when their love relationships end is as powerful as physical pain. On more than one occasion, one of my "love"-addicted clients was admitted to the ER with symptoms of heart failure, but their lab results showed the pain to be "just" emotional. But this pain is a part of healing: you need it to prevent you from wanting to go back or do it all over again with your next lover.

Everybody experiences separation in one way or another when they are growing up, but for some, repeated abandonment, neglect, and betrayal from their caregivers add up to insecure attachment and chronic posttraumatic stress disorder, leaving them deeply wounded. Insecure attachment is the basis of all addictions, especially relationship addictions. Relationship trauma is very deep, and separation from caregivers is one of the first potentially traumatic situations people experience. False beliefs from relationship trauma are rooted deep in all layers of our psyches. It is unlikely that relationship trauma can be healed just by understanding what went wrong. Usually, an experience of a safe relationship is necessary. You, as a relationship addict, are actually right to believe "love will heal" you. Only, you *should not expect such "love" from your romantic partner, but from a therapist.* The purpose of love relationships is life in harmony together, while the purpose of a therapeutic relationship is healing. Only therapists are educated and competent enough to deal with the painful reenactments and projections that happen during the process of recovery from early relationship trauma, while other good-willing people may think that it's about their love gone sour, and leave.

Advice for the addict's family and friends

As with romance addiction, there is no advice for friends and family, for you have no power at all to interfere with or change the addict's affection. Only addicts themselves can change if they decide to. Usually, that would only happen after many disappointments and troubled relationships, when they've finally admitted the responsibility for the mistakes they've made.

18.c. *Codependence and Addiction to Destructive Relationships*

Codependence is a relationship addiction characterized by preoccupation and obsession with relationships with either hurtful, exploitive, narcissistic, violent, dangerous, immature, aloof, or addicted partners. In their relationships, codependents subconsciously reenact the pain of abandonment they experienced in their childhood attachments, in which their parents likely shared similar characteristics to other addicts. Their partnerships are traumatic, full of painful betrayals, dramatic conflicts, and passionate reconciliations—but also surprisingly stable because the codependents fear abandonment and are unable to terminate unhealthy relationships. They need to be needed!

While "love" addicts obsessively try to meet their need to be loved, codependents take it a bit further. Not believing they are worthy of love, but fearing abandonment most of all, they *settle for being needed*. They become caretakers of others and often neglect their own needs altogether. To feel complete, they need another's approval and recognition. Codependent relationships can include romantic, work, social, and family relationships, while "love"-addicted relationships are typically romantic. Addiction to destructive relationships is worth mentioning as a special behavior type of codependence because it leads to physical and psychological domestic violence.

Typical Behaviors (see Exercise 1):
- Constantly thinking about your romantic relationship

- Expecting your partner to change or make your life perfect

- Feeling a loss of identity if a partner leaves you

- Feeling desperate and alone when not in a relationship

- Staying in destructive relationships out of a fear of abandonment

- Trying to control or change your partner to improve the relationship

- Giving up important hobbies, friendships, or activities you don't share with your partner

- Missing out on important commitments (to family, your job, etc.) to fix an existing relationship

- Taking care of your partner, but not yourself

- Choosing emotionally unavailable, married, sociopathic, narcissistic, or addicted partners

- Staying with a partner who abuses you physically, psychologically, or sexually

- Taking pride in staying in a destructive relationship because you feel your partner needs you

- Constantly struggling to maintain the sexual or romantic intensity in your relationship

- Using sex, seduction, or manipulation to attract or hold onto a partner

- Feigning interest in activities you don't enjoy in order to hold onto a partner

- Being unable to enjoy close relationships, even if you want to

- Repeatedly swearing to end the relationship and focus on yourself, but not following through

- Other: ....

History repeating itself

In Part Two of this book, we discussed the effects of addictions on the family and explained that all addictions are **attachment disorders** (see pg. #)—complex defense mechanisms by which people try to escape and numb their painful feelings generated by insecure and traumatic attachment to parental figures in their childhood. In their adult lives, these people often attach themselves to partners similar to those people who hurt them during their childhoods. It's no wonder, then, that traumatized people often choose to have relationships with harmful or dangerous people. In them, they find the perfect actors for replaying their childhood dramas! In psychotherapy, we call this phenomenon **traumatic bonding**. Sometimes it is referred to as the Stockholm syndrome, after a famous situation in Sweden where hostages in a bank robbery developed a psychological alliance with their captors.

Kids love their parents, no matter how badly they treat them; it's the only source of love they know. In an atmosphere of chronic neglect and physical and sexual violence, they believe that this is love and subconsciously keep looking for the same in their adult relationships. When looking for suitable mates, the children of alcoholics often find alcoholics and other addicts. They establish very painful but incredibly stable relationships with them, full of dramatic conflicts and passionate reconciliations. This kind of disorder is so frequently found in the children of alcoholics that in technical literature, we sometimes use the term **adult children of alcoholics** instead of "relationship addict." The attraction to dangerous people is subconscious and intensive. Risk and adrenaline function like boosters, intensifying the experience. Dangerous people display power and seem strong, although, on the inside, they may be weak and prefer to choose submissive partners whom they can control. If the behavior is repeated long enough so that an addiction cycle and system are established, the relationship can become obsessive, pathological, compulsive, and grow into addiction.

You can see how the behavior types of relationship addictions are closely interwoven and overlapping, so it's difficult to draw a line between them. *What they all have in common is their conviction that what they are experiencing is in fact true love, and is a goal worth pursuing regardless of all the troubles that come their way.*

Codependent rescuing and enabling

Addicts of all kinds often have several codependents around them who enable their acting out and try to prevent the natural consequences of their addictive behaviors while at the same time trying to coerce them into changing. This, of course, does not work. All that codependent's "help" really achieves is enabling the continuation of such behavior. This does not mean, as has been falsely argued, that codependents are responsible for the behavior of addicts because they enable it. But many a codependent would rather take the blame than face the fact that they are helpless! They honestly believe they are helping their loved ones by bailing them out, making and accepting excuses for their behavior, and constantly trying to fix their problems.

Codependence was first defined nearly fifty years ago to describe the unhealthy relationships family members have with alcoholics. Disguised as "love" and help, enabling dysfunctional behavior is actually the obsessive, controlling behavior of people who lack self-sufficiency and autonomy. Codependents try to gain a sense of control and prevent abandonment from their chosen partners. Intensity and drama in their relationships, the inability to be alone, controlling behavior, distorted boundaries, perfectionism, low self-esteem, and self-sacrifice to take care of someone else are common symptoms of codependency. The codependent person focuses solely on the needs of another at the expense of meeting their own needs. "If only I could make my husband stop drinking—that would forever solve all my problems!" is a line in the script. They believe their happiness in life depends exclusively on their ability to influence the behavior of the chosen people in their lives. If they succeed, they will be greatly rewarded for all the bad that has happened. The reward is exceptional, "true" love. They cannot think for a moment that they won't succeed, as they don't have a plan B. If they were abandoned, they would be left with a meaningless life. This is the risk that has to be averted at any cost.

Compared to the addict's bad behavior, the codependent may seem almost saintly, always ready to help and sacrifice everything for the sake of true love. Even therapists often fall for this disguise and advise codependents to resolve their problems by simply divorcing the addict—something that a codependent regards as the final betrayal of the sacred bond. But make no mistake; in insisting on their own illusions, codependents are just as compulsive as their partners. Generally speaking, they behave exactly the same as addicts, their drug of choice being the influence they hold over the other person's behavior. They are the ideal psychological partners of addicts and play their share in continuing the addictive drama. Should the addict in their family gather enough strength and start recovering, the codependent's insecurity and fear of abandonment may escalate. They may unconsciously wish for things to return to the way they were, provoking the addict's relapse. This is one of the very good reasons why family involvement is a huge advantage in addiction recovery programs—besides, of course, the fact that they need therapy for themselves.

Codependents and religious gurus

Codependents are incredibly vulnerable to authoritarian leaders who claim they own the ultimate way to love, so they easily fall prey to preachers and religious gurus. A religious guru has tremendous power of persuasion and attracts genuine soul-seekers by the hundreds and thousands, among them, most certainly, some relationship addicts.

God is love! They believe they will find love and God in religious love and devotion to a spiritual leader, but their trust may be bitterly abused. The idea that someone else takes on the responsibility of saving them from things they need to un-

derstand about life, if only they devote their pure, unconditional, and saintly love to them, is a sweet but dangerous trap,
into which codependent devotees of past and present religious
gurus have fallen. What starts as pure, spiritual, and unconditional love and the idea to create a better world gradually turns
into a dangerous oppressive prison. The devotees willingly give
their power over to the guru but are abused by the demands
for unconditional surrender. First, they give up their names
and are forbidden contact with nonconformist members of
their families. Then they surrender their individuality (way of
dressing, occupation, etc.). Next, the guru demands control of
their sexual and marital liaisons, and lots of them are sexually
abused under the pretense of religious rituals or devotion to
the guru, all in the name of "love." In the end, as we have seen
in the cases of Jim Jones and People's Temple in South Africa,
David Koresh and Branch Davidians in Waco, or Shree Ra-
jneesh and his sannyasins in Oregon, there is an armed battle
with the "outside world," such as the one that took 912 lives in
the Jonestown case.

The scope of the problem
We already explained why it's complicated to find relevant
data about the prevalence of different behavior types of relationship addiction. But we can try to estimate the severity
of codependence. According to the 2015 National Survey on
Drug Use and Health,[69] 15.7 million people in the US have
an "alcohol use disorder." Just think of the number of families
whose children are raised to become "adult children of alcoholics," add other major causes of dysfunction in the family
like drug abuse, domestic violence, and mental diseases, and
you will have a rough estimate of the severity of the problem.
In my experience, codependence is among the most common
problems I see in my practice. Roughly one third of my clients
are adult children of alcoholics.

---

[69] "2015 National Survey of Drug Use and Health (NSDUH) Releases," samhsa.
gov, SAMHSA Substance Abuse and Mental Health Services Administration,
accessed December 23, 2022, https://www.samhsa.gov/data/release/2015-na-
tional-survey-drug-use-and-health-nsduh-releases.

Martha's Story

Martha, 42, came to some great insights that she shared with me in a letter:

At yesterday's group meeting, I discovered something important: my own pattern of behavior to dangerous men. Until now, I have only seen parts of it, but have never been able to put them together. The key sentence, in my opinion, seems to be: "If my father does this—then, this is love." As a child, I didn't think that way; I took that behavior to be NATURAL and NORMAL. And then I repeated it in all my own impossible relationships with dangerous men and continued to try even more to get under their skin and do all that I could so that in the end, everything would be alright. Now I can see that until that point, I saw and felt my father, above all, as an injured and helpless person; I overlooked his aggressiveness. That aggressiveness took the form of swearing and threatening behavior, just words, but nevertheless, very frightening. Last time, when we disagreed over something my son wanted, I was astonished as I saw his aggression toward what I was thinking for the first time. I saw how my mother never batted an eyelid. And I also saw how he reacted when I told him how aggressive his reaction was! And all because my opinion about my own son was different from his!

I also very clearly see that all the men in my life also had very distinctive and traumatic childhood experiences with much pain. They all behaved aggressively and disrespectfully toward other people. I always found both things together! The combination was, for me, provocative enough, strong enough. Violence alone drove me away! Vulnerability alone, without potential danger, did not move me! Back there in my childhood, being afraid of somebody was the formula that ruled. If somebody thought differently from him, our father stood up from the table and left the room without a word. In a somewhat softer variation, he demonstratively turned away, nervously moved to another chair, frowned, or pushed his plate away. Very quickly, we all went numb. Such reactions were constantly on show, even for the most ridiculous things, where it was totally irrelevant what anyone thought. If you thought differently to how he did, our father behaved as if you had personally insulted him. He got his way in the sense that I felt guilty and that every one of my thoughts had to be censored.

Now I understand why it was always so difficult for me to express myself verbally and why I had, in such cases, literally speaking, a wholly blocked mind. However, without any such problems, I was able to write. When writing, I wasn't censured, while when speaking, I automatically switched over, and even now, I have to work hard every single time to overcome it . . .

It's also clear that I tried to "domesticate" my perpetrator in every possible way. Reading thoughts, focusing on my father's behavior, constant attempts at preventing his outbursts, relinquishing my own opinion, not being seen and being nonproblematic, caring for others, not having my own needs and wants, not showing dissent, not showing anguish, appearing to be strong . . . nothing was enough. I tried new combinations, I blamed myself, even if I saw that he had made the mistakes.

Advice for addicts

As a joke in recovery circles explains, "You know you're codependent if, when you're dying, someone else's life flashes before your eyes!" There's a grain of truth in this joke: as a codependent, you are so absorbed in trying to fix your addicted family member or partner, you identify with that helper role at the expense of your own identity. In most cases, codependent family members will be the first to seek out advice and come to therapy, but not for themselves! No, they will ask for help so that their family members can change, ignorant of the fact that they have problems themselves. As much as your help is needed in bringing your addicted family member to therapy, you should, as soon as possible, draw healthy boundaries, withdraw your attempts at control, and start taking care of yourself, leaving the addict to take charge of their own recovery and sobriety. I don't expect you, as a codependent, to meet this with approval. You may feel you don't have any problems apart from the addiction in your family. You may reluctantly relinquish control, finding it difficult to understand that your "help" actually enables, and that you are addicted to the act of helping and controlling others. What is most difficult is to focus on your own problems—but this is where recovery starts! By focusing on the addict's issues, you cover up those genuine problems of codependence. You need to take care of your low self-esteem and nonexistent or rigid boundaries, learn healthy self-care, and correct the misconception that unconditional love means that one has to put up with everything.

On the other hand, the "need to be needed" is largely misunderstood even by some therapists, who *try to treat codependence by advising caretakers to emotionally detach from their addicts, thus settling the problem*. In our intimate and family relationships, we are attached to each other in many important ways, and it is healthy interdependence, rather than independence, that we should strive for. As Dr. Carnes has put it in his lectures, splitting up is a "geographical solution" that does not really change anything. It's too easy to find yet another needy addict and complicate your life around them! Real changes always start within, which lays the foundation for changing the circumstances on the outside. Self-help groups for family members of alcoholics or Al-Anon[70] have a long tradition worldwide and are great source of support, wisdom, and help.

Advice for the addict's family and friends

By definition, partners of codependents will have a comparably big relationship problem, whether that be an addiction or something else, and fixing that is the best you can do for

---

[70] AlAnon is a mutual support program for people whose lives have been affected by someone else's drinking. By sharing common experiences and applying the Al-Anon principles, families and friends of alcoholics can bring positive changes to their individual situations, whether or not the alcoholic admits the existence of a drinking problem or seeks help. "Who Are Al-Anon Members?," Al-Anon Family Groups, Al-Anon Family Group Headquarters, Inc., accessed September 15, 2023, https://al-anon.org.

your relationship to be saved. Interestingly, the recovering codependents who try to abandon their superhero roles and set some boundaries are typically met by resistance of other family members, used to being pampered by the codependents. They will try to sabotage their codependent's recovery and get things "back to normal." In my clinical practice, I have found it not so rare to meet a couple made of two codependents or relationship addicts, struggling between the Rescuer and Victim roles, blaming each other for "not loving them enough." If you won't help, at least don't obstruct your partner's recovery. But if you join them in a good recovery program and take on the responsibility for yourself, chances are that the relationship may be restored and even elevated to a higher, more sincere, and intimate level of bonding.

19. Sex-Related Addictions

a. Sex Addiction
b. Co-sex Addiction (Sexual Codependence)
c. Sexual Anorexia

19

Sex-Related Addictions

Introduction

Sex-related addictions are behavioral addictions in which the addict's "drug of choice" concerns sexual behavior or fantasies in some way. Several sexual behaviors—from those as common as watching pornography, to more exploitative ones such as buying and selling sex; engaging in violent, intrusive sex; or having sex with minors—can become obsessive and compulsive to the point of qualifying as addictive. So can behaviors that consist of depriving oneself and others of sex, or avoiding it altogether, as sexual codependents and sex anorexics do. In all cases, the addict is unable to stop acting out their chosen behaviors despite serious adverse consequences, such as poor job performance; loss of trust; the destruction of friendships; the breakdown of the family unit; and in the case of sex addicts, the loss of a lot of time and money wasted seeking out sexual contacts. In pursuing their addiction, the addict with a sex-related addiction usually violates both personal principles and social norms—and as with all addictions, if left untreated, their behavior causes distress and despair in addicts, their partners, and their families.

TABLE 6: The "drug of choice" in relationship and sex addictions

SEX ADDICTIONS	"DRUG OF CHOICE"
Sex addiction	Sex (and the resulting emotional feelings)
Co-sex addiction (sexual codependence)	Control of a sex addict's sexual acting out
Sexual anorexia	Deprivation and avoidance of sexual topics

A brief history of the acknowledgment of sex addiction

In 1983, Dr. Patrick J. Carnes, American expert on sex addiction and internationally known authority and speaker on addiction and recovery issues—whom I proudly call my teacher[71]—presented the concept of sex addiction in his book *Out of the Shadows: Understanding Sexual Addiction.*[72] Three years later, he began a research study in which he examined the lives of 289 sex addicts and 99 of their partners over the following ten years. Many of the participants in this study were highly educated people: priests, doctors, therapists, politicians, and company leaders. But despite their status, they also had one more interesting thing in common: *most of them were victims of childhood abuse, whether sexual, physical, or emotional.* They had grown up in environments full of pain and addiction in the form of alcoholism, compulsive overeating, or gambling. Most of them were also *in recovery for other addictions.* However, they shared that they found overcoming sex addiction difficult, and viewed it as a separate issue.

The study's findings were so profound, a follow-up study was later conducted which expanded the sample base to one

[71] Dr. Carnes founded and taught the International Institute for Trauma and Addiction Professionals courses in which I participated to earn the professional titles certified sex addiction therapist and certified multiple addiction therapist.
[72] Ibid.

thousand people; and afterward, with the aid of the Internet, more than ten thousand. The results confirmed the findings of the first study, and Dr. Carnes wrote a book about the results of this newest research, *Don't Call It Love*, in which he listed the following characteristics of sex addiction:[73]

1. A pattern of out-of-control sexual behavior

2. Severe consequences due to sexual behavior

3. The inability to stop despite adverse consequences

4. The persistent pursuit of self-destructive or high-risk behavior

5. An ongoing desire or effort to limit sexual behavior

6. Sexual obsession and fantasy as a primary coping strategy

7. Increasing the amount of sexual experience because the current level of activity is no longer sufficient

8. Severe mood changes around sexual activity

9. Inordinate amounts of time spent in obtaining sex, being sexual, or recovering from a sexual experience

10. Neglect of important social, occupational, or recreational activities because of sexual behavior

These characteristics probably sound quite familiar to you by now, don't they? They are common to almost every type of addiction, with the only specific difference being the addict's drug of choice—in this case, sex. To us, these characteristics of addiction are now easily recognizable. But at the time, Carnes's work was revolutionary. Though it has since been met with a lot of controversy in the US, it has been widely embraced in Europe, where, in 2019, other experts on this topic became

---

[73] Patrick Carnes, *Don't Call It Love: Recovery from Sexual Addiction* (New York: Bantam Books, 1991), 54-68.

the first to officially acknowledge and define the diagnostic criteria for compulsive sexual behavior disorder in the category of impulse control disorders—found in the *International Classification of Mental and Behavioral Disorders,* compiled and published by the World Health Organization.[74] With this move, doctors and psychologists throughout Europe officially acknowledged sex addiction as a disease.

19.a. *Sex Addiction*

According to *ICD 11*, sex addiction is a behavioral addiction "characterised by a persistent pattern of failure to control intense, repetitive sexual impulses or urges resulting in repetitive sexual behaviour. Symptoms may include repetitive sexual activities becoming a central focus of the person's life to the point of neglecting health and personal care or other interests, activities and responsibilities; numerous unsuccessful efforts to significantly reduce repetitive sexual behaviour; and continued repetitive sexual behaviour despite adverse consequences or deriving little or no satisfaction from it. The pattern of failure to control intense, sexual impulses or urges and resulting repetitive sexual behaviour is manifested over an extended period of time (e.g., 6 months or more), and causes marked distress or significant impairment in personal, family, social, educational, occupational, or other important areas of functioning."[75]

Typical Behaviors (see Exercise 1):

- Constantly thinking about sex, fantasizing about past sexual encounters, or planning future sexual encounters

- Masturbating excessively or compulsively

- Frequently and obsessively consuming pornography in

[74] World Health Organization, *ICD-11 for Mortality and Morbidity Statistics* (World Health Organization, 2023), https://icd.who.int/browse11/l-m/en.

[75] World Health Organization "6C72 Compulsive sexual behaviour disorder," *ICD-11 for Mortality and Morbidity Statistics* (World Health Organization, 2023), https://icd.who.int/browse11/l-m/en#/http%3a%2f%2fid.who.int%-2ficd%2fentity%2f1630268048.

any form

- Engaging in frequent and compulsive sex with prostitutes of any gender

- Engaging in frequent and compulsive anonymous sex with multiple partners to achieve a sexual high

- Being sexual without genuinely intending to have a relationship, and without being truthful about your intentions (**seductive sex**)

- Engaging in multiple affairs while in a committed relationship

- Obtaining sexual pleasure from exposing your private parts and performing sexual acts in front of other people (**exhibitionism**)

- Obtaining sexual pleasure from watching others when they are naked or engaging in sexual activity (**voyeurism**)

- Obtaining sexual pleasure from rubbing against another person while in a crowd (**frotteurism**)

- Being aroused by sadistic activities, such as hurting or degrading another sexually (**sadism**)

- Being aroused by masochistic activities, such as being hurt or degraded (**masochism**)

- Exploiting children, the disabled, or otherwise vulnerable persons for your own sexual pleasure

- Other: ....

How addicts abuse sexual fantasy, arousal, and satisfaction to numb their pain

In his seminal book *Facing the Shadow: Starting Sexual and Relationship Recovery*, Dr. Patrick Carnes identified ten clusters of behaviors typical of sex addiction in which sex addicts frequently and compulsively engage: [76]

1. Fantasy sex

2. Seductive role sex

3. Voyeuristic sex

4. Exhibitionistic sex

5. Paying for sex

6. Trading sex

7. Intrusive sex

8. Anonymous sex

9. Pain exchange sex

10. Exploitive sex

Of course, many people sometimes engage in some of these types of sex, either in romantic relationships or with other consenting adults—even though some of these behaviors can be exploitative, abusive, dangerous, and sometimes even unlawful, depending on where the person lives. Partners might even find fulfillment in some of these types of sex. As with all addictions, it's important to remember that not everyone who engages in certain behaviors is an addict, and not everyone who engages in these types of sex is a sex addict, even if the behavior is harmful—although engaging in a behavior to the point that it causes harm is typically a characteristic of addiction. Indeed, no single specific type of sexual behavior is typical of sex addiction; rather, *what makes the sexual behavior an addiction is not its severity or whether or not it causes harm, but the fact that it is out of control.* Even sex within a loving relationship could be a sign of sex addiction, if that behavior is out of both partners' control!

---

[76] Patrick Carnes, *Facing the Shadow: Starting Sexual and Relationship Recovery* (Carefree, AZ: Gentle Path Press, 2010), 57.

Sex addicts engage in sexual behaviors not primarily for the sake of the act or for their partner, but to achieve the sense of oblivion that follows the sexual act. Intimacy or a relationship is not the goal; in fact, the actual relationship can be secondary, nonexistent, or even just a fantasy. The other person can be totally irrelevant or reduced to an "object," impersonal body, or image. A person's body can be used for arousal, just like an inanimate thing, like an inflatable doll, and concerns about the person's well-being become irrelevant. Instead of intimacy, which they sometimes don't even risk feeling, addicts enjoy the intensity of doing something forbidden. The image in their fantasy and the stimulation of erogenous zones are enough for the sexual release of tension. Such forms of sex bring about physical release, while the spirit and soul remain hungry, thirsty, and cheated. In such circumstances, it is not love that arouses, but instead a fantasy, danger, risk, the forbidden, or the humiliation of another or oneself.

Remember, addicts engage in certain behaviors to repress negative memories and emotions. *Addictions are not about feeling good—they're about feeling less.* Addicts cope with stress, depression, anxiety, loneliness, boredom, attachment deficits, and unresolved trauma by numbing their pain instead of turning to loved ones and trusting others who might provide emotional support. This is the case for sex addicts as well.

What people yearn for, in truth, is love and connection. But sometimes, their "love maps" become so skewed, they don't allow for intimacy. Repressed childhood sexual trauma, for example, may manifest in adulthood as a compulsion to repeat such acts, whether as a victim, perpetrator, or even both. What addicts are unable to deal with, they often act out; such are the laws of traumatic repetition compulsion. And because nothing except love can satisfy their true needs, an intense craving remains, luring them into even more intensive stimulation. Such abusive sexuality can degenerate into sex addiction.

Sex may be the only experience that profoundly affects all three pleasure planes (arousal, satiation, and fantasy) in our neurochemistry. Because our ideas about sex and love are confused and intertwined, some people may think that sex addicts have a very active love life, when in fact, it's quite the opposite. Sex addicts pursue excitement and sexual arousal from images, whether of a person, body parts, erotic images, or even their own fantasies. Remember, *the main difference between the various forms of relationship addictions lies in what they focus on.* Romance addicts are hooked on the rapture of being in love, "love" addicts look for control to prevent abandonment, codependents need to be needed, and sex addicts try to lose themselves in a sexual trance. Regardless of what they believe, none of these addicts actually display any genuine care for the person on the other side! In practice, different types of addiction can intertwine to such a degree that they are each unable to be separated or distinguished from one another. It is not uncommon for sex addicts to be obsessed with watching impersonal pornographic images on the screen while at the same time being addictively dependent on their partners.

Addicts or perpetrators?

What humans consider perverse typically depends on the cultural environment in which they were raised. In ancient Greece, for example, romantic relationships between adult males and teenage boys were socially acknowledged; while even as late as 2003, homosexual acts were deemed criminal in some American states.[77] And according to sharia law in some Islamic countries, if a married person has been proven to have had extramarital sexual relations, they may be sentenced to lashing and stoning to death.

In the Western world, of course, a different code exists, but we should be aware that it is about a cultural agreement. We know that stringent regulations are in place which stipulate that for sexual relations to take place, both parties must be willing participants. If they are mentally healthy adults, and

---

[77] Richard Weinmeyer, "The Decriminalization of Sodomy in the United States," AMA Journal of Ethics, American Medical Association, November 2014, https://journalofethics.ama-assn.org/article/decriminalization-sodomy-united-states/2014-11.

can therefore agree to the act, the state does not interfere. If a child or a mentally handicapped person is involved, however, that person's willingness to engage in sex is immaterial, as they are in an inferior position and usually don't understand what they are getting themselves into.

More often than not, addictive sex has to do with abuse (of oneself or another person) and the denial of the freedom of choice. A man forces his girlfriend into sex; a woman in miniskirt uncrosses her legs, revealing her underwear to her coworkers "by chance"; a man pushes his way through a crowd in a train station to be able to secretly touch women; a gymnastics coach gains the trust of his young protégés and takes advantage of his power over them by leading them into sexual acts. It's not just about the abuse of others. Sex addicts can also hurt and humiliate themselves, for example, through masturbation to exhaustion, or through cutting or pinching their bodies to enhance sexual excitement.

So, are sex addicts also sexual predators, pedophiles, and so-called "sex maniacs"? Not necessarily, for some of the behavior mentioned above can be performed between consenting adults. But what about the more severe forms of behavior, wherein an abuse of power is present? In those cases, we cannot speak of partners, nor about mutuality, even if the victims seemingly accept or even encourage the behavior. In such cases, the addict's behavior encompasses criminal acts, or sexual attacks on others.

Some people may believe that introducing the concept of addiction is really just an excuse that allows sexual predators to get away with their actions. To clarify this matter, we must distinguish between sex addicts and sexual predators. People who do not know much about sex addiction usually suppose it concerns "sex maniacs" or people who entertain forbidden and perverse forms of sex, like pedophiles, sadomasochists, and sex offenders. But we shouldn't get these expressions mixed up. Not all perpetrators of criminal acts against others' sexual integrity are addicted to sex. Sometimes sex offenders are also sex addicts, and sometimes they are not. The difference is that addicts, because of disease processes in the brain, have lost the power of choice and thus cannot hold themselves back, leading to *feelings of shame after the act*. Others perpetrate sexual crimes for different reasons, and feel no regret. They are psychopaths who have no regard for others, and who believe they can do whatever they want without considering others' consent or well-being. Their only regret is in getting caught—not in having undertaken the act itself.

Of course, even if a person is drunk or otherwise not in complete control of their behavior, criminal acts are still illegal, and therefore punishable under the law. Addiction does not eliminate accountability—after all, an addict can choose to get treatment instead of hurting other people. But as long as society tolerates addiction, addicts' responsibility for their disease is at least partially shared. After all, for any addiction to develop, several factors must be present—some of which are not merely personal, but social. Therefore, *in addition to punishment*, society should offer therapy to those addicts who have crossed the line and committed offenses or criminal acts because of their addiction.

Although I have no tolerance for perpetrators of sexual and other violence, I should also note that a strong correlation exists between sex addiction and childhood trauma: surveys of people with sex addictions show that during childhood, 72 percent were physically abused, 81 percent were sexually abused, and 97 percent were emotionally abused.

Shame

"If I had to choose between addictions, I would certainly prefer sex addiction!"

I frequently hear this sentiment from my audience when the topic of sex addiction comes up at my lectures. When I explain sex addiction is not about having a lot of sex, but rather the inability to abstain from sexual behavior that is abusive, impersonal, and shameful, they change their minds. Sex is certainly not an area in which you want to be out of control!

Whenever I lecture on sex addiction, a kind of unease permeates the room. Some of my listeners appear embarrassed, as if they can hardly wait for me to change the topic—but many of these same listeners also secretly enjoy the weird details of the stories I tell. Most listeners rationalize that this sort of affliction only affects "other people." However, there are always some people in the audience who can relate. They prefer to remain quiet and attract as little attention as possible, but they often feel I'm speaking directly to them, and know their darkest secrets. Deep down, they are convinced such things only happen to them—that they are sinners, or at least somewhat perverted—and that if other people knew what they did behind closed doors, they would be appalled and avoid them at all costs.

Sex addicts live double lives. In public, they can be respected and well-known; in private, they regularly participate in sexual acts of which they are ashamed and which would surprise their loved ones. Fortunately, the recent public movement opposing sexual harassment and sexual assault, #MeToo, has exposed many influential public figures' secret harassment of young prospective performers. It's a welcome beginning to the end of such hypocrisy.

Unless they realize they have the disease of addiction, sex addicts feel a great deal of shame at their behavior. They're ashamed of what they do, and even more ashamed that they cannot stop doing it, especially if everyone around them seems to have no problem controlling their urges. To reduce these shameful feelings, they may deny the consequences of their behavior, give numerous justifications for it, ignore their problems, distort reality, and blame others. Though they may rationalize their actions using the phrases "boys will be boys" or "people have needs," they nevertheless experience their own sexuality as a source of shame, especially those sexual acts that contrast with their personal principles. Unfortunately, when acting out escalates into addiction, it also becomes the addict's primary coping mechanism; *to numb the shame generated by their sexual acting out, they must do more of the same!* That is why sex addicts need help to reduce their shame and relearn how to take responsibility for their actions. Introducing the concept of addiction as a disease can help them separate themselves from their behavior and regain control over it.

Cybersex addiction

One form—or rather behavioral pattern—characteristic of sex addiction is **cybersex addiction**, which is also discussed in the chapter about addiction to electronic media. Nevertheless, it is also a type of sex addiction to which all the previously mentioned characteristics apply.

Cybersex addiction typically manifests itself through symptoms such as an inability to control the amount of time spent seeking sexual stimulation online, a preoccupation with porn (even while engaged in other activities), a reliance on porn to avoid dealing with serious personal issues, the onset of withdrawal symptoms when this is not possible, crossing the line to illegal forms of porn, hiding the addiction from others, and risking seriously damaging consequences. Cybersex addicts read erotic stories; view, download, or trade online pornography; visit adult fantasy chat rooms; engage in cybersex relationships; masturbate while engaged in online activity that contributes to their sexual arousal; and search for offline sexual partners and information about sexual activities.

In the previous chapter on cyber addiction, we noted that the Internet is everywhere, affordable, easily accessible, and seemingly anonymous. It responds to the user's every wish. Some Internet-enabled devices can even track users' eye movements to determine which images best capture and maintain their interest. Armed with the information about their preferences, these devices can bring users' personal fantasies to life by offering suggested viewing material that users can access with only a few clicks. For someone used to arousing themselves by looking at vivid photoshopped erotic images, the stimulation presented by real, ordinary people can fall below an arousal threshold artificially heightened by perfect, tailor-made pornography. This can lead to problems achieving sexual arousal without the aid of pornography—and that can be a problem for people in committed relationships.

Is cybersex cheating?

With the development of the porn industry and social media, society has been forced to reexamine its thoughts on the boundaries of physical and emotional infidelity. Does thinking about a movie star while having sex with your wife count as cheating? What about watching a striptease? What about erotic and pornographic pictures in magazines? Movies and videos? No? What about a real-time video session with a woman who may be on another continent and whom you'll never meet, but who responds to your wishes? Where do you draw the line, and how far would you go if the circumstances were "right"?

Currently, it depends on who you ask. The courts in Canada, for example, have ruled that cyber-infidelity, if entirely virtual and exclusive of real-life sexual encounters, does not meet the legal definition of adultery and cannot be used as grounds for an immediate divorce. In the US, opinions vary across different states. Courts in several states have decided cybersex can be legal grounds for divorce, while in many other states, it has not been accepted as sufficient grounds for divorce on its own. Even people who have online sexual encounters do not all agree whether or not their actions constitute cheating on their partner. One study found that 60 percent of people having cybersex with a person other than their partner did not consider themselves unfaithful, while 40 percent admitted they believed they were cheating.

People whose partners have had online affairs tend to have much more uniform views on cybersex. One study found 55.9 percent of partners suffered emotional trauma as a result of infidelity associated with cybersex.[78] The majority of them agree that the *emotional impact of a partner's cyber infidelity* is similar to real-life cheating, and is morally wrong. Basical-

---

[78] Jennifer P. Schneider, Robert Weiss, and Charles Samenow. "Is It Really Cheating?: Understanding the Emotional Reactions and Clinical Treatment of Spouses and Partners Affected by Cybersex Infidelity," *Sexual Addiction and Compulsivity* 19, no. 1–2 (2012): 123–139, doi: 10.1080/10720162.2012.658344.

ly, cheating is anything you cannot share with your partner, whether a real-life affair, digital intimacy, or even lying about other essential facts about your relationship.

The scope of the problem

A lack of empirical evidence on sexual addiction is the result of the disease's complete absence from versions of the *Diagnostic and Statistical Manual of Mental Disorders*. However, people who were categorized as having a compulsive, impulsive, addictive sexual disorder or a hypersexual disorder reported having obsessive thoughts and behaviors as well as sexual fantasies. Existing prevalence of the rates of sexual addiction-related disorders range from 3 to 6 percent.[79] The number of people in the United States living with sex addiction is currently estimated at twelve to thirty million. Both men and women can be affected, though little research exists on female sex addiction. Men have a significantly greater number of sexual partners (fifty-nine) compared to women (eight).[80] In a study conducted in 1991, which I have already quoted,[81] Dr. Patrick Carnes studied the stories of nearly one thousand addicts and their families. A review of his findings allowed him to compile a list of the severe consequences of sex addicts' sexual behavior: sexually transmitted diseases, including AIDS; loss of marital relationships (40 percent) or rights to their children (13 percent); abortions (36 percent) and unwanted pregnancies (42 percent); severe financial consequences (58 percent); loss of work and career opportunities (27 percent); diminished job productivity (79 percent); exhaustion (59 percent); physical injury (38 percent); and even near death experiences. A full 58 percent of these sex addicts admitted to pursuing activities for

[79] Laurent Karila et al. "Sexual Addiction or Hypersexual Disorder: Different Terms for the Same Problem? A Review of the Literature," *Current Pharmaceutical Design* 20, no. 25 (2014): 4012–4020, https://www.ingentaconnect.com/content/ben/cpd/2014/00000020/00000025/art00004.

[80] B.R. Sahithya and Rithvik S. Kashyap. "Sexual Addiction Disorder—A Review With Recent Updates," *Journal of Psychosexual Health* 4, no. 2 (2022): 95–101, doi: 10.1177/26318318221081080.

[81] Patrick Carnes, *Don't Call It Love: Recovery from Sexual Addiction* (New York: Bantam Books, 1991), 14–15.

which they could have been arrested, and 19 percent actually were arrested.

Chrissy's Story

If you still believe sex addiction is a myth, that a lot of sex is good for one's health, and that everyone can decide for themselves the terms of how they act out sexually, I invite you to read the following true story. What Chrissy, 32, in therapy for sex addiction and codependency, told me perfectly illustrates how this type of addiction often begins in the early stages of childhood, long before any signs of adverse sexual behavior appear. Almost all the elements of addiction can be found in her story.

What does it mean to me to be a woman? To not be too intelligent—especially in the company of men. Whenever I wanted to be smart, my father always commented that I was stubborn. He let me know that I made him feel uncomfortable and threatened. It made me think that I mustn't be too smart because I would lose the attention I couldn't live without. I instead pretended to be stupid. He called it stubbornness: "Who would want to be with someone so stubborn?" I hoped that someone would want me. But I believed that no one would want me the way I was. Then I stopped thinking and just did what he wanted me to. Every time I tried to say something honest, I first asked myself if that would hurt him or not. Then I preferred to say nothing and pretended to be stupid, that I had no idea. And I stopped thinking. Everything I was and everything I had inside was a little quieter every time because it was overpowered by his "clever way of thinking."

My father always paid attention to the way I looked. He looked at me in such a way that sexual tension could be felt. And I knew that there was something there he liked. And if he didn't, then I began to think that I had to show myself off; I then learned that this was something that men liked and that there was nothing else. He looked at me in an inappropriate way, the same way he looked at waitresses at bars when my mother wasn't there. There was simply too much energy. When he looked at me, he looked at me from top to bottom, then once again. It could be felt. Oh, how you look good! He had that kind of hug, as if he would suck me in, but didn't care how I felt about it, even though I pushed him away. As if I was his property. As if I didn't have the right to decide.

Later, I thought that I had to allow men to do just that. And even his kiss was the same . . . it wasn't innocent, like a kiss you give a child. He licked his lips and sucked onto me in such a way that I just kind of fell into him. It was disgusting. As if my body wasn't allowed to be mine. As if he sucked away my energy. And if I didn't let him, he would have been offended and say that there was something wrong with me. Every time, I succeeded in pushing him away, at least a little. Later, I wasn't able to do that with other men.

I remember having a fight with him when I was four or five years of age. If I disagreed with him, he told me to go to my room. And if I resisted, the tension in him grew to such a degree that it could be felt in the air, as if it was only going to take just a little bit more for him to completely explode. And I would be guilty of that. I never really knew where that point was . . . where he could still have control over himself, and where he couldn't. And I always looked for that point. When he could no longer control himself, he ran after me into my room and beat me, which felt more like relief than pain. And something sexual could be felt in the air. As if he was enjoying it, smacking me across my bottom. To me, the bottom is a part of the body, which has a sexual connotation. There was a lot of that. And after such tension, there was always silence.

At seven years of age, I began to fantasize about older men who, against my will, did with me whatever they wanted . . . sexually. The more I imagined about it, the more I liked it . . . and the more it relaxed me, the easier I fell asleep. It was as if I needed more of those fantasies every single time. It was as if I had grown to like someone doing those things to me, even though it was totally perverse and terrible. But I liked it, simply because in the end, I was able to calm myself down. At home, there was no affection, and it was the only way I could soothe myself. No one ever spoke to me about feelings, ever.

Somewhere around fourteen years of age, I went on holiday with my parents, and it was there that I had my first experience with a man. He was around thirty-five. It began with him sitting next to me after everyone had gone to bed. We stayed and watched television in an area that was freely accessible to everyone. There was something in the air, and I could feel something was going to happen. I really liked it when he stroked my hair so gently, which was something that almost never happened at home. At that moment, I felt I had to give him something in return to be worthy of his company. It was something spontaneous, and I liked it. But from his side of things, all too quickly, it was heading in the direction of sex. I didn't even know what was going on. All of a sudden, he was all over me, touching me. . . . At some point, I got so excited and couldn't stop myself, or maybe I just didn't think about that possibility. I don't know. I wasn't thinking about what was going on. Then I began to feel scared, because at any moment, someone could have entered. But that turned me on even more. The situation was becoming extremely intense. He had power over me because he was older. . . . My father was older, and I was never allowed to say no to him. I didn't even think I could say no. The fact that he was older was, of course, a fantasy for me—that he could also do things against my will. Everything fit together perfectly. The fear that somebody could walk in, the anxiety and tension connected with what my father would do to me, and every moment that followed. What could he do, that I would become even more aroused? The tension would not let off. He was the first, and I felt something powerful. Before it got to where it was headed, I fled, because I was, all of a sudden, very afraid.

When I was seventeen, once again, it happened in the

same way. I was in a park, and it was dark. At any moment, someone could have walked by. He was older, around forty. I didn't care who he was and what he looked like. All I had in my head was: Was he stronger than the other guy I had a similar experience with, will someone walk by, and how much further will I let him go? I was sitting in the park, pretending to be studying, as I had my books with me. And I noticed some older guy was sitting on the next bench, watching me . . . sexually. I began to look in his direction. I couldn't stop. It was as if I was hypnotized, and I went there. . . . There was no need for him to drop a hint. He didn't have to say a thing, not even a word. . . . Again, I crossed the line, and everything went too fast. When it went too far, as he began to undo his belt, I became scared and afraid and fled.

Every time, I was more and more allured by what would happen next. I already had a very good idea of what men liked. And I already knew how to behave to bring this out in them. I threw sexual energy in their faces, wore mini skirts and blouses showing cleavage because I knew this excited them. I knew I had this power, and in that way, I got their attention. So, that's the way I behaved. I felt that men liked it. I came to realize that men are sexual creatures. And if I wanted their attention, I had to act in a way to arouse their sexuality. This is something I had to give them to be worthy of their company.

Once I said to myself, about my father: "One day you'll see who I am. Because you don't want to see me as I am, and because you take a right, to do with me whatever you want . . . you'll see, and you'll be sorry!" And this is what I used when dealing with men: "You'll be sorry! When I take you so far, and mess with you, and provoke you, you'll hardly be able to control yourselves . . . you'll be totally crazy about me. . . ." In the end, I decide—at least I thought I was the one who decided if, in the end, it would lead to sex. That I have that power, to stop and say no. At least I had the power for some time, but that didn't mean that it all depended on me. I was physically weaker than them, and I could have drawn the short straw.

I was always searching for boundaries. I did this with my father, in the same way . . . whether he would contain himself or whether he would explode. And so, I searched for that limit within me. How far could I take them so that they would still be able to keep it all together? And how much adrenaline would I need, when I wouldn't be able to hold them back anymore, or when they didn't want to play my way anymore. And in that way, I got them. Because I could get it to go so far that they went completely crazy, they could hardly contain themselves. The more they were on the edge of control, the more I felt this power of mine, and the more I liked it. Because I was angry at my father for not having control over him. And here with this new guy, I thought I did.

But I didn't. Because he said that he wasn't going to play that game anymore unless I came to see him. And when he said that, fear grew inside me. And I felt I wasn't worthy and that now he can decide if I will get his attention or not. And if he tells me to come and see him or it will be the end of us, that means I have to go. Because if I don't, the attention will be once again taken from me. Just as my father had once said to me. And again, I felt worthless. I felt I wasn't worthy of love unless I went there and that something happened. To my own detriment, I went there for those reasons. And I went, even though I knew something bad could happen. When I got there, it was all over. He shut the door, he was stronger . . . I said, "No, no, no" a thousand times. But he didn't want to hear it. He knew he had all the control and power—and he took it. And I felt it fade away, that I no longer had control and that I wasn't allowed to have it.

And then I just lay there. I wasn't able to move my arms nor legs. As if I wasn't even in my own body, as I wasn't able to do anything with it. I felt that I could observe the room from somewhere below the ceiling and see my body and everything happening to me from a different angle. As if I had left my body because I was no longer able to move. I don't know how long it lasted. It seemed to be an eternity that I lay there and could hardly breathe.

When I came to, the first moment was so terrible, and if I were to admit to myself how bad it really was, I wouldn't have been able to stand it mentally. And I said to myself: "It was nothing." The first words which I heard in my head. Nonstop: "It was nothing, it was nothing. . . ." In a second. And I gathered up my clothes and got dressed and said to myself that it was nothing. I was kidding myself the whole time, that it was nothing. It was just so that I could survive mentally. Because otherwise, I would have gone crazy. Even more terrible was the fact that it was the strongest adrenaline rush I had ever experienced. Precisely the same as what my father achieved when he beat me. And that's exactly what happened to me because I provoked it into happening. I now know that what happened to me wasn't my fault. But I was responsible because I went there, even though I knew what could happen to me.

Three days later, when I still couldn't believe what had happened, I went back. Again. For the same thing. Because I probably needed something even stronger. But this time around, I didn't resist anymore. This time, I went because I wanted to experience it again. Because it was, in the end, such a release, such quietness in my head, that I probably wanted to experience it again. And if my brother hadn't suspected, I probably would have gone a few days later again. And again, and again and again.

And I don't know where it would have ended. When I wasn't able to go there, I experienced such anxiety . . . even though I felt that what I was doing wasn't so bad. I wasn't able to clearly understand why I actually went there. I thought I would be able to hide it from everyone, that it would go to the grave with me. Everyone does it. Everyone around me told me so. For a long time after, I continued to kid myself that I could hide it, and that it was nothing.

Advice for addicts

In my clinical experience, sex addiction is one of the toughest addictions to recover from—in part because it's simply too easy to hide, even from a sex partner. It's also easy for sex addicts to rationalize their behavior with common phrases like "boys will be boys," or "I have needs"—or even to blame it on a spouse who does not seem to want to put in the effort to fulfill all of the addict's abundant or transgressive sexual desires.

If you believe you might be a sex addict, you might already have caught yourself making some of these excuses. You may also have discovered it easy to find people who side with you against your spouse, rationalizing their own fantasies as they do so. Even some therapists may suggest "decent" porn could help improve addicts' sex lives, and that the less interested partner should make an effort to spice things up in the bedroom to satisfy the sex addict and maintain their interest.

However, if you're reading this book, deep down, you know that the problem is you—and ultimately, only you can do something to truly shift your mindset and improve your situation. Find a therapist educated in sex addiction, find a Sex Addicts Anonymous group, and start your recovery before your addiction can further drive away the people who care for you. You'll find a detailed plan on how to begin in Part Four of this book.

Advice for the addict's friends and family

Discovering your partner's chronic infidelity is typically a traumatic experience. You may experience all sorts of reactions, from disbelief to shock to anger at your partner—and at yourself, for being so naïve. At first, you may feel shame and want to keep your partner's infidelity secret. Then you might want to let everybody know you've been betrayed, and punish your partner. You may regret this later on, if you decide to give your partner another chance and they start treatment, you might come to find you regret some of your responses. In therapy, you may concentrate on the addict's problems and forget that you, too, need help.

If you are a long-term sexual partner of a sex addict, you

may already have begun to adapt your sex life to your partner's. Unfortunately, you may also have found that this tends to bring you all sorts of problems, from emotional trauma and distress, to being pushed out of your comfort zone, to sexually transmitted diseases and other complications of infidelity. You may have experienced a degradation of trust in your partner and the relationship, or even may have found you have begun to compromise your own values and beliefs. You may find your partner's addiction causes you sexual trauma, especially if you experienced prior sexual abuse. However, you may also find yourself being swept up in the addict's behavior, and developing a form of sexual codependency yourself. We'll discuss these and other problems in the next chapter, on co-sex addiction—so read on!

Friends, siblings, coworkers, teachers, and other well-meaning people may also notice the out-of-control sexual behavior of the addicts. If you are one of these people, you may feel there's not much you can do. It is very unlikely you would seriously confront a sex addict because you may think it is none of your business. Feeling powerless, you may choose to ignore it or even play it down like recklessness. The best you can do, however, is to talk to them and mention that therapy is available.

19.b. *Co-sex Addiction (Sexual Codependence)*

Co-sex addiction, or sexual codependency, is a particular form of sex addiction that can also be thought of as a relationship addiction: a compulsive attachment to sex-addicted partners whose own addictions are out of control. However, unlike other types of codependents, sexual codependents behave a bit differently: they believe they can control their partner's dysfunctional sexuality, and therefore end up taking the blame for anything that goes wrong in the relationship. The co-addicted partners therefore try to adapt to the behavior of their sex-addicted mates, often with devastating consequences to themselves.

Typical Behaviors (see Exercise 1):

■ Dressing and behaving seductively, even if you do not

want to, out of a belief your partner is being unfaithful because you are not attractive or sexually proactive enough

- Trying to get revenge on a cheating sex-addicted partner by being unfaithful yourself

- Believing you must behave or dress in a certain way to control your sex-addicted partner's sexual drive

- Withdrawing sexually as a way to control your partner's sexuality

- Believing the sex addict's promises that "it won't happen again"

- Ignoring your friends when they tell you of the sex addict's acting out

- Lying about, rationalizing, or covering up the sex addict's behavior

- Obsessing over the sex addict (e.g., constantly looking for clues to their acting out, checking their spending habits or where they have been and for how long, etc.)

- Experiencing memory loss, unpredictable behavior, or destructive acts against yourself or others, produced by preoccupation with the sex addict

- Experiencing accidents, destructive acts perpetrated against yourself or others, or other dangerous situations produced by preoccupation with the sex addict

- Experiencing severe mood changes—from hope to fear, from grief to self-pity, from anger to guilt, and back to hope again—in progressive cycles, leading to a state of numbness

- Ignoring your own sense of sexual boundaries, morals, or ethics to please your sexually addicted partner and prevent abandonment—for example, agreeing to a three-some, swinging, or imitating a porn scene when you don't actually enjoy these acts

- Being afraid to admit you don't enjoy certain sex acts

- Other: ....

Powerlessness

In their early childhoods, and usually as a result of their relationships with their dysfunctional caregivers, sexual codependents learn they cannot rely on other people to take care of them unless they first "rescue" them from their own mistakes. As adults, they still believe in the same fantasy. Consequently, they are often drawn to sex addicts who present the same visible dysfunction as those caregivers—the perfect match for their codependent rescuing behavior.

The result is usually a mess. Since sexual fidelity is one of the major conditions for establishing a feeling of mutual trust in partnerships, sexual acting out by the sex-addicted partner creates havoc in their relationships with their codependent sex partners, who set out to control the addict's sex life in the hope of preventing further betrayals and emotional abandonment. The sexual codependent puts all their efforts into controlling what ultimately cannot be controlled; and when the sex addict continues to act out, the codependent ends up feeling **powerless**.

At first, the sexual codependents may deny these feelings. Since they need to feel in control of their partner's behavior, they'd *rather take the blame for everything that goes wrong than experience powerlessness over it.* Sooner or later, however, they must admit everything they tried for the sake of "love" simply did not work. With some guidance, this admission can be a good starting point for the beginning of their own recovery.

The scope of the problem

The prevalence of sexual codependence is as uncertain as that of codependence. Partners of sex addicts, especially women, often suffer emotionally when they discover their partner has a sex addiction or has committed infidelity. As many as 80 percent develop depression, while 60 percent develop an eating disorder. Partners of people with sex addictions are also much more likely to contract a sexually transmitted infection from their partner—65 percent of sex addicts admitted that they routinely ran the risk of venereal disease.[82]

Rebecca's Story

My client Rebecca, 35, told me about her life with her sex-addicted husband. Her story illustrates how a sexual codependent can adapt to a situation they feel powerless to improve:

> *My husband is a long-distance truck driver. I met him at a friend's bachelor party. We got drunk and ended up in bed, where we stayed for much of the following weeks. Although my friends warned me that he was the type who has a mistress in every town he drives through, I was too smitten with his lavish affection to really care. When we get married, I thought, my love and regular sex will make him appreciate peaceful family life! Boy, was I wrong!*
>
> *Three months later, I was pregnant, and we got married. I gave birth to our son, and a year later, to our daughter.*
>
> *When I think back, I see that the problems began as soon as my body started showing signs of pregnancy. He completely lost sexual interest in me. At first, I thought it was normal, as my body was getting huge. If he was even home, he stayed up most nights until dawn, watching porn and masturbating. I felt guilty for making him do that, but with two babies crying all night, I just couldn't make myself feel sexual. I was even happy that he was home and not with someone else.*
>
> *After some time, I gathered the strength to get on a strict diet and shape up. I loved him and tried to win him back with sexy lingerie, or imitating some scene from the porn he was watching, although I felt ridiculous doing it. But*

---

[82] Ibid.

nothing worked. He blamed me for never doing anything right. Believing him that he couldn't relax in the presence of children in the next room, I paid for an expensive retreat, but he got drunk every evening and never touched me. Finally, I blackmailed him into visiting a therapist, expecting expert help would make things right. But the therapist sided with him, and they both ended up blaming me for not being spontaneous enough. Supposedly, the proof of his "normalcy" was that he had no problems regularly masturbating. I felt like I was going crazy and tried even harder, but nothing changed. He was either away for work, or too tired, or simply not interested. Slowly, I realized that I was going to live in a sexless marriage. I felt powerless.

Five years into our marriage, a woman contacted me saying that I should know he had given her a sexually transmitted disease. My whole world collapsed. When I confronted him, it turned out he had multiple one-night stands and some lasting affairs while away on his trips. This was his way of life even before he met me, and it continued after we were married. His friends knew, but nobody was sincere enough to tell me. I felt so stupid learning that he solicited prostitutes and regularly went to strip clubs, while I was begging for a little of his attention. . . . How could I not see it coming?

Advice for addicts

The sex addict and co-addict relationship is a closed system in which two people voluntarily participate. As I have already stated, the behavior of sexual codependents differs from that of other types of codependents only in their specific adaptation to the sexual acting out of their addicts, with hope that they might control it. Although you are unequivocally not to blame for your partner's addiction, and most certainly not the consequences of it, you do carry responsibility for the shared relationship problems. If you leave the relationship, chances are that you may find another similarly affected partner. A useful anecdotal "rule of the thumb" says that anybody who stays in a committed relationship with an active sex addict for at least two years will probably have to adapt in some way. Therapy is needed to change that.

Entering into and remaining in a long-term relationship with a sex addict profoundly affects the codependent's love and sex life as well, and both partners need expert help to enter recovery. Marital relationships typically imply some form of shared sexual acts as an integral part of the marriage. But expressing love and sexual feelings in an out-of-control fashion can be as problematic as being inflexible about them. You should not assume you are the healthier one in their relationships and must admit you cannot take matters into your own hands. Both partners need therapeutic help.

Advice for the addict's family and friends

As for friends, relatives, and other people besides partners who would like to help the co-sex addict, there's really not much else to do other than talk the addict into consulting a professional. Although the media is full of advice on sexual matters, and people seem to love reading this advice, they seldom act on it. Addiction is beyond the point where any unsolicited and unprofessional advice can do much good. If you do not understand the mechanisms of addiction and presume the addicts should just stop or curtail their behavior, your advice can even do harm by offering superficial excuses like "boys will be boys" or "just give him what he needs."

19.c. *Sexual Anorexia*

Sexual anorexia is an obsessive state characterized by the mental, physical, and emotional avoidance of anything sexual. Like anorexics who starve themselves or diet obsessively to control their weight, sexual anorexics gain a feeling of power and control from their compulsive disownment of anything sexual. Obsessively avoiding sex can then become their coping mechanism for dealing with other life problems and stresses. It can also be a reaction to a sex-addicted partner, such as an attempt to control the partner's out-of-control sexual acting out.

Typical Behaviors (see Exercise 1):

- Avoiding situations where sexual proposals may happen

- Feeling shame and disgust at nudity and provocative pictures, situations, or words in the context of normal social situations (e.g., on billboards or in movies)

- Dressing "down" to avoid being seen as sexually provocative

- Considering yourself sexually unappealing and rejecting any sexual interest from others as a result

- Choosing jobs that allow you to avoid public interaction out of anxiety and fear of embarrassing yourself in front of others

- Feeling unworthy of the relationships you desire, and refraining from ever attempting to enter into one

- Missing out on important commitments to family, work, and other important areas of your life in order to avoid exposure to sexual topics

- Being unable to enjoy intimate relationships, even if you want to

- Spending a great deal of time anxiously studying others for signs of approval or rejection

- Other: ....

Don't rock the boat

Like other addictions, sexual anorexia has serious consequences. For sexual anorexics, sex becomes a hidden enemy that must constantly be kept at a safe distance, even at the price of denying an essential part of themselves.

How does the sexual anorexic come to fear something that should be so positive as intimacy and genuine contact with another? Human sexual energy, or **libido**, has the potential to evoke deeply repressed feelings. Like a torrent that washes over a riverbed, taking with it anything in its path, sexual energy often spills over any obstacle and uncovers whatever emotion lies underneath: happiness, sadness, fear, anger, and even memories of past sexual experiences or abuse. An intimate sexual experience can trigger repressed memories of incest or sexual abuse, stirring up feelings the survivor wants to escape—an especially dangerous outcome for addicts, who have learned to act out to forget their pain—or even convincing them the abuse is being repeated. They might become angry and bitter. Indeed, this is one more reason abuse survivors avoid potentially loving partners—they're afraid to abandon their defenses and start trusting again.

Physical sexual abuse may not be the only reason people can become sexual anorexics. For most people, sex is a part of the human experience. In expressing our sexualities, we express parts of ourselves. However, many people are taught they should not feel sexual feelings because those feelings are shameful. Their "love maps" tell them they should hate their bodies and sexual feelings and enjoy them only in secrecy, or not at all. Whenever an important part of the human experience such as sex is embarrassing, hated, or disrupted, it can turn against the person and become harmful. People, especially women, turn the shame they feel at their sexuality against themselves, and begin to hate their own bodies. Studies have shown that people who have been abused in this way have learned double standards about their sexuality and their sex organs like, "Sex is dirty, and you do it only with the one you love." For them, sex is embarrassing, dirty, and secretive—but also incredibly important. They have learned to direct their anger, pain, and fear toward sex, and avoid engaging in it so as not to bring up these harmful feelings.

The scope of the problem
Dr. Patrick Carnes in his book *Sexual Anorexia*[83] tried to define

---

[83] Patrick J. Carnes, *Sexual Anorexia: Overcoming Sexual Self-Hatred* (Center City, MN: Hazelden, 1997).

sex addiction on a continuum, putting sexual anorexia parallel to the "acting in" side. In fact, *both seemingly mutually exclusive states can exist simultaneously* within a person or within a family. Both diseases often arise from a background of childhood sexual trauma, exploitation, neglect, and other forms of abuse. According to Dr. Carnes, sexual anorexia is not inhibited sexual desire, sexual dysfunction, being cold and unresponsive, guilt, shame, or religious belief. It is simply the emptiness of profound deprivation—the silent suffering.

Chrissy's Story, continued

Follow on with my client Chrissy from the previous chapter on sex addiction, who eloquently explains how one can obsessively want and avoid love and sex at the same time:

> *I never had any experience with closeness, that real intimacy. At home, it just wasn't there. It was never to be felt. And if someone had come my way and touched me . . . I don't know how much of that I could have taken. Because I have never had contact with myself, or with those close to me in that manner, and I wouldn't be able to handle it. It would have been unpleasant for me to be touched in that way, because there wouldn't be any more tension, which I needed. It would have meant too much peacefulness, too much contact with myself, which I wouldn't have been able to deal with—the idea that someone is there because of me, because I'm a human being, a being of worth—not that I would have had to pay for it with sex. I have never been able to deal with that kind of intimacy. It was so awful that if someone had only wanted that, I would have become so tense, I would have forced him into having sex with me. I wouldn't have lasted even two minutes. Too little, too slow, too much contact with myself. I would feel too much . . . not enough drama, not enough tension. Because if I showed myself to the man as I really was, I would again be faced with my innermost belief that I'm flawed. That I'm not worthy. Who would want to be with me if I only wanted to talk about intimacy?! He would see that I'm not worth*

it, and would immediately leave. Sometimes I said to such guys: "What's wrong with you? What do you want from me? Stop, stop it!" And that's why it was so uncomfortable for me. He wanted to know who I was. I have no idea who I am! I really don't know. You tell me who I am, because I don't know. If a man asked me who I was, I would break down and cry my eyes out because there was too much contact with myself. I didn't know who I was, because I was never allowed to be myself, but only someone others wanted me to be. That is what I learned. And if someone would say: "Who are you?" I would disappear. I don't know! I would become so nervous, I would leave. I preferred to leave rather than get to the point that I thought he would leave me. No, I did that myself. Yes, they were nice guys, even the right guys; but the timing was not so right for me, being as I was at the time.

It's terrible when you don't want sex and you can't gather the strength to set boundaries. As a child, you believe your existence depends on allowing others to take advantage of you, because you want them to love you. If it only takes sex for them to love you . . . then this is what you give. And it's terrible that you can't say no anymore, that you can't stop yourself. I wanted to be able to stop, because my heart was breaking. But I couldn't. And I don't know how anybody could think being addicted to sex is any good. Because of it, everything gets messy. You think you're only worth that, and you give it, because nobody ever knew how to compliment you. No one ever knew how to see you. Is it so difficult to praise a child? Is it not possible to say, "You look great"? How then is it possible for a child to learn that it's good if you look good and know how to attract a guy's attention?

No, it's not good! It's terrible! Because then you feel so dirty knowing you forced such a situation into existence. But if you believe you have no choice, then it is what it is. It's bothersome for others if they don't know how to see this. I don't know what good there is in that. That your heart breaks, that you can hardly breathe. That you don't know what will hurt you more: being totally alone, or the adrenaline you feel at that time. I don't know what's worse.

All of this simply comes from loneliness because you think you have nothing else . . . everything you have is just sex. And you wave it around. If you don't give them that, then you'll really be lonely. Then you won't even have those who just see the sexuality in you. You won't even have them—let alone the others, who in any case were never there. And if they won't be around, then you'll be really lonely. . . .

Advice for addicts

Sometimes people can't distinguish between their wants and needs. Sex is something people *want*, but don't necessarily *need*. A harmonious sexual life is certainly one of the desired characteristics of psychological wellbeing, but deciding to be asexual does not mean that there's something wrong with you. In fact, many mature and religious people choose celibacy and decide to redirect that energy into spirituality or religion. On the other hand, if this choice is compulsive, obsessive, maybe a result of unresolved sexual trauma in your history, you should find an expert to help you deal with it. The same advice is in place if your aversion to anything sexual is the result of the relationship dynamic with a sex addict.

Advice for the addict's family and friends

Since sexual anorexia is about silent suffering in isolation, friends and family can do little to help. Spouses of addicts who are not satisfied with their asexual marriages and want to change should seek expert help.

20

Does That Mean We're All Addicted?

This is the usual query I hear in response to my explanations of behavioral addictions. After hearing about dozens of examples of ordinary people who have fallen into the trap of addiction, listeners sometimes start to worry. They can see they have repeatedly done almost everything I describe as indicating the presence of an addiction, and start wondering whether they have already crossed the line. However, they usually dare not ask me whether they're addicted themselves. Instead, they ask, "Does that mean everyone is afflicted by some sort of addiction, even if only mildly?"

Of course not! Although people can indeed become addicted to just about anything that brings them instantaneous pleasure and relief, or that numbs pain, not everyone who pursues those goals via various avenues is an addict. Though an addict's "drug of choice"—be it prescription drugs, alcohol, nicotine, or behaviors—can vary, and the addict often finds new avenues to pursue oblivion as the old ones lose their power, several different studies conservatively estimate that just about everywhere in the world, in every culture, just 6 to 10 percent of all people eventually become addicted to a substance.

In the United States, alcohol is the most common addictive substance: 17.6 million people, or one in every twelve adults, abuses alcohol or suffers from alcohol dependence, and

several million more engage in risky patterns of binge drinking that could lead to more serious problems. More than half
of all adults have a family history of alcoholism or drinking
issues, and more than seven million children live in a household where at least one parent is dependent on or has abused
alcohol.[84] Other studies have found that about 12 percent of
the population have alcohol addiction, and 2 to 3 percent are
addicted to illegal drugs.[85]

So, although these numbers are large, it's clear not everyone has a substance addiction—as we might expect. But the
actual prevalence[86] of *all* addictions—both substance- and behavior-based—is difficult to calculate, especially since most
addicts have more than one. A very reliable study[87] combining
data from eighty-three studies and considering eleven types
of addiction—tobacco, alcohol, illegal drugs, eating, gambling,
the Internet, love, sex, exercise, work, and shopping—found
addictions in 15 to 61 percent of American adults. And while
that figure certainly doesn't encompass the entire population, it
is an awfully large number—don't you think? Just imagine how
much pain, misery, and betrayal that figure encompasses—the
amount of health, money, and time lost, and the broken relationships and traumatized children. The toll is terrible, especially when you consider that the effects of these addictions
drag on and on, from one generation to the next.

One might imagine these numbers might be inflated due to
the ease with which many Americans can access substances or
perform behaviors commonly thought to be addictive. However, most interestingly, addiction affects the same percentage of

---

[84] "Facts about Alcohol." NCADD National Council on Alcoholism and Drug
Dependence, Inc., NCADD, 2023, https://ncadd.us/about-addiction/alcohol/
facts-about-alcohol.

[85] Kathleen R. Merikangas and Vetisha L. McClair. "Epidemiology of Substance
Use Disorders," *Human Genetics* 131, no. 6 (2012): 779–789, doi: 10.1007/
s00439-012-1168-0.

[86] **Prevalence** is the proportion of a population that exhibits a specific characteristic within a given period.

[87] Steve Sussman, Nadra Lisha, and Mark Griffiths. "Prevalence of the Addictions: A Problem of the Majority or the Minority?" *Evaluation & the Health
Professions* 34 no. 1 (2010): 3–56, https://doi.org/10.1177/0163278710380124.

people living in abundance in the Western world that it does in Africa, where many struggle to feed their children. We can only conclude that there must be something inherent to the human experience that opens the door to the addiction and despair, no matter the resources available to us.

When does a behavior become an addiction?

As an expert in addiction recovery, I have to know and understand the boundaries of addiction—that is, in order to do my job, I must be able to discern when a behavior has transformed into addiction. I have tested these boundaries many times during the thirty years I have worked in this field. Most of the activities and behaviors discussed in this book—eating, sex, shopping, and more—are totally normal, when we engage in them in moderation. But the meaning of "in moderation" can be dangerously stretched to accommodate someone's problematic behavior or use of substances.

Many have tried to determine the boundaries of moderation by using quantitative explanations—for example, by citing an exact number of glasses of wine one can consume per day without being considered an addict. In reality, however, the difference between an addiction and use of a substance or performance of a behavior "in moderation" lies not in the frequency or intensity with which the behavior is performed, nor in how much of the substance is consumed—but in the *purpose* behind that behavior and consumption!

To illustrate this difference, I can cite an example from my own life. When I was still studying, I was a part of a large group of medical students in our twenties. We studied together, and in the evenings, we partied. Of course, we all drank alcohol. Some of us did so merely to relax and be part of the group. Others, however, couldn't wait for evening to come. They didn't stop after the first beer, and almost always got drunk. They drank to get drunk! This was common and acceptable behavior in that group, but later on, many of these drinkers developed alcohol-related problems.

There are three telltale signs that someone's substance use or indulgence in a behavior has crossed the line into addiction:

1. **Continuing to use a substance or engage in a behavior despite negative consequences**

If you continue to drink alcohol despite your wife's threats to leave you—if you continue to gamble despite acquiring debt—if you keep acting out sexually with strangers, although your relationships and health suffer—the line has been crossed, and you can be certain you are in the grip of an addiction.

2. **Withdrawal and cravings in abstinence**

To determine whether you are addicted to a substance or behavior, you can perform a simple test: define the substances and behaviors you suspect might be problematic, and stop consuming or engaging in them for six months. Anybody can stop doing something for a couple of months, but six months is long enough for you to become aware of any difficulty you might have in abstaining completely from a substance or activity. During this time, it's essential that you also abstain from all mind-altering substances—because, craving oblivion, your disrupted neural pathways can easily switch to finding comfort in some other substance or behavior. If you can abstain for six months without experiencing cravings, relapses, slips, and withdrawal symptoms, you don't have an addiction. But make sure you haven't substituted something new for the behavior or substance from which you've decided to abstain, in an effort to escape your troubles!

3. **Using your "drug of choice" to control negative emotions**

Addicts use their favorite substance or behavior to regulate their feelings. Instead of crying, they drink. Instead of feeling angry, they overeat. Instead of expressing rage, they have sex with prostitutes. They can't control their behavior.

The first thing I try to teach addicts in recovery is how to regulate their emotions so they can avoid turning to their "drug of choice" and triggering a relapse. Before they can be expected to stop acting out, they need to be taught alternate solutions to their problems—because they really don't know anything better.

What if you've discovered you may be addicted?

So, what if the above three criteria apply to your behavior? Or what if you've discovered someone you love has problems with addiction? Something must be done.

As we go on to Part Four of this book, we will systematically list everything that must be done to start recovery from behavioral addictions. We'll start by defining and explaining the recovery process, and end with an outline of a personalized recovery program—a plan fitted to your needs and abilities, one that can get you out of trouble. All you need to do then is follow the plan. It works if you work it![88]

---

[88] Another slogan from Alcoholics Anonymous.

21

Exercises for Combatting Behavioral Addictions

Part Three of this book, wherein I explained different behavioral addictions, can be read linearly. Since addictions so often mix and overlap, it's good to have the definitions of the entire range of traps you could fall into at your disposal!

But if you were just looking for quick answers to your questions, you might have skipped the descriptions of other behavioral addictions that don't concern you, and concentrated only on those with which you are experiencing problems. Either way, it's okay. You can always go back if necessary.

In the next set of exercises, you will prepare to take back control of your life.

No matter what type of addiction you have, *recovery begins with abstinence.* This is no surprise. But for people with behavioral addictions, it can be difficult to understand what they need to abstain from. That is why we had to first understand how addictions work, and how they can disguise themselves as "normal" behavior.

But how can one stop engaging in an addictive behavior— which, by definition, addicts are unable to do? This is the paradox you need to understand to take back control over your behavior—for, as a client of mine once eloquently explained: "Sometimes, I just cannot make myself *want* to do the right thing!"

It's true addicts can't always stop, even if they want to—

because the addictive system works automatically, producing intense cravings; and because acting out is the only thing that can satisfy these cravings. The problem needs to be worked around—and it was addicts themselves who found the solution.

In 1935, in his attempts to stop drinking, an alcoholic known as Bill W.[89] discovered two major breakthroughs that have since helped millions of addicts set out on the path to recovery. They are:

- Addicts cannot promise to stop using forever, but they can stop "one day at a time"—and if on each day, they commit to staying sober that particular day, they can make it last, building up a period of cumulative sobriety.

- To stay sober, addicts need the company and help of other recovering addicts who regularly meet to help each other stay clean.

Exercise 8: The list of behaviors you need to stop

In Exercise 1 on pages 23 to 42, you identified harmful behaviors you keep repeating. In Exercise 2, you identified which of those behaviors were the most problematic for you. Then you checked those behaviors for the eleven criteria that define addiction. The resulting list should be *the list of behaviors to which you are addicted, and in which you should stop engaging.*

In the table below, *make a list of all the behaviors you need to stop doing,* and use a pencil to *record the first day you don't engage in that behavior—the day of your sobriety.* This is your new birthday, and you should be aware of it. Later, when you have achieved many days of abstinence, the awareness of your success will help you stay sober—you won't want to ruin it!

Of course, no one is perfect, and you might find it difficult to remain abstinent at first. If you engage in a forbidden behavior on one occasion after a period of sobriety, this is a **slip**. It's

---

[89] William Griffith Wilson (November 26, 1895 – January 24, 1971), also known as Bill Wilson or Bill W., was the cofounder of Alcoholics Anonymous (AA).

not good, but it's not necessarily a disaster. But if you continue to repeat that behavior until you have undone all your previous recovery work and end up back in an addiction cycle, unable to stop engaging in the behavior, this is a **relapse**. After a relapse, you'll have to reset your abstinence date to the date you last acted out. As an example, for a codependent who is trying to recover from her past abusive relationship, a slip may involve driving past her former lover's house or checking his Facebook posts to see if he has found new love. A relapse would involve meeting him again and planning to get back together.

TABLE 7: Exercise 8: The list of behaviors you need to stop

Behavior	Abstinence Date
1.	
2.	
3.	
4.	
5.	
6.	

List your thoughts while working on this exercise:

....

....

....

Exercise 9: Emergency Control Plan

Addiction is a chronic disease—which means addicts can expect periods of improvements and relapses. Although you may be certain this will never happen to you, it's good to know what to do just in case you slip, or even relapse. Life isn't always easy, so it's better to hope for the best and be prepared for the worst.

In my experience, the first time you *really* try to abstain from your addictive behaviors is the easiest, because you are likely to be more confident in your resolutions. After a slip or a relapse, you may find it difficult to rebuild your trust in yourself and your ability to succeed.

The worst thing you can do after the awareness of your failure hits you is give up and succumb to your inner critic—to that voice whispering that you are worthless, bad, or incompetent, and telling you that you'll never make it. This will not help you, but will only give you an excuse to stop trying and "fall off the wagon" completely. Instead, you should gather all your strength to stop acting out and stick to the emergency plan you will prepare below.

One important part of that plan is an **emergency kit**. To create such a kit, prepare a box or a drawer filled with items that remind you why you want to stop acting out. Such items could include:

    a. A list of people you can call for assistance, and their phone numbers

    b. A letter from "sober you" to "acting out you" that you've written in preparation for when you are tempted to slip

    c. A photo of yourself as a child

    d. A picture your child has drawn for you

    e. Something that reminds you of your purpose in life

    f. Something that reminds you that you are a good person

    g. Other emergency measures

You're trying to abstain from watching pornography online. You have put filters on your computer and phone, but suddenly, you get a text message with a new seductive offer. You automatically click on it and start obsessing about it. You know you should erase it immediately, but the craving to look "just once more" becomes irresistible. You know you are seconds away from losing control.

In such a situation, you should immediately go to your emergency kit and avail yourself of its contents. In case you're not at home when you feel tempted to slip, it's best if you keep a copy of your list of emergency measures with you at all times—perhaps in your wallet or purse.

Example:

a. A list of emergency measures

- Call your therapist, a sponsor, or a trusted friend. Tell them about the temptation, slip, or relapse, and arrange an appointment with them as soon as possible.

- Go to a secure place where you will not be able to act out, like a twelve-step meeting, a park, or a church—anywhere you won't be able to access your chosen drug or engage in your addictive behavior.

- Stay with safe people until the craving goes away. Make sure you're not alone until you feel the urge has subsided.

- Engage in a physical activity like running or hiking through the woods for at least an hour.

- Check your emergency kit for further reminders of your resolve to stop acting out.

b. A letter from "sober you" to "acting out you"

Example:

Dear [Name],

I know you're unable to think of anything else but acting out now, and that you feel as if you're going to die if you don't [your addictive behavior] immediately. But remember how bad you always feel afterward, and how disappointed your loved ones will be when they find out you've relapsed—and you know they will find out eventually. Remember they told you they will not be able to trust you if you do it again.

Remember that you are a good person who is trying hard to live your life honestly. Remember the things you love and the people who believe in you, and don't let them down. This feeling will pass, as it always does—and if you don't give up, you'll have a reason to be proud of yourself tomorrow.

Take care of yourself, and go to a safe place immediately. Do it for the child you once were, who is still within you and needs you to take care of him.

I love you.

c. A list of emergency contacts and behaviors

- Call your therapist, sponsor or trusted friend.

Contacts:

....

....

....

- Go to a secure place.

Addresses:

....

....

• Stay with safe people.

Contacts:

....

....

• Engage in a physical activity.

Ideas:

....

....

• Check your emergency kit for additional ideas:

....

....

....

....

....

....

Exercise 10: Accepting responsibility for the things you can change

At this moment, the things that bother you the most are probably the consequences of your out-of-control behavior: your family, friends, and coworkers don't trust you anymore; you've spent money that was meant for family; you're involved with shady people. A plan for repairing the damage will help you sort things out effectively.

At this time, go back to Exercise 5 on pages 97 to 101, where you listed the consequences of your addictive behaviors. Sort them into short-term consequences you can fix in a week; mid-term consequences that will take up to six months to resolve; and long-term consequences, ones that will take years to mend. An example of a short-term consequence might be that you have no more money for rent, having spent it all in pursuit of your addiction. You need to resolve that issue as soon as possible, or your situation will worsen, and you may be evicted. A mid-term consequence might be losing your job—it will likely take you some time to find new employment. But if your spouse has decided to divorce you because you're unreliable, those consequences—including not being able to live together with your children—are long-term consequences.

A **damage control plan** must include:

- the problem—an assessment of where you are,

- the goal—a description of where you want to be,

- the paths that will help you reach that goal, and

- the resources you have to help you get there.

Stick to the plan daily, and use the sources available to you for assistance. If you find the goal you've chosen is too difficult or distant to reach, I suggest breaking it into smaller goals.

Example:

My Problem: *I gained forty pounds due to overeating.*

290

My Goal: *Lose forty pounds in six months.*

Measures Required (with deadlines for enacting those measures):

- *Stop bingeing (immediately)*

- *Stop eating sweets (immediately)*

- *Empty the fridge of tempting foods (immediately)*

- *Only buy items from a list of acceptable foods, compiled with the help of your doctor or nutritionist (immediately)*

- *Eat regularly—five meals a day, and never after 7:00 p.m. (immediately)*

- *Become more physically active—walk (every day; after five weeks, start interval running—five minutes walking, three minutes running, three repeats. Add two repeats every week until you can reach a workout length of forty-five minutes; then progress to fifteen minutes of running and half an hour of walking.)*

Resources/Sources of Help:

- *Twelve-step group (Overeaters Anonymous)*

- *Checkups with your family physician*

- *Find an exercise buddy to train with*

My Problem #1:

....

My Goal:

....

Measures Required (with deadlines):

....

....

....

....

....

....

....

Resources/Sources of Help:

....

....

My Problem #2:

....

My Goal:

....

Measures Required (with deadlines):

....

....

....

....

....

....

....

Resources/Sources of Help:

....

....

List your thoughts while working on this exercise:

....

....

....

PART FOUR:

HOW TO RECOVER FROM ADDICTION

"Serenity is not freedom from the storm,
but peace amid the storm."

—*Slogan of Alcoholics Anonymous*

22

From Information to
Transformation

How do we commence the actual process of recovery?

If you've read the earlier material in this book, you've become well informed on the topic of addiction. You needed this information to correct any misconceptions and prejudices you might have had concerning addiction, and to understand the tasks you must accomplish—whether to help yourself, or to help someone else with their addiction. But if you've realized some of your behaviors indicate you may have an addiction, you'll need to be more than just informed. *You'll need to be transformed.* And this takes more than just learning a few tricks. It takes changing your whole life.

Unfortunately, although we can explain addiction in a way that allows us to understand it, we can't fight it merely by explaining it away—because, ultimately, *addiction is anything but rational.* Rather, it is derived from the irrational parts of our minds, including our sensations, perceptions, memories, beliefs, desires, emotions, and motivations. The mind is not a homogenous structure, and some parts of it are unconscious—like traumatic memories, attachment styles, and certain irrational and immature beliefs one might hold. For this reason, it's quite common for some of our unconscious beliefs to oppose our rational beliefs. For example, if an adolescent had an alcoholic father, they might swear never to marry an alcoholic—but end up falling in love with one nevertheless.

However, some phenomena we experience—like love, for instance—can't be placed in any of the categories listed in the previous paragraph. Is love, for example, an emotion? No—emotions are experiences generated in the central parts of the brain that reflect whether we think something is good or bad for us. But love is much more than that. In psychology, we talk about attachment, but love runs much deeper. For the sake of love, people are even willing to ignore threats to their survival, which is the rational and emotional brain's priority. In this way, love—and similar phenomena such as empathy; compassion; awe at nature, children, or beauty; and religious impulses—can be irrational, though the effect they can have on our lives is certainly very real. To distinguish them from logical thoughts, desires, and emotions, we sometimes call these feelings **spiritual.** Most people experience moments in their lives when they have strong spiritual experiences—moments known as **peak experiences.**[90] They are intimate and personal, and cannot be explained via charts and tables. But they can be expressed in music, poetry, and art.

While slowly sliding down the addiction spiral, an addicted person often abandons their personal spiritual values, giving them up one by one if ever they prevent the addict from obtaining the quick fix that dulls their pain. Furthermore, in failing to live up to their own standards, addicts often lose their sense of connection to others—to their family, their community, or even their sense of being a part of Nature or the Divine. In this way, we can say that *addiction is the opposite of love,* or even the opposite of spirituality. Remember, we've acknowledged addiction is an attachment disorder, which is essentially

---

[90] "A **peak experience** is an altered state of consciousness characterized by euphoria, often achieved by self-actualizing individuals. The concept was originally developed by Abraham Maslow in 1964, who describes peak experiences as 'rare, exciting, oceanic, deeply moving, exhilarating, elevating experiences that generate an advanced form of perceiving reality, and are even mystic and magical in their effect upon the experimenter.'" "Peak experience," Wikipedia, Wikipedia Foundation, Inc., July 6, 2023, https://en.wikipedia.org/wiki/Peak_experience.

the inability to love in a healthy way.

In recovery, this process of gradual spiritual loss must be reversed. As abstinence begins the healing process and the damaged brain is slowly restored, the recovering addict typically begins to experience profound changes in their emotional energy, behavior, and openness to peak experiences. These changes are not only beneficial, but *essential* to recovery.

The following chapters describe the path that lies ahead for recovering addicts, to prepare them for experiences they may not expect. Spiritual peak experiences are common in recovery, especially after the first year. However, if nobody affirms these experiences or explains them as normal, people who have these experiences may fear they are becoming overly emotional, or even crazy. They may repress these experiences, and even forget them. That's why it's important to recognize that you might have such experiences while you're walking the recovery path. Don't be afraid if they start happening to you.

In the remainder of this book, I want to take you by your hand and guide you through the dramatic changes that are about to happen in your life. However, I also respect your personal boundaries. I am not an authority on spirituality, and so I cannot take an authoritative approach to what is so absolutely personal. Everyone's experiences are different and unique. But I can share my personal experience of the recovery path I've walked, as honestly as I can, in the hope that something within you may resonate with my story. Just take in whatever serves you best, and know that *you are more than just your rationality*— even if nobody has affirmed that to you so far.

If you don't find yourself having peak experiences as you heal, don't worry—that doesn't mean you won't be able to recover. You're just taking another one of the many different paths.

Even so, it's important to know the whole path, so you can be aware of where you're going. In the next chapter, I'll explain the three stages of recovery. This book, *Serenity,* describes the first of these stages. It is to be followed by my next books, *Courage* and *Wisdom.*

23

The Process of Recovery

By now, you have learned how to recognize addiction, begun to understand it, and gotten to know the specific features of behavioral addictions that might be a problem for you. You have learned the misty oblivion of addiction is not your ally, but rather a sneaky enemy ruining your life. Now you're ready to take the first step toward freedom from addiction's tricky trap.

How do you go about this? What do you need to help you heal? How can you free your mind from something that's inside it, growing invasively like a cancer of the soul, destroying everything it touches and reaching out even further, into the most distant parts of your life?

Many approaches to the treatment of addiction exist. A therapist's preferred approach typically depends on what they believe addiction to be:

- Those who believe addiction is a **moral failure** look to punish addicts to make them stop acting out—sometimes even by jailing them.

- Those who believe addiction to be a **personality disorder** don't believe it can be treated, so they instead attempt to mitigate the effect the addict's behavior has on others. They may merely shrug their shoulders and advise, for example, that the spouse of an addict get a divorce.

- Those who know the truth—that addiction is a **disease of the brain** manifesting in the physical, psychological, relational, and spiritual dimensions of human existence—can investigate and offer tailored assistance that works for each of their individual clients.

Since, as this last group knows—and as you have learned—one of the main characteristics of addiction is that it is a **chronic disease**, they also know better than to expect their clients' addictions to disappear or get better without appropriate intervention. On the contrary, if left untreated, they will only get worse. The addictive behavior will become progressively more frequent and extreme. At times, the addict will make some progress, and may even begin to feel they have some control over their addiction. But usually, this only turns out to be some kind of balancing between the acting out and acting in behaviors caused by addiction. *To break the addiction cycle, an addict must completely change their lifestyle, values, and relationship patterns—and then maintain that changed lifestyle for several years.*

The difference between treatment and recovery

If you look for solutions to addictions, you will quickly notice that media advertisements for such solutions often talk about the **treatment** of addiction, or **recovery** from addiction. You may have assumed treatment and recovery are the same thing. But in fact, there is a vast difference between the two.

The principal difference between treatment and recovery is that a person undergoing *treatment* absorbs another person's direct, active efforts to help them. The patient, in this case, is a passive object of a process somebody else—a doctor, therapist, or some other professional—actively implements. On the other hand, *recovery* is the process an addict undergoes when trying to quit using a substance or to stop engaging in a particular behavior, and while continuing to abstain from it.

Treatment and recovery can coexist. For instance, if you

choose to go to a treatment facility or get help from some other professional while trying to curb your addiction, treatment may be a part of your recovery journey. But sooner or later, this stage of recovery will come to an end, and you will be left "to your own devices." At that time, while you may continue to engage professional therapists, healers, medical doctors, or peer support groups to aid in your recovery, you'll be the one holding the steering wheel—and in the end, you can be justly proud of directing your own successful recovery. Best of all, this pride will help you heal your low self-esteem—the root cause of all the troubles that have befallen you.

No matter the difficulties you face during any point in your recovery, you must not lose sight of the fact that this sort of healing is possible. Our bodies, after all, have a wonderful ability to heal physical wounds. We usually take this ability for granted, but when you truly consider all the steps involved in the healing process, it looks like a miracle. Whether or not we do anything to aid in this process, like cleaning the wound, stitching it closed, wrapping it in clean bandages, or just letting it be, it will typically heal in a predictable amount of time. And the same holds true for our souls! Once we stop inflicting wounds on our psyche and give the recovery process the time, energy, and willingness it requires to be effective, healing will take place according to its own predictable timeline—even without the sort of treatment doctors can offer, as helpful as it may be.

When I was in medical school, my classmates and I were taught "*Medicus curat; natura sanat,*" or "The physician treats; nature heals." This means doctors can only *assist* nature in healing wounds of all kinds, by ensuring favorable conditions are present while nature does most of the work. Understanding this fact is also important to understanding the process of recovery: first, it allows addicts to recognize that *everyone has the innate natural ability to recover,* regardless of a doctor's presence; and second, it shows them that *they alone are responsible for providing themselves with everything their bodies and souls need* to support the recovery process.

TABLE 8: The difference between treatment and recovery

Treatment	Recovery
An effort to eliminate, control, or mitigate the *effects* of addiction	Healing and personal growth toward greater resilience
A service offered to addicts by professionals to help them through the first days of sobriety	A process of change undertaken by addicts themselves in pursuit of a life free of addiction
A state in which the professional administering a therapy or program is in charge of its application and responsible for its success	A state in which the addict is responsible for their own sobriety and success
Temporary	Ongoing and lifelong
Residential (treatment facility, clinic) or local (outpatient)	Local; may be accomplished where the addict lives, or in any other location
An attempt to correct the damage already caused by addiction	An effort focusing on the addict's personal growth and future improvement

As a recovering addict, you must take care to remember another, vital point: *There is no definitive cure for addiction,* no pill you can take to wipe the effect of the disease away! While some prescription drugs can assist in the process of getting "clean" from alcohol or other substances—some drugs, for example, help mitigate cravings; and sometimes, addicts might need to use medication that helps lessen depression only for a short time, until the over- or underactive neurotransmitters in their brains begin to settle—these drugs only *help* the body commence its natural healing processes. They don't do away with the addiction.

As a doctor, I prefer to trust the wisdom of nature, and use

medication as a form of treatment only in select cases. I believe tampering with the brain's chemistry by introducing prescription drugs in recovery is potentially dangerous, because
we can never balance the dose of the externally administered
drug as meticulously as nature can regulate chemicals in the
brain. Also, addicts are used to having a chemical or behavioral
solution for every problem—feeling sad? Have a drink! Feeling
angry? Go shopping! Feeling inadequate? Check the number
of "likes" you got on Facebook for posting a funny picture of
your cat! These are the exact patterns of comforting behavior
addicts need to break in order to recover. Adding another drug
to the mix, I've found, usually doesn't help much.

Instead, addicts need to trust the *process*. The Substance
Abuse and Mental Health Services Administration (SAMH-
SA)[91] offers this definition of recovery: Recovery from alcohol
and drug problems is "a process of change through which individuals improve their health and wellness, live self-directed
lives, and strive to reach their full potential."[92] This definition
recognizes that there are many different paths to recovery, and
that every addict can find their own way. And since the same
principles found in the process of recovery from addiction to
substances like alcohol and drugs can be applied to recovery
from behavioral addictions, *you can apply these principles to the
process of recovering from your behavioral addiction.*

Don't lose hope when presented with the complexity of
the process you're about to undertake. Recovery is possible!
Millions of people have managed to turn their lives around by
following these basic, simple principles.[93] If an addict meets
these essential **conditions for recovery**, the body will reverse

[91] The Substance Abuse and Mental Health Services Administration, or SAMH-
SA, is a branch of the US Department of Health and Human Services.

[92] "SAMHSA's Working Definition of Recovery," samhsa.gov, SAMHSA Substance Abuse and Mental Health Services Administration, 2012, https://store.
samhsa.gov/sites/default/files/d7/priv/pep12-recdef.pdf.

[93] According to official sources, only AA had 1,967,613 members and 120,455
groups in 2021, and this is only one of the organizations. "Estimated Worldwide A.A. Individual and Group Membership," aa.org, General Service Office
(GSO) of Alcoholics Anonymous, December 2021, https://www.aa.org/sites/
default/files/literature/smf-132_Estimated_Membership_EN_1221.pdf.

the addictive processes and the addict's brain chemistry will return to normal:

1. **S**trong determination to change

2. **T**ime and energy for the recovery work

3. **A**bstinence and sobriety

4. **R**elationships and support

5. **T**rigger and stress management

Note that the first letter of all these conditions collectively spell START. Of course, *starting* is the most important step of recovery!

The stages of recovery

Recovery is a process of change. While recovering from addiction, people go through certain stages, encountering predictable problems in each stage. The timing of each stage is also predictable, though there may be variations as people begin the process of recovery from different positions. Nevertheless, there are more similarities than differences. This is one of the reasons meeting with other addicts in recovery is so stimulating for recovering addicts—they see the results others have achieved and know they can expect the same for themselves, if only they continue their efforts.

Most of the research on the stages of recovery has been done on recovering alcoholics. From this research, I borrowed the Jellinek Curve,[94] the roller coaster-shaped diagram in the following pages, which represents the degradation of alcoholics' lives as their disease progressively worsens, the proverbial "rock bottom," and the ensuing stages of recovery. Dr. Patrick

---

[94] The **Jellinek Curve**, created by E. Morton Jellinek in the 1950s and later revised by British psychiatrist Max Glatt, is a chart that describes the typical phases of alcoholism and recovery. The point of this research was to show that alcohol addiction is progressive and that there is a "vicious circle" associated with obsessive drinking, with much to lose along the way if addicts don't seek help. The curve shows an addict's life can get worse if the cycle of addiction isn't broken—but through recovery, it can also get better.

Carnes described similar stages in his research on sex addicts.[95]

The initial downward slope of the roller coaster represents the development of an addiction. It starts slowly, with occasional excesses in a future addict's behavior. (To make this diagram personal, write your problematic behavior from Exercises 1–3 above the declining slope.) After a while, a habit forms, and the behavior becomes the method addicts use to regulate their emotions—but it is still controllable. Then the negative consequences start to show, and the **crucial phase** occurs: some control over the behavior is lost, but on a good enough day, a certain amount of management is still possible. Now is the time to quit before serious trouble emerges.

If the person goes on, however, more and more control is lost, and the **chronic phase** begins. This is when the actual disease of addiction appears, and obsessive acting out (overeating, overworking, problem gambling, sexual excesses) or acting in (dieting, self-depriving) commences and continues in a vicious addictive system.

Once the curve reaches rock bottom, it enters the loop of the addiction cycle, and may continue around this loop for an indeterminate amount of time depending on the individual addict's disease progression. The following upward movement of the line represents **recovery**, which starts with the decision to stop the behaviors associated with addiction, followed by appropriate action. As you can see, one can slide *down* the slope easily and without effort—but the uphill climb comes in stages indicated by steps, and must be based in both personal and group effort.

There are the **twelve steps of recovery**, each of which has been designed to help addicts overcome obstacles and achieve an ever-new perspective on the problematic ways of thinking their brains have slid into while they were operating in an addictive mindset. Each step has its own foundation and logic; however, they do not always follow each other as linearly as in this scheme. Any **slip** causes some disturbance—and in the

---

[95] Patrick Carnes, *Don't Call It Love: Recovery from Sexual Addiction* (New York: Bantam Books, 1991), 185–196.

event of a **relapse**, an addict can fall back into the addiction cycle, requiring them to start the process of recovery from the bottom again. Such is the logic of addiction. It is of great benefit to addicts to succeed at their first recovery attempt because the process becomes more and more difficult with every consecutive effort, as an addict's belief in their eventual success and determination to succeed fade.

IMAGE 6: The addiction and recovery roller coaster

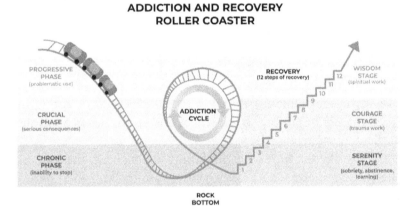

In my and other experts' clinical experience, the recovery work that needs to be done changes with each phase of recovery. In accordance with the wisdom of Alcoholics Anonymous, I have named the stages to match the famous Serenity Prayer.

1. **The Serenity Phase**: Steps 1–3, occurring over the first year of sobriety

    Motto: "Accept the things you cannot change, and achieve sobriety and serenity."

After a period of hesitation and struggle that could last years—or sometimes after only one blissful moment of clarity—the addict decides to commit to recovery. This decision represents the beginning of that recovery. Over the following six to twelve months, recovering addicts focus on achieving abstinence, learning about the disease, and struggling with emotional issues. After all, when the anesthetic effect of their addictive behavior or substance is removed, its consequences are revealed, and the pain that prompted the behavior reappears. In addition, addicts who attempt to achieve sobriety are bound to experience cravings, resistance to which sometimes demands an almost superhuman willpower. Emotional ups and downs will put pressure on them, and they'll have to go through these struggles without the help of their "pacifier"— the addictive behavior or substance they used to use.

At this point, as an addict, you may feel stuck wondering whether or not you should leave your relationship. But this is not the time to get a divorce or quit your job. *Nothing major in the first year!* If you make big decisions, you may find that when the dust settles and the consequences of those decisions come to light, you regret your choices, or feel you have acted out of pressure and made them too soon.

You may also experience setbacks, which may extend this stage beyond the year it would otherwise typically take. Setbacks are usually caused by relapses, or by an addict's failure to recognize and abstain from other addictive elements present in their lives. Some addicts experience compounded addiction, only becoming aware of certain addictive behaviors after they try to abstain from those they have already identified. An addict's greatest struggle in this period is being truthful about the extent and nature of their addiction. If you secretly leave a part of your hidden indulgence unattended, it will likely backfire, as you will turn to it when you have a bad day.

Believe it or not, the first few months of recovery are typically the easiest. You may even be surprised how easy it is to abstain, especially if you never believed you would be able to do so. At this stage, new hope and trust in the program can fuel the recovering addict, imbuing them with positive energy. However, there will be days when your hope sinks, and you won't be able to see the light at the end of the tunnel. This is when you need to contact your rehab buddies to request encouragement and support in maintaining your sobriety.

This book, *Serenity*, is mainly dedicated to the Serenity

Phase of recovery. When we sum up everything we have learned together, we will devote an entire chapter to preparing you for this phase. For now, let's discuss the next steps of recovery.[96]

2. **The Courage Phase**: Steps 4–10, usually occurring in years 1–3 of sobriety

   Motto: "Have the courage to change the things that can be changed."

When you stop engaging in addictive behaviors, your underlying traumatic memories will start creeping back in. This typically occurs spontaneously, after addicts reach a certain level of confidence and safety in a community of fellow recovering addicts, or with their therapist. In this phase, you will likely be faced with all the memories and negative feelings you have spent years or even decades fearing and trying to avoid. During that time, your addiction worked like a lid on a pot, helping you suppress pain by trapping the contents within. Now that the addictive behavior has been removed, the cover is open—and whatever has been hiding down there will reemerge, and must be dealt with.

The Courage Phase of recovery is typically turbulent and stressful, especially for those who begin to remember traumatic events from their early childhoods—events that may even have been perpetrated by their caregivers. As these memories reemerge, you will likely feel anger, sorrow, and profound grief for the abandonment and betrayal that occurred in your past.

You might ask why is it so important to dig out all those old grievances when we can't do anything about them. Actually, engaging with those fears is not about returning to the past, but about the examining consequences the past had on your "mental world map." The past cannot be changed, but the negative and self-defeating beliefs resulting from our traumatic pasts *can*—indeed, *must*—be redefined and transformed. As impossible as this task may seem, you are no

---

[96] The sequel to *Serenity, Courage,* will discuss trauma work in detail, and the third book in the series, *Wisdom,* will discuss the spiritual transformation an addict experiences while undergoing recovery.

longer a child, and aided by what you now know about how the world works, you can identify solutions to your hurts that you could not have recognized as a child.

During this phase, it is important to monitor your physical health. The chronic stress of reliving traumatic experiences can take its toll, and you should take special care to avoid becoming ill. To release the stress you accumulate in dealing with those experiences, you might choose to engage in physical exercise and regular meditation. If you begin recalling childhood sexual abuse or trauma inflicted by your parents, you will likely require expert help in working through that trauma.

Depending on the complexity of the underlying trauma and the level of resistance you offer, this phase may take one or several years, and will go on until your traumatic memories are fully reassembled and processed. There may be some talk of forgiveness, but until your memory has been completely repaired, you may not fully understand what you need to forgive or how to go about doing so. Only after you've gone through the whole process will the idea of offering real forgiveness begin to make sense to you.

Forgiving is the next crucial task of the Courage Phase, which the twelve-step concept and AA community describe as "making a moral inventory of ourselves, dealing with the wrongs we have done to others and making amends to people we have harmed", rather than as "trauma work." In truth, they are one and the same; though at first glance the two acts may feel different, forgiving others and forgiving ourselves are essentially the same process.

3. **The Wisdom Phase**: Steps 11–12, ongoing

> *Motto: "Cultivate the wisdom to know what is your responsibility and what isn't!"*

In the Wisdom Phase, the emphasis of recovery shifts to changes in the addict's family and spiritual changes in the addicts themselves. Addicts who reach this stage may see some of the relationships that were based in enabling their addiction come to an end. When, for example, relationship addicts who used to "need to be needed" to feel good about themselves recover their basic sense of self-worth, they might no longer want to put up with a partner's exploitation or betrayal. However, the quality of their remaining relationships often improves dramatically, allowing for more intimacy and their improved capacity to resolve conflicts. No longer feeling pulled this way or that by the force of their addictions, they achieve stability, and often find themselves becoming less judgmental and more compassionate.

When your relationships start improving, the major problems your addiction brought to your life will finally begin to disappear, and you will be able to see further into your future than you ever have before. At long last, you will be able to formulate goals apart from "just getting out of this mess."

What will you do with your life now that you have outgrown mere survival? Is there a purpose to all the troubles and changes you've been through? Can you forgive all those who have harmed you, now that you know that we grow through adversity? Will you forgive yourself for all those lost years and wasted opportunities? And how might you share with others the insights you've received through your recovery work?

As questions like these start arising within you, you may feel driven to find answers. You'll begin to recognize your responsibilities, and your potential, which is unlike anybody else's. It is the unique impact you can make on this world, and in the Wisdom Phase, you may start to recognize it in yourself: the pull to finish the mission entrusted to you by a "Power Greater Than Ourselves," which the AA community calls God. By sharing your story in the group, or becoming a mentor to a newcomer, for example, you may encourage fellow members who still hesitate—and seeing them thrive will reward you with good feelings.

What about those readers who are not religious, and do not believe in a god?

Maybe you wonder where this is going, feeling that somehow I derailed from the safe scientific way of describing recovery and introduced a new variable, God, as "deus ex machina"[97] or a magical solution. How can you recover if you are an atheist when such a twist of your beliefs is expected?

I can relate to these feelings. As a medical doctor, I was trained to observe the human body and life as marvelous works of nature rather than as miracles created by a deity. My family was not religious, and neither were most of my friends. However, even from a very young age, I believed there was a meaning and purpose to everything. I felt that this meaning involved me personally, and that my answer to life's challenges mattered. You could say that I was spiritual, but not religious.

Until my mid-thirties, I never thoroughly examined this philosophy. Only after the crisis triggered by the addiction in my family and the beginning of my recovery did I begin to turn to a "Higher Power" for help with the things that hurt me. It happened spontaneously, when, in a moment of deep crisis, I asked, "Please, let this turn out well!" Immediately, I felt comforted, as if someone had assured me things would be alright.

I developed a sort of inner dialogue with this entity, and found guidance and comfort in it. Its name did not matter; it spoke to me. However, I soon learned that merely asking for what I thought would be a benevolent outcome did not work. All I could do was let go and accept what might happen— to cooperate with the circumstances of the universe that were dictated by someone other than myself.

Nowadays, many people, especially young people, are put off by organized religion, but still believe there is an organizing principle, making sense of the world and the events. They are *spiritual, but not religious.* My program can work for them too, even if the word "God" is never uttered. For me, being *spiritual means believing that the world and your specific place in it have a*

---

[97] Latin for *"god out of the machine,"* "an unexpected power or event saving a seemingly hopeless situation, especially as a contrived plot device in a play or novel." Elizabeth Knowles, "Deus Ex Machina," Encyclopedia.com, Encyclopedia. com, June 11, 2018, https://www.encyclopedia.com/literature-and-arts/language-linguistics-and-literary-terms/literature-general/deus-ex-machina#:~:-text=deus%20ex%20machina%20an%20unexpected,in%20a%20play%20or%20novel.

meaning and a purpose and feeling responsible for your constant growth as a person. It also means that you feel that we're all interconnected, parts of a bigger picture. Even if you choose to become a vegetarian so as not to contribute to the killing of animals, or if you donate money to the underprivileged, this still means that you feel personally responsible for doing good and believe you are part of the bigger whole. The program will work for you. Just replace the words "Higher Power" or "God" with the term of your choice, like love, nature, meaning, wisdom, fate, or providence.

The Wisdom Phase is ongoing, as recovery never stops. Rather, it seamlessly changes into **personal growth**, allowing you to reach the level you were on before falling into the addiction "hole," and to rise up and beyond. You become a better person—more responsible and conscious, shining your new-found light on everyone around you.

My Story

My own recovery from codependence was difficult, but well worth it. It taught me so much, and made me a better person.[98] To illustrate the recovery journey, I'll share my recovery phases as I experienced them.

> *For years, I'd known things were not well between my husband and me. Our relationship had become superficial, and I was experiencing health problems and emotional outbursts, but attributed them to external, unrelated causes. I didn't consider these problems worth turning my whole world upside down to fix—and so the ground under my feet slowly disappeared, leaving me feeling powerless and alone.*
>
> *My wake-up call came on the day my husband confessed he had become addicted to gambling and had put us in severe debt. Finally, I had reached my "rock bottom." I didn't waste too much time deciding what to do; it was clear we needed help. I got us a meeting with a therapist and into a recovery program the very next day!*

---

[98] I share my story in further detail in my book *Stronger Than Love.*

*The first six months of my **Serenity Phase** were like a honeymoon. I trusted the therapist to hold my husband accountable for his actions, and stopped controlling him. I believed the program would work its magic, and then we'd go on with life as it should be. The only direct intervention our therapist made with me was telling me I should take care of my own problems and leave worrying about my husband's problems to him. But I'd thought my husband was my only problem!*

With the therapist's help, I learned that my submissive, people-pleasing behavior was actually an expression of an addiction called codependency. Taking his words about taking care of my own problems first to heart, I started learning about codependency, examining every resource I could find. I was doing great!

But the honeymoon wore off when I learned my husband had only been pretending to cooperate with the therapist, and was still actively gambling. This betrayal was harder to take than the thousands of betrayals that had come before. This time, I knew I'd put everything on the table to help us succeed, and if that hadn't been enough, I was truly powerless.

At the time, as spouses, my husband and I were financially responsible for each other's debts. After his betrayal, I decided not to enable his addiction any longer. Even though I still cared for him, divorce was the only way to prevent him from taking out any more loans in my name. When I finally filed for divorce, all the dirt, oppression, and manipulation his addiction had brought into our marriage came out. It was a tough year, but my recovery group helped. I took the work of the recovery program seriously, and it worked really well.

*My **Courage Phase** began when I met someone new and fell madly in love. He was stuck in a dead-end marriage with two very young children whom he loved dearly. Thus began my ordeal: I wanted to direct things in a way that would lead to him deciding to divorce, so we could really be together. But the decision was not mine to make! For* *the sake of my own recovery and sobriety, I needed to distance myself from his problems and mind my own. Trying to provide for and take care of my two daughters, pay for therapy, and cover my ex-husband's gambling debts without a dime of alimony was a big enough struggle. Every day, I had to remind myself of my boundaries, responsibilities, and recovery goals, so that I wouldn't enable or rescue the man of my dreams because that would mean a relapse for me. At night, when I lay in bed alone, past wounds reopened and came back to haunt me in the form of profound loneliness. Oh, how I craved to reach out to him—to lose myself in his warm embrace, and make him promise everything would turn out well for us. But I resisted the urge, waiting for him to make the move. And ultimately, those lonely nights brought me to the revelation that my loneliness stemmed from my father having abandoned me when I was less than four years old. Once I understood its root cause, the pain became bearable.*

*My **Wisdom Phase** followed. What I wished for in my lonely nights was granted to me—but not in the way I wanted. After an entire year of struggle, my new partner's divorce came through. This is where my story could have turned out the way I wanted, had it not been for the intervention of the Higher Power: only a month after his divorce, my lover was diagnosed with terminal liver cancer. In the final two months before his death, he moved in with me, and together, we experienced a heightened awareness of each passing day, came to terms with life's beauty and the terror of life unfulfilled, and helped each other understand and accept that we had been given the grace of love, only to have it taken away almost immediately. With his help, I transformed my own emerging relationship with God into a leading pillar in my life, and grew into a stable and dependable anchor for my children and my clients to turn to for guidance and reassurance.*

When my loved one passed away, grief took what remained of my fantasies and burned them to ashes. I realized life was too precious to be wasted on daydreaming. I was done avoiding life; I had to live for the both of us. I discovered that my ability to help people, when put into the proper perspective, was a blessing—but I also realized I needed to understand and respect the difference between enabling or rescuing and helping people. I could only help those who took their share of the responsibility for their own well-being. I trained to become a psychotherapist and built myself a career out of writing books on behavioral addictions. In this line of work, every day, I meet people who claim they want my help—but some of these people only want my attention, and I must distinguish between them and those who are ready to actively work to get better. I take clients who are willing to work, and with every correct choice I make between enabling and helping, I become stronger and wiser. Remember, in small enough doses, poison can be a medicine; and medicine taken incorrectly can be a drug. I have learned to know the difference between them.

In the worst moments after my partner's death, a friend put a book into my hands: A Course in Miracles, published by the Foundation for Inner Peace. It called to me more strongly than any book ever had before. Over years and years of practicing the daily meditations in this book, my dialogue with God has changed from a silent whisper to a clear inner voice I never ignore—which I further developed when I discovered another book, A Course of Love by Mari Perron and Dan Odegard. Every day at sunrise, I take this book in my hands, read a few paragraphs, then close my eyes and sit still. And it speaks to me. This is how I nourish my soul, and I will never again let it go, for I've fought too hard to find it.

23.a. *Strong Determination to Change*

Everybody has a breaking point—a moment when they realize their helplessness and become willing to accept help. The recovering addicts in Alcoholics Anonymous call this "rock bottom," the point in their lives when they felt they were at their lowest. For some addicts, rock bottom may mean a dramatic drop in their overall quality of life; while for others, it could mean experiencing a series of more mild negative consequences of their addiction—a few drops too many in a cup that is already full. Many addicts find their rock bottom in an eye-opening event or occurrence that finally convinces them that they have a problem and need to get professional help.

Rock bottom can be much lower for some addicts than it is for others. Your breaking point might come when you see the look in your child's eyes when you forget to pick them up from day care because you've been gambling. Or it may come in the form of your second wife finally deciding to divorce you because of your sex addiction. Under the influence of distorted thought patterns caused by neurotransmitters that make you feel good, and supported by your devoted enablers, you may have felt you were the master of the universe, able to get away with anything. In the process of becoming addicted, driven by your cravings, you crossed many a line—but now, you've crossed one too many. Now that you've hit rock bottom, the consequences of your behavior are catching up with you.

"To cease smoking is the easiest thing I ever did. I ought to know because I've done it a thousand times!" This famous phrase, which has been attributed to Mark Twain,[99] reflects the fact that the difficulty in "quitting" any addiction is not in making the decision to stop engaging in an addictive behavior, but rather in sticking to that decision when things become difficult and the cravings and withdrawal symptoms start wrenching at your gut. Then denial sets in, tempting you to draw the line a little further away. If the consequences of their addictive behaviors are grave enough, addicts will be able to keep their promise to quit for days, weeks, or even months. Indeed, before making their final decision to quit, most addicts have already stopped for some time, and used this success as proof they were actually not addicted. But the reality of addiction is this: *a recovering addict can make a thousand good decisions, but it only*

---

[99] Quoteresearch, "It's Easy to Quit Smoking. I've Done It a Thousand Times," Quote Investigator, Quote Investigator, September 19, 2012, https://quoteinvestigator.com/2012/09/19/easy-quit-smoking.

takes one wrong decision to ruin everything.

Ceasing to abuse substances or behaviors may seem impossible—but in reality, that's the easy part. However, even successfully doing so *doesn't mean you've been cured of addiction.* Most people who decide to stop acting out—even addicts— can do so for extended periods provided their resolve is strong enough and their circumstances favorable. But life is long, and presents many challenges. *The real challenge is to endure when times get tough.* Sooner or later, something always happens that might prompt the vicious addictive system to start spinning again, if you are not careful. It's like living on a minefield and trying not to set off the bombs. The only sure way out of trouble is to remove the hidden mines—which is done neither quickly nor easily. After a while—usually six months to a year into recovery—an addict's external environment often starts changing for the better, and the pressure of the negative consequences of their previous behaviors wears off. That's when you will need an inner source of motivation to help you maintain your willpower. You will need to embrace the truth that you alone are worth the trouble of changing your life for the better and making it into what you want it to be.

Often, it is difficult for a person with low self-esteem—as addicts are by definition—to put so much effort into self-improvement. They feel they're not worth it. This is why **spiritual changes** are needed. Whether you believe in a god, in the wisdom of nature, or another system that helps you make sense of this world, your beliefs—including a foundational belief in your own inherent and innate goodness, as you were originally created to be—must be the source of your strength to fight your cravings and stay on track—because you *are* worth it. And when you resist the temptation, you will be proud to have endured—which in turn will boost your feelings of self-respect, and further motivate you to continue your recovery.

Ultimately, personal spiritual transformation is at the heart of change for the better—and as such, it is the essence of recovery, which (don't forget!) necessitates the reversal of fundamental beliefs based in insecure attachment patterns formed in childhood. For a child, their father should be a figure who guarantees safety. To reforge a healthy, secure attachment style, the adult, then, must look to a "Father in Heaven" or similar higher power—a power greater than oneself—as the authority that can guarantee all will be well.

The expressions **Higher Power** and **Power Greater Than Ourselves** were coined by Alcoholics Anonymous and similar recovery groups that allow religious people and nonbelievers to benefit from their healing principles. This reflects the beliefs of AA cofounder Bill Wilson, who underwent a dramatic spiritual experience while in the depths of his addiction—an experience that led him to believe reliance on a higher power is essential to recovery. In his own words:[100]

"My depression deepened unbearably and, finally, it seemed to me as though I were at the bottom of the pit. I still gagged badly on the notion of a Power greater than myself, but finally, just for the moment, the last vestige of my proud obstinacy was crushed. All at once I found myself crying out, 'If there is a God, let Him show Himself! I am ready to do anything, anything!'

Suddenly the room lit up with a great white light. I was caught up into an ecstasy which there are no words to describe. It seemed to me, in the mind's eye, that I was on a mountain and that a wind not of air but of spirit was blowing. And then it burst upon me that I was a free man. Slowly the ecstasy subsided. I lay on the bed, but now for a time I was in another world, a new world of consciousness. All about me and through me there was a wonderful feeling of Presence, and I thought to myself, 'So this is the God of the preachers!' A great peace stole over me and I thought, 'No matter how wrong things seem to be, they are still all right. Things are all right with God and His world.'"

While Bill W. hoped others would come to the same conclusion that there exists a Higher Power that can be summoned to help in one's recovery, he wanted to leave the door to recovery wide open to all, "regardless of belief or lack of belief." Ultimately, it is left up to the individual to decide how

---

[100] Alcoholics Anonymous World Services, *Alcoholics Anonymous Comes of Age: A Brief History* (New York: Alcoholics Anonymous World Services, 1957), 64.

they wish to define this power—for it is important that their definition be personal and powerful, so as to give them the greatest opportunity for success.

You certainly don't need an experience like Bill's to end your addiction—but if one happens to you, don't fear that you may be losing your mind. Our minds are able to deal in more than just rationality, and we have certain capacities that we may not be aware of unless in extreme danger. Recovery, trauma, and extreme situations shatter our minds to the core, and may bring out things we never knew were part of us. I've heard about such experiences many times from my clients, and have experienced some myself. The results of these "divine interventions" were always helpful—so don't fight them.

23.b. *Time and Energy for the Recovery Work*

Addiction does not happen overnight—and it will not disappear overnight, either. Recovery is a long process, as the body and brain, like everything in nature, take time to heal.

How long does it take for the brain to heal?

The science related to understanding how the brain recovers is relatively new: not so long ago, it was thought that the brain does not change at all after reaching maturity. We now know that is not the case. Over the course of my more than thirty years of work in an institution for rehabilitation, I saw evidence of this with my own eyes in patients who were admitted after having had a stroke—a temporary interruption in blood flow to the brain that causes massive damage. When they were first admitted, these patients were unable to speak, walk, or move their arms. After a couple of months, they regained some of these abilities; and after a year or so, they were often very nearly back to normal, though some residual changes could be observed. Their progress clearly showed that their brains underwent very intensive repair in the first year following their strokes.

In recovery from addiction, you can expect rapid improvement in your thinking and reasoning abilities within the first year of sobriety, and some additional progress during the next two or three years. (The research into the effects of recovery on addicts was originally done on alcoholics, but I can confirm this timeline of recovery with my own experience of recovery from codependence, as well as my clients' experiences.) The first three months are troublesome, full of intense emotions and hardship; but a newfound belief in your ability to abstain and in the support of the recovery program will help you through. After a year of sobriety, your thought processes will have changed. Your thoughts will seem much brighter and clearer, as if you had stepped out of a fog. And after that, you will continue to improve, though at a slower pace.

When I began working with people in recovery from behavioral addictions, my colleagues and I thought different therapy or peer support groups should exist for various behavioral addictions: there should be a group for gamblers, one for food addicts, one for codependents, and so on. However, in my case, I simply didn't have enough clients to create so many different groups, so I had to adapt and put all of them together in one group. It proved to be a great idea: not only did they thrive in such a "generic"[101] group, they also found that—once they mastered sobriety—their recovery needs and experiences were comparable.

Putting them all into the same group had another beneficial effect. Most people actually experience more than one behavioral addiction at a time. They may, for example, oscillate between overeating and sex addiction; and beneath it all, there may be a hidden relationship addiction. Abstaining only from the behaviors inherent to the sex addiction would leave all the repressed sexual energy to be poured into the relationship addiction and overeating. The behaviors associated with those addictions would then escalate, and the recovery process would not even truly begin. To cover all these addictions as necessary in separate groups would mean going to three different meetings—but in my "generic" group, all three behaviors would be addressed, and healing could begin.

Ultimately, my experience with this group showed me recovery needs to start with a thorough analysis of all the be-

---

[101] In recovery language, meaning *nonspecific*.

haviors that contribute to a person's addiction cycles, followed by the development of a plan for abstinence. We have already created the list of behaviors from which you need to abstain in Exercise 8 on page 284.

When is it safe for a recovering addict to "use" again?

This is the question everyone seems to ask. If you ask me, the answer is *never*! What the brain learns well enough for it to become automatic is never completely forgotten. The only thing we can do to "forget" the experience of addiction is *never to walk that path again*—not even in your imagination, and if possible, not even in your dreams. Because each time you walk it, your brain remembers it, and it feels like you never stopped.

Do you doubt it? If so, try to imagine how long it would take you to completely forget how to drive a car, dance, or do something else one learns well enough to do it automatically. Even after years of not driving, once you got inside a car and felt the steering wheel in your hands, it would only take you a couple of minutes to remember everything about how to drive it. Addiction, too, is a learned behavior that has become automatic after years of use. *Don't push it!* In the face of such a powerful automatic response, it's better to be on the safe side, and avoid engaging in the behavior altogether.

The idea of lifelong sobriety may be too much for an addict, and may contradict the assertion that addicts can't promise to stop forever. That is why it is helpful to introduce the concept of "*taking one day at a time.*" If a goal like lifelong sobriety seems too difficult to achieve, break it up into more achievable components. You may not be able to promise to avoid a behavior forever, but you can promise to avoid it for today. And tomorrow, you can make the same promise again.

23.c. *Abstinence and Sobriety*

For a person to recover from addiction, abstinence and sobriety are necessary. When addicts stop using addictive substances and behaviors, their brains will, in time, recover; and their neurotransmitters will revert to their "default settings," allowing them to feel pleasure and reward in ordinary, everyday situations.

However, one should not confuse recovery with abstinence from a drug or behavior. **Abstinence** is only a prerequisite of recovery—not its final goal. If a person is abstinent, it means they are, at that moment, "clean," or free of the drugs, alcohol, or behaviors that defined their addiction. **Recovery**, however, is the entire process of change, restoring the addict's body-mind-soul-relationship system to what it would have been if not for the addiction. Considering the amount of time and effort that must be given to do the work to achieve that, the outcome can be even better than the addict's state before the addiction began.

Sobriety includes abstinence, but encompasses much more than just ceasing to drink or to abuse drugs. We have learned that the brain can achieve a "high" through various substances and behaviors. To be sober means to be without this influence. It is essential to understand that. You may not be an alcoholic, but "just" a codependent; however, if you get drunk, you won't be sober, and the next thing you'll do is dial your ex-partner's number and ask him to take you back! So, as an addict, you need to abstain not only from your "drug or behavior of choice" (for help identifying these, see Exercise 1 on page 23 and Exercise 8 on page 284), but also from *other drugs that can change your brain function*, as well as from the ***triggers*** *that might set the addictive system into motion*, like stress or intense emotion. To live a sober life, you need to change your life in a way that guarantees you can avoid all these challenges.

That being said, it seems much easier for people with chemical addictions to set safe boundaries than it is for people with behavioral addictions to do so. Recovering alcoholics know they mustn't touch alcohol or other mind-altering substances, and that they must avoid triggers like stress and bars—and that's it. But someone with a food addiction *can't* stop eating altogether, so they must define their own personal boundaries when it comes to their emotional eating. Recovering behavioral addicts of various kinds will often be surrounded by people eating sweets, watching porn, gambling, and staying in unhealthy relationships, and these people will all tell the recovering addict this behavior is normal. Consider this, however: it is thought of as normal for most adults to drink alcohol in moderate quantities, too—but not for a recovering alcoholic. For them, drinking any amount of alcohol, even in moderation, is simply not safe. As a recovering behavioral addict, you have to accept responsibility for your own recovery and create boundaries around activities people typically consider normal, just to stay safe—even at the cost of being excluded from some fun social events. And to do that over the long period of recovery—and even over an entire lifetime—takes determination, and a strong will.

Slips and relapses

If you engage in a forbidden behavior on one occasion after a period of sobriety, this is a **slip**. It's not good, but it's not necessarily a disaster. But if you continue to repeat that behavior until you completely lose control and end up back in the addiction cycle, unable to stop engaging in the behavior, this is a **relapse**. By definition, addiction involves slips and relapses, and it's naïve to think you won't experience them. This is what the first of the twelve steps of recovery teaches: *don't be arrogant and believe that this can't happen to you!* It's better to be prepared for the worst, while hoping for the best.

To prepare for a sudden "attack" in which you find yourself unable to stop engaging in an addictive behavior—after all, it's a slippery slope, they say!—you have to understand the way your addictive system works. In Exercise 6, on page 101, we identified the elements of your addiction cycle. Recheck the exercise to prepare yourself so you know in advance when the ball starts rolling. As we know, this cycle begins long before you actually start acting out and abusing substances or engaging in certain behaviors. It may start with something someone says, the loss of something important to you, or just exhaustion and stress creeping in after long hours at work. Eventually, however, your willpower will fail, and you'll lose sight of your recovery goals. You'll feel vulnerable and entitled to comfort yourself in the way that has worked well so many times. You may even feel hostility toward the people helping you remain abstinent, whom you may perceive as not allowing you to ease your pain. Then the cravings will set in, and before you know it, you'll succumb. *Just a little bit!* you may think—but all too soon, you reach the point of no return. You go right back down the roller coaster, and nothing can stop you.

If you're familiar with how your addiction works, you can catch the reins and resume command before you reach this point. But after that, if you haven't stopped, you'll go into a full-blown relapse.

To combat a crisis of this sort, it's good to keep items that remind you of your decision to recover nearby at all times. Place a childhood photo of yourself; a list of your friends', recovery buddies', group mentor's, or therapist's telephone numbers; a card featuring a recovery slogan or a positive affirmation; and a letter from your healthy self to your "inner addict" into a box. Recovering addicts call this box and its contents your "First Aid Kit," and you should keep it somewhere you can easily access it in an emergency.

Withdrawal

Withdrawal is the physical and mental reaction addicts experience when they abruptly stop using addictive substances or engaging in addictive behaviors. It is an extremely uncomfortable feeling of anxiety and excitement, and it's a consequence of the changes in the levels of neurotransmitters present in the brain.

The body has many mechanisms that maintain levels of chemicals and other parameters, like temperature, for example, within certain boundaries. When something changes these parameters, we feel unease, which can escalate to pain and other negative feelings. These feelings act like flashing red lights that signal something has gone wrong. When addicts stop particular behaviors or quit using addictive substances, the resulting lack of dopamine produces an intense, unpleasant withdrawal experience. Addicts in withdrawal start trembling, shivering, itching, and sweating; feel uneasy, fatigued, tense, and irritable; think obsessively about their "drug" or behavior of choice; and experience insomnia, headaches, disorders of sexual drive, physical pain, suppressed or exaggerated appetite, nausea, increased heart rate, breathing problems, depression, anxiety, and even flu-like symptoms. And make no mistake: the withdrawal symptoms that come with abstention from the behaviors associated with codependency and "love" or sex addiction can be as bad as the symptoms of withdrawal that come with abstention from drugs. They may even be worse, because during withdrawal, relationship addicts psychologically reexperience all the losses they felt in their childhoods.

But there is one important thing to keep in mind: withdrawal symptoms are *temporary*. If you don't give in to them or relapse, after a while, they subside. Although complete abstinence can be extremely difficult or even impossible to achieve in the case of some behavioral addictions, such as food addiction, in most cases, addicts typically find it works best. They find moderate use, even to quell terrible withdrawal symptoms, is far riskier and more detrimental to the process of recovery than the temporary withdrawal symptoms they suffer under complete abstinence.

Cravings

As we already explained in the chapter about problems at the level of the brain, an addictive craving is an intense desire for something—a desire so sharp, you feel your very survival depends on fulfilling it. For example, you may have just finished a delicious lunch filled with healthy macro- and micronutrients. But even though you're full, you still crave something sweet for dessert. This craving is obviously not a result of hunger, but rather your brain calling for something that will release dopamine into your reward system, seeking comfort and a sweet taste. This craving won't go away if you have some more chicken—and once ignited, this flashing red light in your brain leads you to obsess over finding something sweet to put in your mouth.

Addicts have figured out that turning away from these cravings within three seconds is a good way to get rid of them without succumbing to them.[102] Usually, they choose to turn

---

[102] "S.L.A.A. Terminology." slaadfw.org, accessed December 27, 2022, http://www.slaadfw.org/terminology.html.

these sorts of thoughts over to their Higher Power, asking it to please remove the unwanted thought. In other words, the simple act of thinking about something else, even for a moment, usually helps—sometimes only for a short while, but with practice, for an increasingly long time.

Daria's Story

Daria, 34, in recovery for codependency after having been married to a drug addict, describes her cravings and withdrawal symptoms:

My husband had a business trip last week, and he told me that he was coming back on Thursday, but today is Friday and there's no sign of him. His phone is dead. I've left a hundred messages. I want to call the police or the hospital to see if there's been an accident, but he has strictly forbidden me to contact the police because he said this would just give them a reason to investigate his business. I called his friends, and they couldn't tell me anything. I'm afraid of my own thoughts. I would rather see him dead than with another woman. We've played this game so many times, and I always fall for the same promises. He promised not to take drugs, and I believed him, but now all the newfound hope for our relationship is going down the drain, leaving me alone, powerless, and as angry as hell. . . .

I don't know what's happening to me. I feel such anxiety and despair, but most of all, there is this aggression, and I don't know where it comes from. I'm afraid of these feelings. I want to explode and act out, but I know I shouldn't. But it would make me feel better, for I could get rid of the burden I'm carrying; the burden—I don't even know what is. I feel physical pain in my chest, and I can't breathe. I don't know what I'm angry at, or why I'm so angry; I just want it to stop. I want to run away. I'm terrified of seeing my daughter, knowing she feels my pain, seeing her walk on eggshells around me. I don't even recognize myself anymore. I'm terrified of the fact that I've been fighting this same thing for five years and that I've spent most of my time during these five

years wondering if he's going to come home or not, if he'll re-
lapse and leave us, if he's with someone else, and whether he
actually loves me or is just using me.

23.d. *Relationships and Support*

Relationships are important for everyone—even for those who
avoid them and claim they can live on their own. They are the
invisible, yet very real, fabric that glues all of us together. They
define who we are and our roles in the grand scheme of things.
We're in different relationships with our family and friends,
our coworkers and neighbors, our fellow citizens, and—as citizens of the Earth—with all people. But that's not all. We're
in relationship with every living being, having the capacity to
destroy their habitat and cause their extinction. Maybe you believe that you're in a relationship with the Power Greater Than
Ourselves, and you call it Love. Relationships are important
for everything. For recovery, too!

Recall that when we discussed the problems addiction creates at the family level (Chapter 10), we said addiction is an
attachment disorder. Then we discussed the attachment styles,
arguing that people who have learned it's unsafe to attach to
their families of origin keep looking for love in the wrong places when they grow up, finding violence and betrayal instead.
But they still think it's love, even though these relationships
don't have many positive features. They're stuck with the people who cause them pain, but they are too afraid to leave, so
they choose to numb the pain of betrayal by indulging in drugs
or behaviors that change their awareness.

Relationship styles are extremely basic, in addition to being
one of the first things we ever learn—so changing yours from
one that lends itself to toxic shame and addiction to a healthier
one that will enable you to progress and grow means metaphor-
ically turning the foundation of your entire belief system upside
down. Not an easy task, for sure! You know precisely what you
should do—but the whole time, alarm bells are ringing inside
your head, warning you that you're heading in the wrong direction. That it's unsafe to trust people. That you're vulnerable and

exposed. That you're going to be abandoned, which is the same as death. Yes—for an infant, it certainly is. But now you're an adult, and you should be able to choose freely what you want to change about your relationship with the world.

You can't accomplish that alone. You need a firm anchor, a safe connection to the people who have made these changes themselves and know exactly how it feels to do so, but who remain firm in the belief that people are good, that the world *can* be a safe place, and that love conquers fear.

Twelve-step groups, principles, and community

The story of the founding of Alcoholics Anonymous is a perfect example of the power of healing relationships.

It began eighty years ago, when the organization's two legendary founders, Bill W.[103] and Dr. Bob[104]—both longstanding alcoholics—first met to help each other stay sober through the night. They found that together, they could accomplish what each had unsuccessfully attempted many times before. This idea, along with adherence to some spiritual concepts, led to the foundation of Alcoholics Anonymous, the first massively successful addiction recovery program. Soon, alcoholics and their wives and children heard about their success and wanted to participate. To organize their program for their new followers, Bill wrote out twelve steps for recovery. Though they may sound archaic and odd at first, they convey the essential ideas of the process of recovery. Out of respect for the text that has helped millions of people recover, and still works after eighty years, I have left the text as it was first conceived by Bill W., in half an hour on a feverish night when he was working on the first draft of the famous Big Book of Alcoholics Anonymous. These are the **original twelve steps of recovery,** as published by Alcoholics Anonymous:[105]

---

[103] William Griffith Wilson, also known as Bill Wilson or Bill W., was the co-founder of Alcoholics Anonymous.

[104] Robert Holbrook Smith, also known as Dr. Bob, was an American physician and surgeon who cofounded Alcoholics Anonymous.

[105] "The Twelve Steps," aa.org, General Service Office (GSO) of Alcoholics Anonymous, 2023, https://www.aa.org/assets/en_US/smf-121_en.pdf.

1. We admitted we were powerless over alcohol—that our lives had become unmanageable.

2. Came to believe that a Power greater than ourselves could restore us to sanity.

3. Made a decision to turn our will and our lives over to the care and direction of God *as we understood Him.*

4. Made a searching and fearless moral inventory of ourselves.

5. Admitted to God, to ourselves, and to another human being the exact nature of our wrongs.

6. Were entirely ready to have God remove all these defects of character.

7. Humbly asked Him to remove our shortcomings.

8. Made a list of all persons we had harmed, and became willing to make amends to them all.

9. Made direct amends to such people wherever possible, except when to do so would injure them or others.

10. Continued to take personal inventory[,] and when we were wrong[,] promptly admitted it.

11. Sought through prayer and meditation to improve our conscious contact with God *as we understood Him,* praying only for knowledge of His will for us and the power to carry that out.

12. Having had a spiritual awakening as the result of these Steps, we tried to carry this message to alcoholics, and to practice these principles in all our affairs.

Today, Alcoholics Anonymous is the largest recovery community in existence, claiming an estimated 2.1 million members worldwide, including 1.3 million US residents; its recovery principles have provided the foundation for twelve-step groups for other behavioral addictions not affiliated with the main organization. These spin-off groups exist in most major cities throughout the world, and though they are not explicitly endorsed by Alcoholics Anonymous World Services (AAWS), which oversees the organization's copyrights, AAWS does grant them permission to use the twelve steps—with the words "alcohol" and "alcoholics" exchanged with the name of the spin-off group's focus substance or behavior.

Twelve-step groups traditionally operate entirely on their own, outside the jurisdiction of official medical organizations. This has caused some controversy, and occasionally, even competition between these groups and official medical treatment programs. While I'm not going to enter this debate, I will say that the mere fact that so many people successfully recover by adhering to these principles makes them deserving of respect. People differ, and should have various recovery programs to choose from. Furthermore, twelve-step groups' only purpose is to help addicts stay sober and support them for the rest of their lives. No money is collected, and no business funds them, so no profit or power is gained from the movement, and no conflict of interest can be expected.

That being said, let me stress that twelve-step groups are **peer support groups**. Some people, if not most, will need **therapeutic intervention** at some stage of their recovery in addition to a support group. Most therapists, including myself, encourage their clients to go to twelve-step meetings as well as therapy. We know working with clients is much easier when they are stable and supported by their peers in these organizations.

Marital and family problems

Our most important relationships are those we have with our family members, and it is in the family that we act out everything we believe love is or should be. There, we are open and vulnerable to hurt, betrayal, and abandonment. And yet, when things go wrong, we are strongly motivated to stay and hope for better.

Addicts and codependents are a "match made in heaven"—

both needy, with low self-esteem, and desperately searching for a safe haven and secure attachment. When these people meet, they subconsciously recognize each other's neediness and believe the fallacy that "the power of my love will heal their wound, and then they'll never let me go!" After years of trying and failing, their enchantment with each other turns into a curse and a self-fulfilling prophecy. They stop trusting and realize their worst fears of being neglected and abandoned have come true. They have failed each other so many times, and their childhood wounds are wide open. They may come to believe that the only way out is through separation and divorce. But if they don't understand what has befallen them, they may repeat their mistakes in their next relationships.

The destiny of love relationships affected by addiction depends on whether it's possible to restore trust and respect between the couple or not. This is what marriage and family counselors try to do. But it's hard. After all, how can you trust someone who has let you down so many times? Even if you try to substitute control for trust, living with an addict may not get any easier. After all, how much proof of a partner's reliability does someone need before they can start trusting again? And like Daria from the previous chapter, will you not suddenly fall into the bottomless pit of despair again if one day your partner doesn't show up at the expected time?

Children of addicts need and deserve help for their own problems, but their struggles often go unnoticed unless they start acting out themselves. We have discussed this in Chapter 10: Problems at the Level of the Family; as well as Chapter 18.c: Codependence and Addiction to Destructive Relationships.

23.e. *Triggers and Stress Management*

Triggers, in "recovery jargon," are the cues, catalysts, and re-minders of past acting out. If you are an addict, certain situations, people, and behaviors may be dangerous and harmful triggers for you, prompting addictive behavior that can lead to a relapse, induce cravings, or threaten your moral attitude and jumpstart the addiction cycle.

To protect your sobriety, you need to set proper boundaries when it comes to these triggers. However, the boundaries nonaddicts consider "normal" are not safe enough for you. For addicts, triggers are like allergies: healthy people can eat peanuts as much as they want, but for someone with a peanut allergy, it's dangerous even to put a peanut-tainted spoon in their mouth. Similarly, most people drink alcohol in small quantities from time to time, but they don't get drunk, because they know when they need to stop to avoid getting drunk. *For an alcoholic, however, no amount of alcohol is safe to consume, because their brain will immediately remember the old addictive shortcuts, and they won't be able to stop in time.* Many people have had ideas about teaching alcoholics to drink in moderation—I know of many failures, and no successes. Since alcohol is not necessary for life and is "needed" only by alcoholics, I see such attempts as a form of addictive denial.

To determine what constitutes a trigger, we must examine our "mental world maps," which we discussed in Chapter 16, when we explained *addictions to risk, money, and work.* In our minds, words' meanings are interconnected. Each concept is connected to several other concepts, forming a sort of network. If you let your mind drift freely along these networks, the stream of thoughts that results can take you quite far from your original ideas. If you think of something as important to you as the source of an addict's addiction is to them, you could no doubt identify a lot of apparently harmless words connected with that concept. The same goes for memories of past events. They're also interconnected, and bound together with memories of smells, music that was playing at the time, physical feelings, and so on.

IMAGE 7: The network of meanings in a gambler's mind

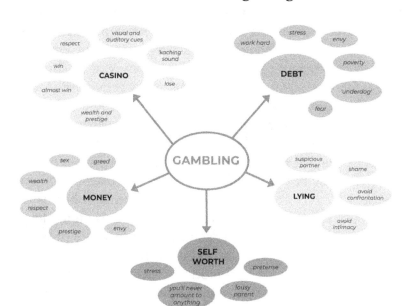

Experiences of past substance use or acting out behaviors are engraved in an addict's memory alongside feelings of pleasure. *When part of this network is activated, the whole network linked to it will be triggered.* You may merely pass the street that houses your favorite bar, or hear some music about codependent "love"—and the next thing you know, you won't be able to think of anything else, leading to intense cravings to repeat the addictive behavior and probably ending with you drinking or dialing his number. So, anything that may evoke such a response needs to be avoided.

How long do you need to take care to avoid your triggers?

The experience for which many an addict has paid dearly is that this "hypersensitivity" never ends. This part of the addictive system is never wholly deactivated. When triggered, you'll feel the old cravings as if no time at all has passed. Even after decades of sobriety, it takes only one drink or one moment of yielding to these addictive cravings—and before you know it, you're back at the beginning.

Stress

Stress is the sensation of strain and pressure we feel when confronted by something threatening, whether in our environment or in our own thoughts and feelings. The body responds to stress by activating its systems for alertness and reacting to danger. This can be positive, allowing us to better rise to the challenges we face. For example, feeling mild stress before an exam or public appearance can actually help us perform better. But some people may feel they're not ready to cope with these challenges, and for them, this stress may be negative. If this negative stress becomes chronic, leaving the person without enough time to recover between stressful events, it begins to have a negative influence on the body. If this goes on too long and exceeds the body's coping ability, the individual's physical and psychological health may begin to suffer.

Stress-related health conditions include memory and sleep problems, depression, skin conditions, high blood pressure, obesity, heart disease, digestive issues, and autoimmune diseases like thyroid dysfunction. Additionally, high levels of stress are common triggers of relapse in *all* addictions! The changes one experiences while under pressure tamper with the same neurotransmitters that govern addiction. Yes, some people behave like they're *addicted to stress!* People who go bungee jumping or parachuting or who drive dangerously to make themselves "more alive" are actually behaving in ways that make their bodies release adrenaline. Many of them are even proud of being "adrenaline junkies." We covered that in the chapter about addiction to risk. Other people seek out highly volatile or dangerous relationships to achieve the same effect, claiming they feel no attraction to safer candidates. "No adrenaline, no chemistry!" they sometimes say.

To avoid relapsing, you must lead a life as free of stressors as possible. Of course, it's unlikely your life will ever be entirely stress-free—but this makes it all the more important for you to keep your stress under control and take the time to stay sober, healthy, productive, and happy.

Exercise 11: Your list of triggers and stressors

To be on the safe side and attempt to stave off potential re-lapses, you will need to set your own personal boundaries for dealing with the triggers and stress.[106] For example, to avoid triggering their addiction, food addicts may find they mustn't keep any sweets in the fridge, go food shopping without a list, read recipes, or cook for others.

List the boundaries you need to respect to guard against triggers and relapses. Be thorough and state the facts, making sure to include guards against potential triggers like working excessively, not getting enough sleep, and so on.

Example: To avoid triggering my addiction to food, I will:

- *never go shopping when hungry*

- *buy only items on the list*

- *avoid the sweets section*

- *empty the fridge of anything off-limits*

My boundaries with triggers and stressors:

....

....

....

....

....

---

[106] However, as you complete this exercise, it's still good to compare notes with others who have been successful in long-term recovery.

....

....

....

....

....

....

List your thoughts while working on this exercise:

....

....

Trauma Work

In Greek, the word **trauma** means "wound." In English, as we've previously noted, this word is commonly used to describe an *event that causes so much distress, a person can no longer cope with it—which results in that person experiencing an overwhelming amount of stress.* The expression is also used to describe the physical and emotional consequences that a person undergoes due to such an event. **Physical trauma** is an injury, such as a wound, resulting from an accident or attack. In contrast, **psychological** or **emotional trauma** describes distressing changes in the mind of the person who has been traumatized. Trauma may result from a single distressing experience, or from recurring instances of emotional overwhelm that can be precipitated over weeks, years, or even decades. Finally, in addition to short-term consequences like stress, pain, and emotional distress, trauma can also lead to serious long-term consequences.

Not all, but a great majority of people who have problems with addiction also suffer from the negative long-term consequences of trauma. They are not necessarily aware of this at the beginning of recovery—but when they have remained sober for some months or a year, they may start remembering painful situations they lived through, most often in their early childhoods. Although some people blame therapists for "putting these ideas into their clients' minds," this happens spontaneously. It's logical: Many times, we have said addictions are born from a person's attempts to numb themselves to negative emotion or escape a painful reality. When addicts stop using numbing substances or engaging in addictive behaviors to suppress their pain, the repressed feelings return to the surface, bringing with them the whole memory network of traumatic events that caused them. This is good because it's necessary for recovery. Addicts *drink, use addictive substances,* or *act out* to *avoid feeling the emotions connected to trauma.* To recover from their addictions, they need to accept that they have to stop trying to forget. They need to remember.

But remembering is also very stressful. **Traumatic memory** is different from ordinary memory—it is raw, unprocessed, and disconnected from other memories (not feelings!). Often remembering a traumatic memory feels more like reexperiencing it than recalling a memory. To fully recover from addiction, you must reprocess and integrate these rediscovered raw memories into the narrative of your life. To do this, you will likely need the help of a therapist. This is *not* a do-it-yourself job—especially if the trauma was severe, or if you were very young when it happened.

Because traumatic memories that spontaneously reemerge are a great source of stress, they are a potential threat to your sobriety. So are other sources of great emotional turmoil, like a divorce or the breakup of a significant relationship. As you enter recovery, it becomes your job to control your memories of trauma and the sources of stress to which you are exposed until you are ready and able to process them with a therapist. For this reason, you need to take your potential past trauma into account even before you may be ready to deal with it.

To do that, you need to lead a healthy life across the physical, emotional, relational, and spiritual dimensions of human existence. The personalized plan you will create will help you stay healthy and weather some of the crises you can expect in the future, when traumatic memories emerge and triggers present themselves in spite of your best efforts to create boundaries. The plan consists of many activities—indeed, as many as possible—and needs to be reasonable, well-designed, and include many healthy behaviors to replace your bad, addictive habits.

Most recovering addicts have some better days when they make healthier decisions. But as time goes by and they start forgetting the troubles that led them to want to recover and make these good decisions, they begin to drop the healthy habits one by one. Having a concrete plan will hold you accountable for staying on track.

For any addict who wants to stay in recovery, a healthy personalized recovery plan is necessary—for the rest of their life!

Grace's Story

See how my client Grace, 48, in therapy for codependency, addiction to food (overeating), and addiction to work, successfully weathered a crisis with the help of the information she learned in my recovery program:

> *This Friday, my boss told me they plan to add six more hours to my already overburdened weekly schedule. Supposedly they cannot find another solution to the problem. I was so shocked, I wasn't even able to negotiate, so I just waited, stunned, for the work to come my way. I was waiting for the boss to realize this simply couldn't work, and fix it. Seriously! Is she my "mother," and should she take care of her "child"? Of course not! The "child" would have to take care of its "mother" and sacrifice herself in the process. But I'm*

*done putting myself last. I'm going to take care of myself!
I'll go to the union representative if I have to. I know my
body can't handle any more of this. I've told her I already
have a thyroid condition. Enough is enough!*

*My feelings were everything from anger and power-
lessness to sorrow and rage. No, I will not agonize in advance! I wanted to cry, but I couldn't. I kept myself busy doing housework so I wouldn't have to think about it. When
my husband came home at midnight, he advised me to let
it out by crying, but I couldn't. I only slept a couple of hours,
and woke up feeling severe pain in my back. I went for a
walk, and it was a bit better. Then I decided to go to the
gym, although I wasn't feeling great and had no energy or
motivation to work out.*

*I started with the punching bag. It felt so good! I vi-
sualized my boss, and I wanted to vent all the rage I felt
for her. But after a moment, she was replaced by the image
of my father. In an instant, I was crying like there was
no tomorrow. I was hitting the bag from the deepest part
of my soul. My anger went from my body to the bag and
was replaced by overwhelming sorrow. I was mourning the
father I never had. The father who would take care of me
and create a strong and self-conscious me. I would respect
myself. I would be really strong, not out of the need to survive, but from taking care of myself. He would always take
care of me, be there for me. He would hug me, and I would
feel his strong, deep love and acceptance. For him, I would
be the best and his favorite. I would be the way he wanted
me to be. Something that would bring fulfillment to his life.
He would accept me entirely. When I would bring home
my future husband, he would accept him as one of his own
family. My children would be his favorite grandchildren.
He would accept and love them dearly. He would want to
be in their company. He would be THE FATHER.*

*My body was tense right down to its very essence. I just
wanted to move and take it out on, on, on . . . something.
I was pounding without stopping and crying, crying, and*

crying even more. Tears were flowing and I was sobbing out loud. I wanted to drag myself into a corner, feeling it was more than I could stand. But then I would vanish and disappear from this world. So I kept pounding . . . with all my might! Needless to say, I can still feel the consequences. My entire body aches. But in essence, it's a good feeling. I can feel myself. This is ME!

In the beginning, I felt shame for crying in front of all those people, but only for a moment. Then it didn't matter anymore. I couldn't be bothered with feeling shame on top of everything else. I was just pounding, pounding. A friend from my support group encouraged me to keep going, to get to the bottom of it. I felt I was far back in the past. It felt good, and everyone accepted me. No one thought I was weird. It was clear to everyone that it was completely normal, even good, that I was letting it out. I felt at home. The coach encouraged me to accept my sorrow as if it were completely normal. Oh, but it is normal! Why should I have to hide it? This can't be wrong or shameful. It's just that the pain has to be released!

And oh, how it got released! Later, I was absolutely exhausted, as if I had nothing left inside. I was trembling from the cold and from exhaustion. I took a hot shower, wrapped myself in a bathrobe and made some tea, and just sat there. I told my husband everything. I wasn't in a hurry, although everything was waiting for me. It was time just for me. I am important! I knew my body was overburdened, but I didn't even feel it. All I felt was the sweat pouring off me. I didn't even feel my own body. I was scared. How could I have not felt that? I have to take care of my body. It's important. How new this is to me! All the things I have ever done to my body and never felt it! I just kept on and on, more and more . . .

The group meeting in the evening felt really good. They saw me at the gym and asked me how I felt. Now I was calm enough to talk about my feelings. I felt accepted—in everything, without judgment or them pitying me. They cared. And understood. Oh, how good it feels. On my evening walk, I felt my posture was different. I was taller, my spine was upright, and I felt stronger in the core. I walked differently. I really did release a heavy burden, and made some room—for me!

I've decided not to give in. I'll go to my boss and quite calmly explain that her plan won't work. I won't listen to her trying to coerce me into backing down by explaining that it's the only way. They need to find another way, not at the expense of my health. I know my rights, and I value myself too much to give in. I'll be calm and dignified. I'll take care of myself.

24

Your Personalized Recovery Program

As a medical doctor with four decades of experience in rehabilitation, a psychotherapist who has worked in recovery from
behavioral addictions for thirty years, and a recovering codependent who has maintained sobriety for thirty-five years, I
can help you create your own personalized recovery program
out of whatever resources are available to you. I guarantee it
will work if you work it![107]

Throughout this book, you have found several suggested
methods that may help you recover. But these are only measures
and exercises to help you weather a crisis. They're not enough
to keep you safe and help you change long-term. *Change is a
process that takes time and effort, not just a decision that "from now
on, things will be different."*

For change to occur, a long-term recovery program is necessary. A carefully developed plan will help you endure the bad
times when they inevitably come, giving you a structure to adhere to when your willpower begins to fail you. Like Ulysses,
who asked his friends to tie him to the mast to prevent him
from following the deadly songs of the Sirens into the ocean,
you must find something firm to anchor yourself in times of
crisis. This program is something solid to which to tie yourself!
This is the difference between good advice and real help, and the

---

[107] "It works if you work it!" is a recovery slogan in AA groups.

difference between failure and success: the presence of something to hold onto when you begin to falter.

There are many different **commercial recovery programs** available to choose from. But not everyone will have the time to abandon their regular lives and go on a retreat for a month— or the money to afford such a program. And even if you did, after the program ended, your problems wouldn't magically be gone—so you'd still need to take responsibility and make sure your recovery needs were met. The program I propose in this book will consider everything commercial recovery programs offer, but *you'll be in charge* of finding the right professionals within your own reach and organizing them into a network to fulfill your needs. You alone can take on the responsibility to create the circumstances necessary for your success. There'll be no one but you there in the wee hours of the night when your cravings start yelling inside your brain and every cell in your body cries out for oblivion—*just this once!*

Finally, people are different, so to accommodate different kinds of people, recovery programs must be different, too. Indeed, to achieve maximum effectiveness, they must not only be merely different—they must be *personalized.* One size does not fit all. The needs of a sex-addicted, high-profile lawyer in a competitive firm may be very different from the needs of a codependent schoolteacher in suburbia. But in recovery, they'll go through similar stages and face similar challenges, so their programs will have something in common.

The elements of your personalized recovery program and where to find them

Let's start with the definition of addiction: a disease with consequences across all four dimensions of a person's life—the **body**, the **mind, relationships**, and **spirituality**. Everyone has these dimensions, and the personalized recovery program we create will be oriented around them. But we're also very different when it comes how much we develop each of these dimensions. Our best, most developed characteristics—and our possibilities for improvement—can vary greatly.

Like a frog, which always leaps into the water when threatened, people tend to have a favorite dimension to which they automatically retreat when things go wrong. For me, it's the mind. I tend to find my way out of trouble by thinking my way out, and I also overuse that pathway as a defense mechanism when I daydream and fantasize.

Take some time to reflect on which of the four dimensions you most trust to get you out of trouble. Is it the body? Do you take pride in your fitness, relying on it and knowing it has never failed you? Is it the mind, as it is with me? Is it relationships, in which you tend to rely on others to rescue you? Or is it faith in the divine order that gets you through? Whichever dimension you choose, this is the dimension you don't need to worry as much as the other dimensions because it is your **primary strength.**

Usually, a person will have two **intermediate strengths** as well. Mine are relationships and spirituality, both of which are quite important to me. You can do yourself a favor if you consistently put effort into upgrading your skills in these categories. You can, for example, learn how to strengthen your relationships by reading self-help books, improve the quality of your friendships, and establish a circle of reliable friends to help you through the tough times.

But *what will make the most difference to your recovery is the energy you invest into your least developed strength.* The weakest link decides when a chain breaks or how far the whole system can progress. This is why you must be mindful not to neglect your least developed dimension or omit it altogether.

For me, the body is my weakest dimension, so turning to it to get out of trouble is the *last* thing I'd do spontaneously. In fact, I would prefer to think of ways to avoid it. But during my own recovery, I learned that *the things I tended to avoid were precisely the things I had to put most of my efforts into changing.* After all, sometimes you just have to run! So I run, and I exercise. And when I start neglecting my body, I know I'm heading for troubled waters.

Your personalized recovery program elements are:

- **Body:** Regular exercise, balanced diet, sleep and rest, play, yoga and martial arts

- **Mind:** psychotherapy, learning about addiction, journaling, emotional regulation

- **Relationships:** therapy groups, support groups, marriage and family counseling, friends and family, work relationships

- **Spirituality:** meditation, creative expression or art, prayer, religious and spiritual communities

Make sure you don't exclude any of the dimensions, and be sure to put most of your efforts into your weakest one.

TABLE 9: The elements of your personalized recovery program

ELEMENTS OF YOUR PERSONALIZED RECOVERY PROGRAM	
BODY	a. Regular exercise b. Balanced diet c. Sleep and rest d. Play e. Yoga and martial arts
MIND	a. Psychotherapy b. Learning about addiction c. Journaling d. Emotional regulation
RELATIONSHIPS	a. Therapy groups b. Support groups c. Marriage and family counseling d. Friends and family e. Work relationships
SPIRITUALITY	a. Meditation b. Creative expression or art c. Prayer d. Religious and spiritual communities

24.a. *Body*

The body is a beautiful tool we use to experience and connect to the world around us, and to express the one inside us. I like to think of my body as a materialized image of my soul. But many addicts hate their own bodies for reflecting all the imperfections and mistakes the addicts have made.

Have you read the novel *The Picture of Dorian Gray* by Oscar Wilde?[108] It's about a handsome young man with a corrupt soul who is granted a wish to stay forever beautiful—but the scars and impurities resulting from his immoral behavior show up on his portrait. Dorian becomes obsessed with the ugly changes in the painting and decides to destroy it, but the cuts on the painting become wounds on his own body. He is found stabbed to death, old and ugly, while the portrait is immaculate. Similarly, addicts hate their own bodies because their bodies display evidence of their addictions (especially in the case of substance addictions!), sometimes letting everyone who sees the addict know of their problems. They want to destroy this evidence by destroying their bodies. This thinking has to be changed. Don't kill the messenger!

Below, you'll find ways to care for your body while you recover from addiction.

a. **Regular exercise**

Regular exercise is an essential part of a healthy lifestyle. You'll find it helps you better deal with your cravings and withdrawal symptoms, as well as instills more confidence in you. It will also mitigate the effect stress hormones have on you, so the stress of recovery won't be too difficult for your body to withstand, nor lead to stress-induced diseases. If you are otherwise healthy and physically able, you should aim to engage in at least half an hour of rather intensive aerobic exercise—for example, jogging, walking uphill, or riding a bike—every day. At least three times a week, try to include a longer workout, like an hourlong gym session

---

[108] Oscar Wilde, *The Picture of Dorian Gray* (Harlow, UK: Pearson Education, 2008).

or a hike. If you are an exercise addict, you'll need to keep your exercise moderate. Get rid of the stopwatch and the charts, and instead learn to listen to your body telling you when enough is enough.

b. **Balanced Diet**

Maintaining a balanced diet is important. We usually associate diets with efforts to manage body weight, but actually, a diet is simply a collection of recommendations for healthy nutrition in the broader sense. When you implement a diet only for the purpose of losing weight, you expect that one day, when you reach your goal weight, you will again change your eating habits, and may even resume eating as you did before. The type of diet discussed here, however, refers to a pattern of eating implemented not necessarily or only for the purpose of losing weight, but rather to maintain good health. Such a diet is not temporary, but rather followed for life.

According to WHO standards,[109] a healthy diet balances energy intake, usually calculated in the form of calories, with energy expenditure. In general, under these standards, total fat should not exceed 30 percent of a person's total energy intake, free sugars should constitute less than 10 percent of total energy intake, and salt intake should be less than 5 grams per day. It's recommended to consume five portions of fruits and vegetables per day. Here is an example of how your plate might look when taking into account all these healthy principles. Of course, if you have a disease that requires management via a special diet, like diabetes, you should follow your doctor's or dietitian's recommendations when determining what constitutes a healthy diet in your case.

---

[109] "Healthy Diet," World Health Organization, WHO, April 29, 2020, https://www.who.int/news-room/fact-sheets/detail/healthy-diet.

IMAGE 8: Healthy eating plan

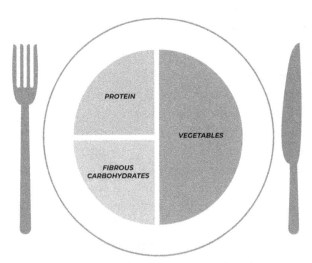

Improper diets, lack of food, a deficiency of essential elements and minerals, bingeing, and starving all create stress in the body—which, when under stress, redirects its energy to "fight or flight" mechanisms and slowing cell growth and repair. That is why I recommend you implement changes in your diet gradually, so as not to kick your body into a stress reaction and compromise your sobriety. Try to change one thing a week—for example, start by reducing carbs and supplementing more vegetables, while the overall calories stay the same. The next week, try reducing fats, and so on.

Of course, if you're a food addict, you'll have to abstain from the foods that are most likely to trigger your addiction. But even if you resort to emotional eating only on occasion, you'll feel better if you avoid sugary, starchy food and substances that induce food cravings, like chocolate.[110]

---

[110] As diabetics know, changes in blood sugar can produce emotional highs and lows that can be controlled by diet. The measure of how much a certain food can elevate blood sugar after a meal is called its glycemic index (GI). The mood swings of addicts, especially food addicts, can be controlled by avoiding food with a high GI, as these can trigger cravings and lead to relapse. Rachael Ajmera, "Glycemic Index: What It Is and How to Use It," Healthline, Healthline Media, December 14, 2020, https://www.healthline.com/nutrition/glycemic-index.

If you need to lose some weight, make sure you don't do so too drastically by skipping meals or trying all sorts of "wonder diets." Instead, consult a dietitian to learn the best way to achieve your weight loss goals.

c. **Sleep and rest**

Sleep and rest are natural ways to replenish your energy. Recovery is a difficult process that will drain you of energy, but as fatigue and stress can trigger relapses in addicts, you'll have to make sure you have enough rest. Establishing a good sleep routine takes time but works wonders in increasing your energy. Make a plan that allows for at least seven hours of sleep each day, and stick to it. You might consider buying a simple activity tracker that offers sleep control options. If you have problems falling asleep, establish a daily routine that will help you do so, and avoid experiencing too much stress, excitement, or emotional turmoil right before bedtime. You should also avoid consuming food, caffeine, and alcohol in the evenings, as this can lead to difficulty falling asleep.

Unfortunately, in our hectic, workaholic-enabling environment, some people may try to do extra work at the expense of sleep—even though they are chronically sleep-deprived. Don't do this—it can only backfire! When you work through fatigue, you suppress the signals your body is giving you that you're tired, perhaps with the aid of caffeine. Because you refuse to listen to your body, you can go from tired to exhausted without noticing. Eventually, you will come to a breaking point, and stress-related diseases will result, starting with thyroid dysfunction and high blood pressure. You may also end up burning out, after which you might need months or even years to recover. As you can see, working *too* hard is not a good investment!

d. **Play**

Play in this context means a having fun while doing an activity that requires a lot of motion. Engaging in playful activities like dancing or playing basketball will reduce the time it takes you to recover from stress, and you'll likely meet new friends for your support network.

Often, addicts feel they don't have time for play—but after they stop spending endless hours engaging in addictive behaviors like watching porn or trying to get noticed by their "Prince Charming," they're often surprised to find themselves with plenty of time. Use it well!

e. **Yoga and martial arts**
Yoga and martial arts often incorporate slow, thoughtful, balanced movements that offer an excellent way to reshape your body from a knotted, stressful mess into an elegant, sleepy cat stretching out in the sun. Doesn't that sound good? When we discussed trauma, I stressed that unprocessed traumatic memories are suppressed and stored in the body, burdening it with tension and pain that is difficult to release. In addition, thoughtful attention to breathing is an excellent way to reduce stress and regulate negative emotions.

These disciplines are very popular, so you'll likely be able to find a group of practitioners almost anywhere. I highly recommend you take the time to fit these activities into your schedule.

YOUR PLAN: THE BODY

List the activities you've decided to do regularly to take care of your body, and the resources you need to stick to your plan. Then incorporate these activities into your daily schedule.

Example: I have decided to start working out regularly and eating according to a healthy diet plan. I'll check out the gyms in my neighborhood and enlist in one I like the most. I'll check my workout equipment and find running trails. I'll find reliable sources for advice on my diet on the Internet, and consult with my doctor or dietitian for advice on my medical condition. I'll also commit to sleeping at least seven hours a night.

a. **Regular Exercise**

What I'll Do   Resources

....

....

....

b. **Balanced Diet**

What I'll Do   Resources

....

....

....

....

....

....

....

....

c. **Sleep and Rest**

What I'll Do   Resources

....

....

....

d. **Play**

What I'll Do   Resources

....

....

....

....

e. **Yoga and Martial Arts**

What I'll Do   Resources

....

....

....

24.b. *Mind*

By "the mind," I don't just mean the human capacity to reason—even though most people are convinced any problem can be resolved with reason, and this is usually how we go about trying to do so. But emotions are part of the human psyche, too. They are the *alternative system to intelligence,* informing us about our environment. There is no telling which of the two systems is better. In fact, people work best when both mental systems are in balance and well aligned.

But often—and certainly in the case of addicts—people's mental systems are not in balance. From a very young age, many children are taught by their families of origin to repress or ignore some emotions. Remember the dysfunctional rules addicted families have prohibiting the expression of one's feelings? If you've been trained not to pay attention to part of your mind in a similar way, it's time to unlearn those wrong instructions and reclaim your full potential. You're an adult now, and you can't count on finding a new family to help you learn healthier thought patterns.

In adulthood, people can create new families with their chosen partners. Many people hope these unions will bring new opportunities for changing the rules and roles that they learned in childhood, which brought them so much misery. But instead of acting as a chance for a new beginning, addicts' partnerships often inadvertently recreate the toxic environments of their families of origin. Why is this so? It's because they find precisely what they're looking for: they're looking for love, and by definition, love is the kind of relationship they had with their parents. Therefore, instead of finding a solution to the problem, they find another stage on which to play out the dramas of their childhood. Using your spouse as a therapist to help you work through your childhood issues is a bad idea because you'll tend to blame them for the problems you have.

Instead, you need a professional to help you work through these early traumas. A person you voluntarily allow to have power and authority over you because you respect their experience may be a **psychotherapist**, but not necessarily—a

mentor, counselor, teacher, priest, or social worker may be able to fulfill this role. Provided they are mature enough to understand what this entails and do not abuse the power you give them, you can create a therapeutic relationship with any of these professionals. However, *if your childhood experiences involve sexual, physical, or emotional abuse, you will best be served by a seasoned psychotherapist.*

a. **Psychotherapy**
Psychotherapy is undertaken in cooperation with therapists: licensed professionals who are highly skilled in establishing a **therapeutic relationship** with their clients. In this position, they have some power to guide people through life, and the educational system that grants their licenses ensures they are qualified and reliable enough to be entrusted with that power. Therapists help people in highly vulnerable situations, and can cause a great deal of harm if they are not trustworthy. For this reason, *you must choose a therapist you can trust, and establish a therapeutic relationship that feels safe.* Research and experience have proven that the therapeutic modality (a type of treatment) in which a therapist is experienced is less important than having the *good rapport and trust* you can develop in a good therapeutic relationship. For addicts, it is good to find a therapist with experience in addiction treatment. If your therapist doesn't have this experience, they can still help you, provided you take care to find *other trustworthy people (such as a sponsor from a twelve-step group or a counselor)* who are able to hold you accountable for your actions and alert you to the warning signs that your addiction is once again trying to take control.

b. **Learning about addiction**
Learning about addiction does not require a therapeutic relationship, which means that you can do it on your own. However, this also means that any new knowledge you gain may not reach the depths of the psyche where the toughest of problems are hidden, and thus the knowledge you need may not be available in times of crisis. Learn-

ing new facts will diminish the power of false prejudices you may have about yourself and others, making you more open and able to make accurate, mature decisions. These days, people mainly obtain information online, where plenty of excellent resources exist for those who want to learn about addiction. But there is also a downside to finding information online: nobody really checks if what they tell you is accurate. Remember, *popularity is not a substitute for quality!* Books can be a little better; most traditionally published books have been checked by editors who guarantee they make some sense. Still, it's not impossible to find a published book containing total nonsense. When I started learning about addiction thirty years ago, finding good books on the subject was a challenge. Nowadays, it's a challenge to discriminate between what is valuable and what is just rubbish. In such cases, I advise you to select books based on their author's reputation and credentials.

c. **Journaling**
Journaling is a tool you can use to reclaim responsibility for your life and create a narrative of your life that makes sense. This process of coming to understand yourself is one of the great gifts of recovery. Many an addict's psyche is fractured, shattered into parts that may not be entirely coherent or even aware of each other—after all, human memory is naturally unstable, and trauma, defense mechanisms, and addictions can make you forget the promises you made and truths you understood yesterday. It might be that today, you only remember how terribly you miss your ex-husband, forgetting the terror you felt yesterday when he drunkenly beat you. Some addicts can even lie to themselves, genuinely convincing themselves of falsehoods. This is possible because one part of their psyche is not in contact with others, and the memories stored there are otherwise forgotten. This disconnect from troubling thoughts, memories, or bodily feelings is called *dissociation*.

Journaling can help make an addict's fractured, addicted

psyche feel more coherent. Sometimes, you may be surprised to read what you wrote yesterday, feeling very different now that an addictive mood has passed. Rereading what you have written will help you consolidate your experiences with addiction and recovery. What's more, journaling can also be a very efficient way to prepare for your hours with a therapist so that you get the most out of this valuable time.

d. **Emotional regulation**

Emotional regulation is also important to achieving mental well-being. Learning how to act when fearful, angry, stressed, happy, or sad is part of our early programming in our families of origin. If your family was dysfunctional, however, you have likely learned some dysfunctional ways of reacting to your feelings. *Addictions are themselves dysfunctional methods of regulating emotions.* When you stop engaging in your addictive behavior, you'll need a more practical way of dealing with your emotions. Drowning them with alcohol, purging them by vomiting, or suppressing them through overstimulation with porn must remain off-limits.

What can you do instead? Performing conscious breathing[111] or using the Emotional Freedom Technique[112] may work for you, or you might choose to talk to a trusted friend. In addition, as we have already mentioned, meditation (especially mindfulness) and physical exercise are excellent ways to regulate emotions.

---

[111] **"Conscious breathing"** is an umbrella term for methods that direct awareness to the breath. These methods have the primary goal to build mindfulness and control stress and traumatic response.

[112] The **Emotional Freedom Technique (EFT)** is an alternative treatment for physical pain and emotional distress, also referred to as "tapping" or "psychological acupressure." According to its founder, Gary Craig, the cause of all negative emotions is a disruption in the body's energy system which is described essentially like the ancient system of meridians known in Traditional Chinese Medicine (TCM). Similar to acupuncture, tapping is applied on acupuncture points to balance disturbances in the meridian system and thus calm down the negative emotions. "What Is EFT? - Theory, Science and Uses," The Gary Craig Official EFT™ Training Centers, Gary and Tina Craig, 2023, https://www.emofree.com/eft-tutorial/tapping-basics/what-is-eft.html.

YOUR PLAN: THE MIND

List the activities you have decided to do regularly to take care of your mind, and the resources you need to stick to your plan. Then incorporate these activities regularly into your daily schedule.

Example: I need to find a therapist I can trust. To find one, I'll check online ads, select a couple therapists, and meet them to see how they usually work and how I feel around them. I'll also read at least one article a day online about my condition. I'll visit a library and see if I can find some additional reading on emotional regulation. I'll start writing a journal, documenting my sobriety date and other important changes in my thinking.

a. Psychotherapy

What I'll Do   Resources

....

....

....

....

....

b. Learning about Addiction

What I'll Do   Resources

....

....

....

....

....

....

c. **Journaling**

What I'll Do   Resources

....

....

....

....

d. **Emotional Regulation**

What I'll Do   Resources

....

....

....

....

24.c. *Relationships*

Repairing relationships is an essential part of psychotherapy. To recover from addiction, you'll need to be surrounded by a "safety net" of people you trust, who will provide the consolation, support, and feedback you'll desperately need.

Unfortunately, it is likely that when you enter recovery, most of the people in your personal network will be angry at you for having let them down while you were in the throes of addiction. They may even be a part of the problem! Your family is probably your first choice when it comes to support, but they can be both resentful *and* a part of the problem. If you can get them to cooperate, it will be to your advantage. *However, the best people to help you set sane boundaries for yourself and others will be other recovering addicts.*

A group of people is much more than the sum of the parts. Something happens when people sit in a circle and decide to open their hearts to each other. A beautiful, warm feeling of safety, intimacy, and connection envelops the group. When people are in tune with each other, their emotions resonate, and they feel empathy for one another. Secrets shared in such a group lose their tinges of shame and become forgivable. That is why *a safe, empathic peer group that is ready to really listen and share is the best therapy for addicts.* Such a group can offer exactly what you needed way back in your childhood, when you turned to substances or bad behaviors to compensate for the lack of what you needed. In this sense, love truly heals.

For this reason, *a therapy or support group is an absolutely essential component of a good recovery plan.* You should not attempt to omit it from your personalized plan—even if you instinctively shy away from sharing your shameful secrets with others. To recover, you'll need their help!

a. **Therapy groups**

Therapy groups are the best tool therapists can use to help heal addictions. Such groups are always formed by therapists, and usually consist of ten to twenty of their clients, whom they also see individually. The therapists conduct the group's meetings, and may do so in a directive way, or by letting things evolve more spontaneously. Ultimately, however, they are the ones responsible for ensuring whatever happens in group meetings is safe and follows the desired path. A therapy group is like an orchestra: each member plays their own tune while following the conductor's baton; but together, they play a beautiful melody that is deeper and more complex than each member's melody could be by itself. For these reasons, group therapy can rightfully be called "healing people with other people."

b. **Support groups**

Support groups are mainly different from therapy groups in that they don't have a therapist to direct them and guarantee the group will be steered toward and support the growth and healing of all its members. Without this guidance, support groups must instead have strict rules that govern each member's conduct, including the conduct of those who take on leadership roles. First and foremost, the group must be safe enough for members to feel comfortable sharing their innermost secrets. This safety is typically guaranteed by anonymity. In some of these groups, each member will also be required to sign a confidentiality agreement.

Another difference between therapy and support groups is that support groups can sometimes become much larger than therapy groups. They may be *open* to strangers who can decide to join at any time or *closed*, consisting only of members who have known each other for years; twelve-step groups are typically open to anyone who wants to join, but a study group, for example, may choose to stay closed.

Another difference is that therapy groups usually dissolve after the therapist believes the work is done. In contrast, support groups can continue to meet indefinitely, provided their members agree to do so—and as such, you can find lifelong support there. All twelve-step groups are support groups, and they usually do not require membership fees, though donations are accepted. By contrast, you will have to pay to join a therapy group. Some twelve-step groups have existed for decades, and **sponsors**[113]—seasoned members of the group who have experience with long-term recovery—may function as well as therapists in directing the group and aiding its members. However, they are not qualified to "treat" outside the narrow range of support and sharing, and should not attempt deep, significant psychotherapeutic interventions like reframing or confrontation.

Nevertheless, I encourage clients who attend my therapy groups to join a twelve-step support group for their primary addictions as well. Most people with behavioral addictions are family members of alcoholics, which qualifies them to join Al-Anon.[114] Not all of them take my advice, but I've observed that those who do also do well in their recovery, and the people they meet in their support group may become their friends for life.

The downside of support groups is that nobody is responsible for the course they take, or for any power struggle that emerges between members who may want to lead the group in different directions. As such, the quality of any individual support group can vary based on many factors. It's best to go to a couple of different meetings before deciding where you feel safest.

---

[113] "An AA booklet defines a **sponsor** as 'an alcoholic who has made some progress in the recovery program and shares that experience on a continuous, individual basis with another alcoholic who is attempting to attain or maintain sobriety through AA.'" "Examining the Role of AA Sponsors in Alcohol Recovery," Practical Recovery, Non 12 Step Drug Rehab and Alcohol Treatment, 2023, https://www.practicalrecovery.com/examining-the-role-of-aa-sponsors-in-alcohol-recovery/#:~:text=An%20AA%20booklet%20defines%20a,to%20help%20the%20newcomer%20get.

[114] **Al-Anon Family Groups**, founded in 1951, is a worldwide fellowship that offers help for people who have been impacted by another person's alcoholism.

TABLE 10: The difference between therapy and support groups

	THERAPY GROUP	SUPPORT GROUP
Leadership	therapist	shared
Safety guaranteed by	therapist	anonymity; a contract (occasionally)
Stance toward new members	closed	open or closed
Cost	varies	typically free (donations accepted)
Duration	limited	ongoing
Activity and purpose	treatment	recovery

c. **Marriage and Family Counseling**

Some therapists are specially educated to help families and couples understand and resolve conflicts and improve their relationships through marriage and family counseling. Marriage counseling gives couples tools they can use to communicate better, negotiate differences, problem-solve, and even argue more healthily. These tools can help you and your loved ones restore trust and better establish personal boundaries. They can help save your marriage; or if not, at least help you separate without unnecessary battles that are seemingly about the children and alimony, but are in fact about unresolved grievances within the relationship. It's worth investing in these tools, since nothing costs as much as a nasty divorce!

If you're codependent, in addition to marriage counseling, you should have a therapist or a group that will help you work through your codependence. Initially, a conflict of interest may appear to exist between marriage counseling, which often advocates you "**stay**" and fix your relationship; and codependence recovery programs, which suggest you should "**go**" and leave the relationship so you can avoid the addictive "substance"—the relationship itself. In my opinion, "should I stay, or should I go?" is not the right question to be asking at the beginning of recovery from codependence: unless there is physical and psychological violence involved, simply leaving your partner typically resolves nothing.

I advise my codependent clients to put all their efforts into their own recovery first, and to postpone dealing with other issues until they are through the emotionally challenging Serenity phase. *"Nothing major the first year"* is excellent advice from twelve-step programs. However, improving communication in a marriage and restoring broken boundaries will help everyone involved, regardless of whether you stay or go in the end.

d. **Friends and Family**
Improving communication and restoring broken boundaries are also important for the friends and family of addicts. If possible, while their addicted relative engages in recovery, they too should have some support group or a therapist to whom they can go and speak. Meeting families with similar problems regularly and sharing their experiences can also be of great help.

Some people believe talk of marital and addiction-related problems is too much for kids, but *these kids live in the middle of the battleground of the addicted family every day.* Talking about problems does not make them any worse, and can actually help kids learn how to resolve them or obtain appropriate help.

In some cases where divorce really is the best solution for the couple, parents nevertheless justify staying in an unhealthy marriage "because of the kids." While I agree that separation and divorce may be traumatic for children, many of my adult clients tell me they wished their parents would have divorced so the constant arguments would have stopped. In these cases, a counseling session that enabled all of them to speak their truth could have saved them from many misunderstandings.

Of course, this kind of therapy must be age-appropriate. Since addictions start developing at a very young age and teenagers are at the greatest risk, delaying the involvement of children is not a good strategy. My clients who work as teachers tell me they sometimes open discussion on these topics in the classroom, and that kids are eager to participate. They're interested in social problems and very observant of what goes on around them, and really appreciate it when an adult conducts a relevant conversation with them about addiction, sex, the Internet, and other topics that interest them. Discussion of such topics in a safe environment, like a school or a choir, can help a child who lives in a dysfunctional family learn that sources of help exist for them, if their problems become overwhelming.

When addicts sober up and resume their responsibilities, they are usually faced with remorse and guilt for the things they did or failed to do for their families while in the throes of addiction. Confrontation with the negative consequences of their addictive acting out adds to the burden of shame they are already feeling, threatening to push them back down the slippery slope into addiction. According to the twelve-step model of recovery, a lot of recovery work is about *forgiving yourself and making amends* to those you have harmed, including family and friends. In Steps 8 and 9 of most twelve-step programs, recovering addicts are encouraged to make a list of all the people they have harmed, become willing to make amends to them all, and make those amends directly whenever possible, except when doing so would hurt those people or others. This work, which is also spiritual, is the only real balm for the addict's low self-esteem, which ultimately underlies all addictions.

e. **Work relationships**

Most people spend a lot of time at work, and so they often form important work relationships with the people they work with. Although we may believe work relationships are less essential than familial relationships, their influence on our behavior and well-being is nevertheless considerable.

When we discussed issues related to money, work, and time, we learned that our use of these resources mirrors our sense of self-esteem. Those with positive self-esteem value theirs and others' time and don't show up to work late or stay there for long hours unnecessarily. They know they need time to rest and play, to be with their family, and to sometimes do nothing, too. They are flexible in their planning and aware of their priorities. *Overworking, being tired, and lacking sleep or the time to eat a proper meal* are all behaviors that may trigger a slip or relapse—so you need to avoid them. You may argue that in your line of work or under your current boss, that's impossible. But *everything is impossible until it's attempted!* I have heard many stories of successful negotiations with seemingly unsupportive bosses from people who just needed to set proper boundaries. But if this does not work, you must value your recovery enough to start looking around for a long-term job solution that will better help you maintain your sobriety.

YOUR PLAN: RELATIONSHIPS

Repairing **marital** and **parental relationships** will likely require expert help—so you need to identify the sources of such help that are within your reach, and choose the ones that best suit your needs. It's difficult to advise which **therapy group** is best for you. Preferably, you'll go to a couple of their meetings to see where you feel the safest. **Support groups** that work without therapists and offer regular meetings and friendly advice are a good choice to help you resist temptation and work through crises. Their advantage is that they are available regularly, their support is not time-limited, and they are free of charge.

Other, less important relationships, such as those you have with your **friends** and **extended family**, may also have been damaged by your addiction, but they will usually either improve or dissolve without expert intervention. Friends and friendly family members who are ready to help you with support or advice, can be a great help. Choose those you can trust, tell them about your problems, and ask if they're ready to take a phone call at odd hours if necessary.

Most people spend a lot of time at **work** where they forge meaningful relationships with bosses and coworkers. Addictions will damage work relationships, too. In recovery, this needs to be repaired. List the problems below that you have at work that may prevent you from staying sober, like excessive stress; triggers; overworking; bullying; inconsiderate or toxic coworkers or bosses; inability to set proper boundaries for rest, regular meals; and so on. Then think of short-term and long-term solutions to these problems

Here, list activities you can participate in to develop a safe, supportive network of relationships. Then, contact the chosen people and groups and select those with whom you feel safe. Incorporate regular meetings with them into your schedule.

Example:

Relationships

Marital relationship: *I will find a couples therapist and attend meetings with my spouse.*

Extended family: *It seems that I always relapse after family gatherings because I'm disappointed to see my father drunk. I will try to avoid them or go only in the company of a safe person. I will go to a couple of Al-Anon meetings to see if I fit there.*

Work: *I will try to negotiate not to work overtime so that I have time for my recovery work. I will skip office parties where alcohol and sweets are offered.*

a. **Problems in marital relationships: sources of help**
List the contacts of the available therapists and select one.

Therapists and therapy groups in my region

Type of group and
overseeing therapist   Contacts

....

....

Marriage counseling and
couples groups   Contacts

....

....

b. **Problems with extended family and friends:
sources of help**
Support groups in my town

Type of group: twelve-step,
other   Contacts

....

....

Supportive friends
I can call anytime   Contacts

....

....

....

....

c. Problems in work relationships: a list of what I can do to reduce the work-related stress

....

....

....

24.d. *Spirituality*

We have said spiritual transformation is at the heart of change for the better and is therefore the very essence of recovery. We've also argued that one does not need to be religious to be spiritual. *Believing there is something sacred within you and everyone else and that we are all interconnected through that holy spark at the center of our beings is crucial to recovery.*

People who have long been caught up in addiction suffer tremendous degradation of their moral values and concepts. Instead of knowing love, intimacy, and connection in their relationships, they know more about control and the fear of abandonment. They need to relearn—or possibly even experience for the first time—the trust, respect, intimacy, vulnerability, and positive regard that are necessary parts of healthy relationships.

For people like the children of alcoholics, who have been traumatized by the very people who were supposed to love them the most, this world is a scary place full of dangers, with no one to turn to for help. These people's most pervasive feelings are powerlessness and helplessness. When they were kids, they felt pressured to prematurely assume some adult responsibilities, like taking care of younger siblings or grandparents, in order to survive the constant crises and danger within their family. But to a small child, facing the grown-up world with all its responsibilities and hardships feels as impossible as climbing the highest of mountains. They do it—the survival instinct is strong—but *the feeling of being powerless—of being small, inadequate, inept, faced with tasks too big to handle—stays with them all the way to adulthood as a traumatic memory, and reappears with every hardship in every important relationship they face.* They need to be better than others—perfect and always alert—just to survive. This breaks them down, and they may resort to substances or behaviors to comfort and numb themselves. They may also question their faith: "If there is a God," they often ask themselves, "why doesn't He intervene and stop the suffering and abuse?" Their experience has caused them to lose trust not only in their family and those around them, but in a higher power.

How can victims of abuse be persuaded that the world is safe for them now, and warrants their trust? The answer lies in realizing that trust does not come from collecting enough proof one is safe—for life is in many ways unpredictable, and no matter how much proof one collects, unexpected events and tragedies can still occur. Ultimately, trust comes from the *belief*—which one must consciously *choose* to adopt—that the world is safe enough, that people are basically good, and that the world they see makes sense. For someone from a troubled family, these assertions are challenging to accept. Still, until they do, any hardship they encounter will undermine their feeling of safety—and their recovery.

What is a "sense of self"?

How do we know who we are? Are you just this body you see and feel, or just the mind you experience? Or is there something more, something that connects you with others—love, perhaps? The feeling of being human? An appreciation for life and this beautiful planet? We are here so briefly, and then gone—what sense does it make? And what is the difference between a life full of struggles to be good, even perfect; kind; connected—and a life of acting out all your desires to the fullest, regardless of the harm this might cause? We'll all die, anyway!

To answer these questions, I will speak again from my personal experience. Within my deepest awareness of myself, there is a spark of the Divine, which calls itself "I am!" It wants to express itself and be known. It wants to connect with others, recognizing similar sparks within them longing to be known. It is the source of my tenderest feelings for the beauties of this world, and the source of creativity that drives my endeavors. As a codependent, I had almost let it die, not appreciating it and believing I was actually only my roles: the good girl, the Rescuer, the mother, the daughter, the wife. But now, I know all these roles are just uniforms we put on. When I put on my white lab coat, everyone recognizes and knows me as a doctor. But without me inside, this coat—like all these roles—is nothing. The spark is everything. It is the essence of me.

I care for my spark by meditating every day, and by reading

books by renowned spiritual teachers and letting them reso-nate within my soul. I often go out in nature, surround myself with beautiful things, or stroke my cat or dog. Sitting by the fire and watching the flames is one of my favorite ways to feed this spark. And most of all, I try to share what I feel with my family; with my clients; and with you, my reader. By sharing love, one often gets more of it. When you respond to my shar-ing, I feel deep satisfaction, and a feeling that I have connected with someone else in the best way I know.

a. **Meditation**

Meditation is much more than useless daydreaming, as some uninformed people may believe. It is a regimen for training the mind, and a necessary part of most spiritu-al disciplines. Standard, everyday consciousness usually touches only the more superficial layers of the psyche. But our wounds and the prejudices derived from them are hid-den in much deeper layers—layers to which we usually do not have access, but which nevertheless influence our ex-periences. To heal those wounds and correct our false con-cepts, we must become aware of them. Most therapeutic techniques try to reach this goal, but indirectly. In medi-tation, however, we train our minds to contact these layers directly and instill in them a sense of peace and safety.

Meditation is not autohypnosis or some sophisticated technique you must learn, but it does work best if *practiced daily*—as does anything involving the brain.

In our everyday lives, we are aware of what goes on around us, and spend most of our time using reason and judgment, the functions of the brain's frontal cortex (see page 55). We plan, compare, judge, and decide what the world means to us, and we are usually able to choose be-tween various courses of action available to us. But at the same time, most of our thought processes operate outside our conscious control, as do the processes that control our bodies. Gaining awareness of these gives you a couple of precious seconds to say "*NO*" when you feel yourself drifting into a relapse. You can use your awareness of these processes to consciously decrease your stress levels—an important ability, as stress is one of the primary triggers for relapse. And in the long run, with training, you also can awaken within your mind the long-forgotten spark, the inner voice speaking on behalf of your own divinity and your connection to God—as you understand him.

Many different meditative routines exist. Some are simple, consisting only of sitting still while slightly tightening and then relaxing the muscle groups from head to toe. These methods work well for releasing stress energy, which is caught in tense muscles. You can also relieve this stress through running, completing an exercise routine, doing yoga, or even listening to spiritual music.

More complex meditative routines are best learned from a teacher. These can involve different tricks for silencing the "chatter" of the conscious mind, like repeating a mantra or visualizing intrusive thoughts being caught in a flytrap. Lately, **mindfulness meditation** is becoming increasingly popular, not only for recovery purposes, but for aligning oneself with the Universe. Taught in one-week courses, it involves being conscious of one's breathing and observing the mind as it wanders. The Internet offers many sources of guided meditation from which you can benefit a great deal. In your effort to connect to both the deepest part of yourself and to the broader world, you should look for the source and method that best suit you.

Instructions for Meditation

The best times to meditate are first thing in the morning or at night before going to bed. At the latter time, in preparation for sleep, the mind turns inward, toward its deeper layers.

Sit comfortably in a quiet, partially darkened room where no one can disturb you. Keep your spine upright and your feet flat on the ground. I do not recommend sitting with legs crossed in a lotus position unless you are used to it. If you have low blood pressure or are frequently dizzy, you can meditate while lying on a bed, but you may become sleepy in this position.

As you sit still, try not to think about anything. If any thoughts intrude, try to calmly let them go and leave your mind empty. This will get easier with practice. If you like, you can listen to guided meditation via the Internet. There are plenty of resources for Safe Place Guided Imagery[115] on the Internet, and you can easily find one you like and follow the instructions. I recommend you meditate for ten minutes first thing in the morning and another ten minutes before bedtime. After a while, your body and mind will learn how to relax and calm your emotions quickly. However, if you experience disturbing or frightening thoughts during meditation, please finish immediately with a positive image, and talk about it with your therapist.

b. **Creative expression or art**

Creative expression or art in any form is the expression of the deepest parts of our souls. You can sit, close your eyes, and let your hands work a block of clay. You can dance like nobody's watching. You can write a poem about your experience—which will be described in poetry much differently than if you were to describe it rationally. The aesthetics and the quality of the craftsmanship of the final work do not matter. When we create art of any kind, our "heart of hearts" is speaking—our innermost, core essence: the long-forgotten source of love and grace within us. Find a way to nourish this source, and you'll be richly rewarded.

c. **Prayer**

Prayer, like meditation, is the conscious turning toward our spiritual core. It involves asking for help and guidance, giving thanks for the gift of life, and wishing everyone the best. It acknowledges a "Power Greater Than Ourselves" that is in charge of all things, developing and playing out our lives

---

[115]You can listen to the recorded instructions for Safe Place Guided Imagery on my website, www.sanjarozman.com

according to a plan we do not consciously control, but that we trust has love at its core. It also involves acknowledging that despite our efforts, the world does not exist so that all our wishes will come true—but it is nevertheless good. After all, some things we cannot control may turn out even better than they would have if we could force them to go our way.

By acknowledging we do not have ultimate control over things, we release the burden of a responsibility that was never ours, which was in fact only an illusion created to soothe our fears of the future. Stepping down from the pedestal of omnipotence and humbly accepting that we are only human—an admission particularly crucial for code-pendents—is not humiliating; *it is simply the truth!* Being human means making mistakes because we usually do not know exactly what will happen in the future; if we learn from them, these mistakes are not *bad*, but merely errors everyone and anyone might make—which means they can be forgiven. Forgiving yourself for the mistakes you have made and making amends with those you have harmed as a result of those mistakes is a necessary step in recovery, and paves the way to changing things for the better. And if you want to move on from the role of a victim and take responsibility for your life, you must forgive the people who have hurt you, too.

Make some room for the things you value that remind you of your connection to God or to your own spirituality: a small altar including a picture of yourself as a child, some shells you collected on your favorite beach, beautiful flowers, crystals and candles, a heart-shaped stone you found while hiking in the hills, a book of poems, a religious text that appeals to you, and so on. Create a sacred space for these items in your room and in your heart. With others' permission, you might even put them in the middle of the circle at your therapy or support group so that while the group is in session, you will be subconsciously reminded of the best part of yourself.

d. **Religious and spiritual communities**

Religious and spiritual communities can be a great source of strength for religious people as they recover from addiction. If you can participate in a group prayer session, you will find that the feelings of connection you develop here are greater than those you can feel by yourself. And praying for a fellow person in need will also bring you deep satisfaction and help you believe in the goodness of others and the world.

Reading spiritual and religious texts by great philosophers or spiritual guides is a great way to align your conscious mind with your core self. For almost thirty years, I've been inspired by the teachings of *A Course in Miracles*; and for the last six years, my experience with the course has been upgraded through regular readings of, and meditation guided by, *A Course of Love*. These spiritual (not religious) self-study texts and the exercises within them have both answered and corresponded entirely with my spiritual needs as I have recovered. I encourage you to try them and see if they resonate with your needs, too.

YOUR PLAN: SPIRITUALITY

List the activities required to meet your need for a meaningful and loving relationship with the Divine. Then, find the contacts within your reach where you can practice such activities. Explore the possibilities, find some that you like best, and make them part of your routine.

Example: I will do a safe place meditation on a specific website every morning before getting up. Every evening before going to bed, I will recite the Gratitude Prayer and give thanks for everything good that happened during the day. Also, I will make it a habit to keep a gratitude journal. I will accept my friend's invitation to a group meditation on Friday evenings. I remember to do something good for somebody every day.

a. **Meditation:** Check the Internet for guided meditations and select some you like for regular use. In addition, list the contacts of meditation classes or workshops and commit to regular attendance.

Meditation class, mindfulness

....

....

Contacts

....

....

b. **Creative expression or art:** Go to a concert, museum, or gallery. Enlist in painting, acting, or modeling classes. List the contacts of artistic classes and explore how you feel while creating art.

Artistic classes

....

....

....

Contacts

....

....

....

c. **Prayer:** Make it a regular habit to thank the people and things you are grateful for every morning, and finish every day with a short review of the day and say thanks for the experience. Explore churches and spiritual or religious groups in your community and see where you feel welcome. At least once a week, go walking or hiking in an area of natural beauty, preferably alone, to feel in contact with nature. Below, list the sacred places you want to visit and the contacts of the people in charge.

25

Walking the Walk

You now have a state-of-the-art, personalized **recovery plan**, and you have firmly decided to stop your addictive behaviors and regain control of your life. Good job! I congratulate you on your honesty and willingness to change your life for the better.

What you have to do now is put the plan into action. Starting now! There is no better time to start than now. Each journey, no matter how long, begins with the first step.

Take it NOW!

Exercise 12: At the Crossroads

Read the following instructions slowly into the voice recorder of your smartphone or listen to the instructions you can find on my website, www.sanjarozman.com. Sit comfortably in a quiet room. Let your arms rest on your lap and place your feet flat on the floor. Then play the recording and follow the instructions. Close your eyes....

Imagine yourself standing at a fork in a road. Behind you is the timeline of your life, full of traumatic events, misunderstandings, losses, betrayal. . . . It breathes despair and loneliness. . . . You don't want to go back there. You're done with all of it!

Where you stand, the road splits into two. One fork goes downhill and continues in line with the old timeline. As far into the distance as you can see, the old story continues to repeat: . . . hope followed by despair . . . faith followed by betrayal . . . passion followed by loss.

. . . Imagine your life going in that direction. . . . Where would you be in a year? . . . In five years? . . . In ten years? . . . At the end? You don't want that!

Return your thoughts to the fork. Look at the other road, the new possibility that is open to you. See it rising steadily uphill. When you look at this road, what do you feel? Do you have some feeling that perhaps you don't deserve to go there? Do you fear the effort necessary to get there? Is there some fear that you're not going to succeed?

In your mind, with your eyes still closed, look around you. You're not alone! There is someone there to help you. . . . Who is it? It may be a friend, a deceased relative, an angel, or Jesus. . . . Let the person become known to you. . . . Greet the Helper and ask them for help. . . . If they have anything to say, listen. . . .

Behind the Helper is a gate. A marvelous arch surrounds it. . . . Go there and see if there are any inscriptions on the gate. . . . Listen to the Helper explain what the inscription means. . . .

Now, go deep into your heart of hearts and find there the sincere wish to change your habits into what they should be . . . a wish that has been there as long as you can remember . . . a vision of life, peaceful and loving, full of meaning and connection to others . . . full of love. . . . Let it resound within you; let it fill your hungry heart. . . . Remember the joy you felt as a child when you mastered some sport or had a great idea. . . . Let that joy fill the emptiness inside you. . . . If anything is stopping you, like the fear that you don't deserve to feel good, kindly ask your Helper to remove it from your heart, and watch them do it. . . .

Your Helper smiles at you, showing you through the gate, and showing you that the vision of your life as it should be is in the distance, along the path on which you now stand! Your Helper invites you to join them on the journey. . . . Feel the strong attraction toward the new direction and the deep joy and serenity that envelops you simply at the thought of going there. . . .

And, when you're ready, step through the gate!

Congratulations! You've made it!

Make the commitment to stay on the path, no matter what.

There are stairs in front of you, going slowly uphill. Take them. . . . Your Helper goes along, and you can always ask them to remove a burden or a troublesome thought, but you must walk by yourself. . . . When negative thoughts, self-doubts, or cravings come to haunt you, you can ask your Helper to remove them from your heart, for they have the power to do that! You can ask your Helper for advice when you're in doubt. . . . You can ask for peace when emotions overwhelm you. . . . You can ask for clarity when you're not sure. . . . You can ask for love when you feel alone!

And you'll be granted your request . . .

At each step, take your time to reflect on your position. . . . Be grateful for having found the path that leads to the fulfillment of your greatest potential. Know that this is the only fulfillment that can ever really and permanently satisfy your cravings. . . . The peace and serenity of knowing you're on the right path are what you've been looking for your whole life.

This is it!

Promise your Helper that you will visit this place often and regularly so that the two of you can continue further and further in the direction of the place where life is the way it should be; and consult your Helper any time you're in danger or tempted to slip back into your old ways. . . .

Finally, thank yourself for the giant step you've just made. Your new life has just begun!

Now open your eyes, reflect on what has just happened, and write your feelings on this exercise on the page below.

List your thoughts while working on this exercise:

....

....

....

The above meditation isn't just wishful thinking or some kind of cheap consolation. Your rational mind might think so—but your deeper levels of consciousness operate differently. Like dreams, myths, and fairy tales, they are vaguer and more fantastic, full of magical beings and unexpected twists of fate.[116] Even if the message feels strange to your reasoning mind, your subconscious will understand and accept it. You need not rationally believe in all I explain here—just follow the instructions, and let it work for you.

The tasks of the Serenity Phase

To move through the Serenity Phase of your recovery, you must complete the following tasks.[117]

1. **Define the problem**: One of the first things we learned about addiction is that it is a disease—not a sign of your inability to run your life, nor a moral failure of which you should be ashamed. However, this disease differs from most others in that your own behaviors can cause it—*or put an end to it.* By first defining the problem and recognizing it for what it is, you will be able to identify how the various elements of your life relate to your problem, and be ready to take the next step.

2. **Define the behaviors you must avoid**: The boundaries of abstinence are highly personal, and differ from addict to addict. What's more, adhering to them requires absolute honesty—with yourself and others.

---

[116] Psychologist **Carl Jung** believed a very deep part of each person's unconscious mind is inherited and shared with everyone, encompassing the soul of humanity. This collective human unconscious is populated by *archetypes*: ancient primal symbols such as the Wise Old Man, the Shadow, and the Great Mother. Jung believed the concept of the collective unconscious helps explain why similar themes can be found in mythologies around the world. He argued that the collective unconscious has a profound influence on the lives of individuals, who live out its symbols and clothe them in meaning through their own experiences. This, he reasoned, is what allows guided meditation to reach the deepest levels of the mind. Carl G. Jung, *Man and His Symbols,* ed. M.-L. von Franz, Joseph L. Henderson, Jolande Jacobi, and Aniela Jaffé (New York: Doubleday, 1964).

[117] Adapted from the thirty-task model in Patrick Carnes, *Facing the Shadow: Starting Sexual and Relationship Recovery* (Carefree, AZ: Gentle Path Press, 2010), 304–316.

3. **Prevent slips and relapses**: Recovery demands you understand how your addictive system works and what drives it, so that you can avoid not only the addictive behavior itself, but also any triggers or cues that might inspire you to indulge in that behavior. To prevent slips and relapses, you must establish boundaries regarding these triggers, and avoid them—often, for the rest of your life.

4. **Build a support structure**: Recovery rarely happens in a vacuum. To progress, most addicts need to be a part of a community of fellow addicts in recovery who will hold them accountable for their promises and actions. After all, you may lie to your spouse, family, and even yourself; but it is much more difficult to get away with lying among a group of recovering addicts who have all told such lies themselves.

   Many addicts find this task of the Serenity Phase one of the most daunting. After all, admitting your shortcomings and flaws to yourself is one thing, but sharing them in public takes much more courage. Nevertheless, doing so is essential, for addiction is a disease of denial. This is why recovering alcoholics must all state their position when introducing themselves in AA meetings: "My name is John, and *I'm an alcoholic!*"

5. **Understand the involuntary nature of your addiction (the "serenity to accept the things I can't change")**: "I can stop whenever I want to!" All too often, this is the refrain of an addict in denial. Such addicts believe their slips and relapses are just unfortunate coincidences, or try to blame them on other people. Only when you experience how truly powerless you are over addiction can you understand that a "mind machine" over which you have no control—the addiction cycle—is steering your destiny toward "rock bottom." Only then can you "surrender" to the process of recovery—and when you

finally do, new possibilities for healing and thriving will open to you.

6. **Understand your responsibility for your addiction and life ("courage to change the things I can")**: In the grip of your addiction, you may have preferred to think, "If addiction is a disease, then I am a patient. As a patient, I am a victim; therefore, I am not responsible for my actions." But this attitude will prevent you from taking back responsibility for your addiction and recovery. Ultimately, you are responsible for your actions even though your awareness of their consequences has been compromised by addiction; just as if you had hit someone while driving under the influence of alcohol, you would not be able to use your drunkenness as an excuse to avoid punishment. Remember, you took the drink! In the end, only taking responsibility for your actions and their consequences will prevent you from doing more harm to yourself and others.

7. **Understand the reasons you developed your addiction, and forgive yourself ("wisdom to know the difference")**: To avoid excessive self-accusations and regret over your addiction and actions, which can only lead to shame—the motor of the addiction cycle—you must understand the meaning of addiction in your life. You must realize that your addictive behavior started developing when you were young and ignorant of how the world worked; and that, in the beginning, it even served a purpose: to help you survive the traumatic events that befell you in your early life. To forgive yourself for your actions, let go of your shame, and break the addictive system, you must also allow yourself to realize all people are fallible, and that we sometimes cause harm to ourselves and others even when we have good intentions.

8. **Achieve emotional sobriety or serenity**: Sobriety does not only mean abstaining from mood-altering substances and behaviors, but also stopping your emotions from escalating excessively. This is not something you can master in only a day or two. That's why the Serenity Phase can take up to a year—or even longer, if relapses occur. Your body needs time to return to homeostasis, and there is little you can do to speed this task.

Be patient. Serenity and patience go hand in hand. As part of your recovery, you must learn the benefits of achieving deep inner peace, and how to enjoy it.

This will be difficult at first. It will feel unnatural. Your whole body will crave drama and excitement. At times, you will forget how hard your life used to be when you were in the throes of addiction, and wish to return to indulging in your addictive cravings. But to continue your recovery, you must remain steady, and wait for those cravings to stop.

9. **Undertake spiritual change—ask for and accept the help of the Higher Power and your own responsibility for change**: Finally, when you have achieved emotional sobriety and inner peace, something sacred can emerge from deep inside. Like the fox who learned how to love in the story of the Little Prince, ready to flee at any sign of disturbance,[118] ancient memories of something divine may start coming to you in your morning meditations. Sit with them, and let them come a little bit closer every day. From these memories, you can begin to establish a personal relationship with the Power Greater Than Yourself. This relationship is the only truly safe anchor in this world that you can rely upon in every circumstance. Allow yourself to become intimately acquainted with it, and let it heal and help you in your recovery.

---

[118]Antoine De Saint-Exupéry, *The Little Prince*, trans. Richard Howard (New York: Harcourt, Inc., 2000).

TABLE 11: The tasks to accomplish in the Serenity Phase and related exercises

Tasks to Accomplish in the Serenity Phase	Related Exercises
1. Define the problem	Exercise 1: What are the harmful behaviors I keep repeating? Exercise 2: What problems do I have as a result of these behaviors? Exercise 3: Is it an addiction or not?
2. Define the behaviors you must avoid	Exercise 8: The list of behaviors you need to stop
3. Prevent slips and relapses	Exercise 11: Your list of triggers and stressors
4. Build a support structure	Chapter 24.c.: Connect to a recovery community; get a therapist and a mentor or sponsor
5. Understand the involuntary nature of your addiction	Exercise 4: What am I ashamed of? Exercise 5: What are the consequences of my addictive behavior? Exercise 6: My Addiction Cycle Exercise 9: Emergency Control Plan
6. Understand your responsibility for your addiction and life	Exercise 10: Accepting responsibility for the things you can change
7. Understand the reasons you developed your addiction, and forgive yourself	Exercise 7: My Addiction Timeline
8. Achieve emotional sobriety or serenity	Work the personalized program daily; meditate; use the tools for emotional regulation; avoid stress and triggers
9. Undertake spiritual change—ask for and accept the help of the Higher Power and your own responsibility for change	Work the personalized program daily; meditate; pray

The Challenges of the Serenity Phase

What obstacles might delay or compromise your progress through the Serenity Phase? If you are sure you have honestly identified and abstained from all your addictive behaviors, the reasons for your lack of progress may be found in these negative beliefs:

1. **The Negative Belief: The problem is with other people!**

   "I only drink because my wife is constantly criticizing me!" an alcoholic might argue, in an attempt to justify his drinking. And when I meet new clients in therapy for codependence, I must first convince them to *let go of control of their chosen partner*—their "drug"—and instead mind their own business.

   Addicts' attempts to shift all the responsibility for their actions onto other people reflects their belief that they are *victims* not only of their own addictions, but of others. But as we have already seen, such a stance can only prevent an addict from changing. Only when the addicts stop believing *someone else* needs to change so *they* can be at peace, and instead start investing all their energy into changing themselves, can they begin to progress in their recovery. Until then, they typically focus on complaining about others who *don't understand how much better everything would be, if only they changed in accordance with what the addict wished!* The addicted codependent might spend inordinate amounts of time vacillating over whether or not to leave their relationship. What they don't understand is that they should take care of the part of the problem that belongs to them, and let the other part take care of itself.

2. **The Negative Belief: I can't trust anyone!**

   Your lack of progress may stem from a belief that the world is not safe. This is one of the first beliefs every person establishes as a young child—so this belief lies in the foundations of the numerous decisions we make afterward, influencing every one of them. If you believe the world is fundamentally unsafe, and that other people are doing things that hurt you, you may feel entitled to medicate your pain with substances and/or certain behaviors. But as long as you believe this, you will not progress in your recovery.

Changing one's foundational beliefs is not an easy task. Trust is tricky to build, and easy to destroy. Worse still, the belief that the world is unsafe can be hard to deny, because bad things can happen to everyone, sometimes unpredictably. The insecurely attached addict basically distrusts everything and attempts to control everything around them.[119] However, the idea that we can control every aspect of our lives is an illusion. Some of the most essential elements of our lives are indeed beyond our control. We cannot, for example, force someone to love us. We cannot decide when we meet our soulmate, or whether we will fall victim to a severe disease. It is more reasonable to believe that, even though things sometimes don't work out the way we wish they would, they will still work out somehow, for better or worse—sometimes even better than we had hoped.

However, sometimes things do not turn out as well as we had hoped. In such cases, it can be difficult for an insecurely attached person to accept events as they have happened, and avoid feeling justified in their belief that the world is ultimately unsafe. They may then turn to their comforting addictive behaviors, and find themselves back in the addiction cycle. This is why it is so imperative that addicts work to change this particular category of negative belief—even if that belief seems logical given the state of the world and the events that occur within it.

When bad things happen, spiritual or religious people

---

[119] See the chapter on insecure attachment, on page 72.

may find a source of relief in their belief in a higher power—a Divine being, Nature, the Universe, or anything greater than themselves. They may believe that "everything happens for a reason," or that while negative events can occur, something good may be waiting just around the corner. For insecurely attached addicts, replacing their negative beliefs about the danger the world poses with beliefs like these can be a big help. In their case, learning to let go and *accept the things they cannot change* is an especially important part of the Serenity Phase—as noted in the prayer itself.

3. **The Negative Belief: I'm not worth it; I'm not important!**

Typically stemming from an upbringing in a dysfunctional family, these negative beliefs are deeply ingrained in the belief systems of the children born into those families. These children are often successful when it comes to survival; but when the battles stop and they should thrive in peace and serenity, they become disoriented. They learned how to escape pain, but forgot where they wanted to go. They panic when they don't hear the drums of the battle to which they are accustomed. They stop striving for further growth, and their traumatic memories catch up with them. Just like Ellen, whose testimony I share below, they're accustomed to a certain ratio of good versus bad in their lives, and feel that's what they deserve. When things go smoothly, they suspect some troubles may be piling up somewhere in the background—so they prefer to sabotage their progress to maintain the ratio of good and bad to which they are accustomed, because—ironically—it makes them feel safe. It's challenging to convince these children of dysfunctional families that they can and should expect better, and even reach out for more. However, in order for them to progress and stop self-sabotaging their own recovery, they must eventually change those negative, deeply ingrained beliefs.

Ellen's Story
While in recovery from codependence and bulimia, Ellen, 42, a mother of two young children, told me her story:

The first couple of months after I entered the recovery program went relatively smoothly. I felt great relief that I had finally surrendered to and admitted my problems and now had help taking care of them. I was absorbed in all the activities that were a part of the recovery program. I started going to the gym regularly, and after the initial muscular pains had subsided a little, it was something I looked forward to. I learned to eat responsibly and not overeat when I was feeling lonely or anxious. I met some new people who understood me and cared about me. Life became almost beautiful. I'm aware that it's not the real beauty of life yet, but rather the abstinence from and absence of addiction. But I still don't have control over my life yet. I don't mean addictive control, but I simply don't feel in charge of my life. There is life as I want it, and there is life as it really is. I should take control and steer my life there. I should be able to take responsibility for what I want and think about how I will get there.

But now, I feel stuck, like I'm standing still. I'm like a sailboat in the absence of wind.

No breeze. No direction. I don't know how to go on and where to go. It feels weird living like that. No drama. Just me, calm in serenity, listening to myself and my feelings. It feels like the old gym lessons at school: after you finished your set of exercises, you sat down until you got a new assignment. It's too calm. I know, serenity and all that—but I don't feel safe in the absence of drama. It feels unnatural. I'm used to overachieving, and I thrive when I need to multitask to get me out of trouble, all at the last minute. Now, all that has gone, and instead of being happy, I started anticipating something that will reinstall the usual trou-

blesome way things work out.

I don't feel safe. I feel the shadows of the past behind me. I fear that somewhere behind the scenes, some evil is accumulating. Something is just waiting to happen and ruin everything. My ex will emerge out of nowhere and start hassling me again. I would love to see him arrested. Does that make me a bad person? Will I get some "bad karma" for wanting such a thing? He has done so many bad things to me, things nobody should endure. I'll only feel safe if he were in prison or on another continent. Somewhere in the background, I feel the troubles piling up. Fear is rising. I worry about my health. I observe the feelings in my body, anticipating symptoms of a disease. I'm ashamed to go to the doctor, who told me so many times that it's only my imagination. But what if I get sick? How am I going to handle the expenses and sick leave? How am I going to care for the kids? I keep doing positive affirmations halfheartedly. If I write "I am successful," something in me vibrates: I don't deserve it! I'm not worthy of being at peace!

Yesterday was really bad. I told my mother about my health problems. She didn't react—didn't show any concern or worry. She just asked if I had gone to the doctor. Then she paid for some classes for my kids. I felt invisible. She never asked how I felt. She didn't care! You can't give your daughter money instead of asking, "How are you? Are you well?" I felt invisible, as if I didn't exist . . . unimportant, invisible, as if I wasn't there . . . but I was aware, and it hurt so much! What would she have done if I had told her I had cancer? Would she have asked me if I had seen a doctor—and then bought the kids some candy? That's how she handles things. But I need acknowledgment that I can live, breathe, laugh, and feel. That I can even have my ups and downs. I can see that in the past I tested her now and then to see if she noticed me, if I mattered. She could never give me the approval I so desperately needed. My disappointment, anger, and projections spilled onto the others around me. I attacked, and blamed, and rejected them. It was ter-

rible. I wasn't even aware of it. But yesterday, I decided to just breathe through the feelings and let the Higher Power take care of them. I believed it was there, and I trusted it would take care of my problems. I knew the cause of my pain, remembering that it was only my projection. And after a while, the pain subsided. I could see that it was all in the past, and that I could break free from all of it.

What Ellen did is precisely what needs to be done in such a situation: she sat down, breathed, and let God take care of it, trusting that He would. As you do the same, the pain will subside, and clarity will replace the struggle.

26

Moving On to Trauma Work

This book can guide you through the first six to twelve months of your recovery. When the layers of oblivion and numbness are washed away and the drive to escape has receded, you will start perceiving the world differently, and new possibilities will unfold.

However, in the process, traumatic memories hidden beneath those layers may start to emerge, and will have to be dealt with. For most, merely remembering and mourning your losses will help them heal. But if the memories become too painful, I suggest you find a therapist to help you deal with them, as this is not something that can be done alone.

If you are a child of a dysfunctional family who has suffered abandonment, betrayal, or violence at the hands of your caregivers, you will likely also discover additional obstacles you will need to recognize and overcome in the course of your recovery, and it won't be easy. Nevertheless, to progress on the path of recovery, you must repair the damage past traumas have done to your life.

Dealing with these traumas and continuing your journey of recovery is the focus of my next book, *Courage*. I invite you to join me in this book as I explain how trauma changes its victims, and discuss what they can do to recover from it. After that, *Wisdom*, the final book in the series, will support your spiritual change as a result of your dedicated work and efforts to achieve a better life.

As the members of Alcoholics Anonymous do before and after each of their meetings, we can return now to the Serenity Prayer and use it as a mantra during recovery. As you ground yourself in the recovery principles outlined in this book and strive to take one more step along the path to recovery each day, I encourage you to repeat its words:

> *God, grant me the **Serenity***
> *to accept the things I cannot change,*
> ***Courage** to change the things I can,*
> *and **Wisdom** to know the difference.*

Say these words thoughtfully, with appreciation for the millions of people who have struggled and are still struggling to take this path from addiction to a better life. Think of these people! Now that you've read this book, they are no longer just the figures you might pass in the street. In sharing their stories, they have let you look into their hearts. They're the cashier in the shop where you buy groceries, the waitress at your favorite coffee place, the mechanic who takes care of your car, the teacher at your yoga class. They are ordinary people, just like you and me, who just want to live their lives as best they can. And in the evening, they all meet and recite these sacred verses, manifesting their collective willingness to grow into lives free of addiction. As a witness to their endeavors, you now know those struggles are the same as yours, and you have become part of their fellowship, whether you attend these meetings or not. A path has been laid at your feet, and you have started walking, step by step, taking one day at a time.

Keep walking! The path does not end here. There are places you need to go to. There are people waiting to meet you. There are experiences that will change you. There are things you need to accomplish, and skills you need to master. Becoming a better person is now your purpose—and creating a better world will be your legacy.

Acknowledgments

Many people contributed to the birth of this book. I'd like to express my gratitude for their patience and passion with which they helped make my work better and bring it to the reader.

My family supported me the whole time, encouraging me and tolerating my temporary lack of emotional availability while I was concentrating on the text. My daughters **Katja**, **Barbara**, and **Jana** are grown now, and they learned to wait for me to return from a busy writing session and resume my responsibilities as a mother. I am especially grateful to Katja, who contributed to the book by crafting the illustrations and the book cover. Discussing concepts with her inspired some of my best ideas.

Kurt Wilkesmann, my literary agent, found me and talked me into the idea of publishing a book in the English language. He was the first to read the manuscript, and the tears in his eyes when he finished were proof I was touching on something important. As a native Anglophone, he helped me express my ideas smoothly. Discussing the manuscript with him was fun, and I learned a lot.

Noah Charney—the American art historian, Pulitzer Prize nominee, and bestselling writer who fell in love with Slovenia and moved here to stay—helped me find my way to a publishing contract via his many connections in the publishing world. Thank you, Noah, for your enthusiasm, and for believing in me.

Working with my editor **Erin Harpst** was fun and very rewarding. Thorough, and professional, she really dug into the work from a "model reader" perspective and helped me notice where I was not precise or thorough enough. Like the proverbial sculptor, she helped remove the redundant marble to allow the masterpiece to shine through. **Ceci Hughes** accepted the task of finishing Erin's work and gave it the final varnish. Thank you both for the patience and attention to details that I overlooked in my eagerness to have the work done.

Robert H. Pruett, founder and president, and the rest of **the team at Brandylane Publishers, Inc.** and **Belle Isle Books**: I appreciate that they believed in my work and did their best to get it out to the people. Even though we were separated by the distance of half the globe, I felt as though we were a team.

Bibliography

The following books and articles have been my sources of inspiration and learning. I've read and reread them so many times now, I feel the ideas within have been imprinted in my mind. The concepts they discuss have become important parts of my "mental world map," helping me find my way out of troubles and into personal growth. Footnotes throughout the book indicate where I used excerpts or direct quotes from their texts.

1. *A Course in Miracles: Combined Volumes.* Los Angeles: Foundation for Inner Peace, 1976.

2. Adams, Kenneth M. *Silently Seduced: When Parents Make Their Children Partners.* Rev. ed. Deerfield Beach, FL: Health Communications, 2011.

3. Ajmera, Rachael. "Glycemic Index: What It Is and How to Use It." Healthline. Healthline Media, December 14, 2020. https://www.healthline.com/nutrition/glycemic-index.

4. *Alcoholics Anonymous: The Story of How Many Thousands of Men and Women Have Recovered from Alcoholism.* New York: Alcoholics Anonymous World Services, 1986.

5. American Psychiatric Association. *Diagnostic and Statistical Manual of Mental Disorders.* 5th ed. Arlington, TX: American Psychiatric Association Publishing, 2013.

6. Augustine Fellowship. *Sex and Love Addicts Anonymous.* Boston: Augustine Fellowship, 1986.

7. Beattie, Melody. *Codependent No More: How to Stop Controlling Others and Start Caring for Yourself.* 2nd ed. Center City, MN: Hazelden, 1992.

8. Bellringer, Paul. *Understanding Problem Gamblers: A Practitioner's Guide to Effective Intervention.* London: Free Association Books, 1999.

9. Berne, Eric. *Games People Play: The Psychology of Human Relationships*. New York: Grove Press, 1964.

10. Boriskin, Jerry A. *PTSD and Addiction: A Practical Guide for Clinicians and Counselors*. Center City, MN: Hazelden, 2004.

11. Bratman, Steven, and David Knight. *Health Food Junkies: Orthorexia Nervosa: Overcoming the Obsession with Healthful Eating*. New York: Harmony Books, 2004.

12. Breiter, Hans C., Itzhak Aharon, Daniel Kahneman, Anders Dale, and Peter Shizgal. "Functional Imaging of Neural Responses to Expectancy and Experience of Monetary Gains and Losses." *Neuron* 30, no. 2 (May 2001): 619–639. doi:10.1016/s0896-6273(01)00303-8.

13. Brownell, Kelly, and Mark Gold. *Food and Addiction: A Comprehensive Handbook*. 1st ed. New York: Oxford University Press, 2012.

14. Carnes, Patrick. *Don't Call It Love: Recovery From Sexual Addiction*. New York: Bantam Books, 1991.

15. Carnes, Patrick. *Facing the Shadow: Starting Sexual and Relationship Recovery*. Carefree, AZ: Gentle Path Press, 2005.

16. Carnes, Patrick. *Out of the Shadows: Understanding Sexual Addiction*. Center City, MN: Hazelden, 2001.

17. Carnes, Patrick. *Sexual Anorexia: Overcoming Sexual Self-Hatred*. Center City, MN: Hazelden, 1997.

18. Carnes, Patrick J. *The Betrayal Bond: Breaking Free of Exploitive Relationships*. Deerfield Beach, FL: Health Communications, 2019.

19. Carnes, Patrick, David L. Delmonico, and Elizabeth Griffin. *In the Shadows of the Net: Breaking Free of Compulsive Online Sexual Behavior*. Center City, MN: Hazelden, 2001.

20. Carnes, Patrick J., and Kenneth M. Adams. *Clinical Management of Sex Addiction*. 2nd ed. New York: Routledge, 2019.

21. Cermak, Timmen L. *Diagnosing and Treating Co-Dependence: A Guide for Professionals Who Work with Chemical Dependents, Their Spouses, and Children*. Center City, MN: Hazelden, 1986.

22. Cheng, Cecilia, and Angel Yee-lam Li. "Internet addiction prevalence and quality of (real) life: a meta-analysis of 31 nations across seven world regions." *Cyberpsychology, Behavior, and Social Networking* 17, no. 12 (2014): 755–60. doi: 10.1089/cyber.2014.0317.

23. Claude-Pierre, Peggy. *The Secret Language of Eating Disorders: How You Can Understand and Work to Cure Anorexia and Bulimia*. New York: Vintage Books, 1997.

24. Cooper, Alvin, Dana E. Putnam, Lynn A. Planchon, and Sylvain C. Boies. "Online Sexual Compulsivity: Getting Tangled in the Net." *Sexual Addiction and Compulsivity* 6, no. 2 (April 1999): 79–104. doi: 10.1080/10720169908400182.

25. Costa, Sebastiano, Nadia Barberis, Mark D. Griffiths, Loredana Benedetto, and Massimo Ingrassia. "The Love Addiction Inventory: Preliminary Findings of the Development Process and Psychometric Characteristics." *International Journal of Mental Health Addiction* 19, (2021): 651–668.

26. Cozolino, Louis. *The Neuroscience of Psychotherapy: Healing the Social Brain*. New York; W. W. Norton & Company, 2017.

27. Cutler, Robert B., and David A. Fishbain. "Are alcoholism treatments effective? The Project MATCH data." *BMC Public Health* 5, no. 75 (July 2005): doi: 10.1186/1471-2458-5-75.

28. Kasl, Charlotte Davis. *Women, Sex, and Addiction: A Search for Love and Power.* New York: HarperCollins, 1990.

29. Dayton, Tian. *Emotional Sobriety from Relationship Trauma to Resilience and Balance.* Deerfield Beach, FL: Health Communications, 2010.

30. Dayton, Tian. *Trauma and Addiction: Ending the Cycle of Pain through Emotional Literacy.* Deerfield Beach, FL: Health Communications, 2000.

31. Dayton, Tian. *The ACOA Trauma Syndrome: The Impact of Childhood Pain on Adult Relationships.* Deerfield Beach, FL: Health Communications, 2012.

32. De Saint-Exupéry, Antoine. *The Little Prince.* Translated by Richard Howard. New York: Harcourt, Inc., 2000.

33. Dixon, Stacy Jo. "Average daily time spent on social networks by users in the United States from 2018 to 2022." Statista.com. Statista, June 2, 2022. https://www.statista.com/statistics/1018324/us-users-daily-social-media-minutes.

34. "Eating Disorder Statistics." ANAD. National Association of Anorexia Nervosa and Associated Disorders, 2023. https://anad.org/eating-disorders-statistics.

35. Fisher, Helen. *Why We Love: The Nature and Chemistry of Romantic Love.* New York: Henry Holt, 2004.

36. Gentile, Douglas A., Hyekyung Choo, Albert Liau, Timothy Sim, Dongdong Li, Daniel Fung, and Angeline Khoo. "Pathological video game use among youths: A two-year longitudinal study." *Pediatrics* 127, no. 2 (2011): e319–329. doi: 10.1542/peds.2010-1353.

37. Haymond, Bryce. "AA Co-Founder Bill Wilson's 'First Vision' Account." Thymindoman.com. Accessed September 6, 2017. https://www.thymindoman.com/aa-co-founder-bill-wilsons-first-vision-account.

38. Herman, Judith. *Trauma and Recovery: The Aftermath of Violence—from Domestic Abuse to Political Terror.* New York: Basic Books, 1997.

39. Hite, Shere. *The Hite Report: A Nationwide Study of Female Sexuality.* New York: Seven Stories Press, 2003.

40. Hite, Shere. *The Hite Report on Men and Male Sexuality.* New York: Alfred A. Knopf, 1981.

41. Horney, Karen. *Our Inner Conflicts: A Constructive Theory of Neurosis.* New York: W. W. Norton, 1992.

42. *International Statistical Classification of Diseases and Related Health Problems, 10th Revision, Fifth Edition.* World Health Organization, 2016. https://apps.who.int/iris/handle/10665/246208.

43. Jung, Carl G. *Man and His Symbols.* Edited by M.-L. von Franz, Joseph L. Henderson, Jolande Jacobi, and Aniela Jaffé. New York: Doubleday, 1964.

44. Kaplan, Debra L. *For Love and Money: Exploring Sexual & Financial Betrayal in Relationship.* Self-published, CreateSpace, 2013.

45. Karpman, Stephen B. "Script Drama Analysis II." *International Journal of Transactional Analysis Research & Practice* 10, no. 1 (2019): https://doi.org/10.29044/v10i1p21.

46. Karila, Laurent, Aline Wery, Aviv Weinstein, Olivier Cottencin, Avmeric Petit, Michel Reynaud, and Joel Billieux. "Sexual Addiction or Hypersexual Disorder: Different Terms for the Same Problem? A Review of the Literature," *Current Pharmaceutical Design* 20, no. 25 (2014): 4012–4020, https://www.ingentaconnect.com/content/ben/cpd/2014/00000020/00000025/art00004.

47. Lancer, Darlene. *Codependency for Dummies.* Hoboken, NJ: John Wiley & Sons, Inc., 2015.

48. Longstreet, Phil, and Stoney Brooks. "Life Satisfaction: A Key to Managing Internet & Social Media Addiction." *Technology in Society* 50, (2017): 73–77. https://doi.org/10.1016/j.techsoc.2017.05.003.

49. Maté, Gabor, and Peter Levine. *In the Realm of Hungry Ghosts: Close Encounters with Addiction.* Berkeley, CA: North Atlantic Books, 2010.

50. Mellody, Pia, Andrea Wells Miller, and J. Keith Miller. *Facing Codependence: What It Is, Where It Comes from, How It Sabotages Our Lives.* San Francisco: HarperSanFrancisco, 2003.

51. Mellody, Pia, Andrea Wells Miller, and J. Keith Miller. *Facing Love Addiction: Giving Yourself the Power to Change the Way You Love.* San Francisco: HarperSanFrancisco, 2003.

52. *Mending a Shattered Heart: A Guide for Partners of Sex Addicts.* Edited by Stephanie Carnes. Carefree, AZ: Gentle Path Press, 2011.

53. Milkman, Harvey B., and Stanley George Sunderwith. *Craving for Ecstasy and Natural Highs: A Positive Approach to Mood Alteration.* Thousand Oaks, CA: SAGE Publications, 2010.

54. National Research Council (US) Committee on the Social and Economic Impact of Pathological Gambling. *Pathological Gambling: A Critical Review.* Washington, DC: National Academies Press (US), 1999. https://www.ncbi.nlm.nih.gov/books/NBK230631.

55. Norwood, Robin. *Women Who Love Too Much: When You Keep Wishing and Hoping He'll Change.* New York: Pocket Books, 2008.

56. Norwood, Robin. *Letters from Women Who Love Too Much: A Closer Look at Relationship Addiction and Recovery.* New York: Pocket Books, 1989.

57. "Origin of the Serenity Prayer: A Historical Paper."
    aa.org. General Service Office (GSO) of Alcoholics
    Anonymous, July 30, 2009. https://www.aa.org/sites/
    default/files/literature/assets/smf-129_en.pdf.

58. Olson, David H., Candyce Smith Russell, and Douglas
    H. Sprenkle. *Circumplex Model: Systemic Assessment and
    Treatment of Families.* New York: Routledge, 2014.

59. Parnell, Laurel. *Rewiring the Addicted Brain with EMDR-
    Based Treatment.* New York: W. W. Norton & Company,
    2019.

60. Perron, Mari. *A Course of Love: Combined Volume.* Nevada
    City, CA: Take Heart Publications, 2014.

61. Roberts, Kevin. *Cyber Junkie: Escape the Gaming and
    Internet Trap.* Center City, MN: Hazelden, 2010.

62. Roth, Geneen. *When Food Is Love: Exploring the
    Relationship Between Eating and Intimacy.* New York:
    Plume, 1992.

63. Roy, Alec, Bryon Adinoff, Laurie Roehrich,
    Danuta Lamparski, Robert Custer, Valerie Lorenz,
    Maria Barbaccia, Alessandro Guidotti, Erminio
    Costa, and Markku Linnoila. "Pathological
    Gambling: A Psychobiological Study." *Arch Gen
    Psychiatry* 45, no. 4 (1988): 369–373. doi: 10.1001/
    archpsyc.1988.01800280085011.

64. Rozman, Sanja. *Sanje o rdečem oblaku.* Ljubljana, Slovenia:
    Založba Dan, 1993.

65. Rozman, Sanja. *Zaljubljeni v sanje.* Ljubljana, Slovenia:
    Založba Dan, 1995.

66. Rozman, Sanja. *Peklenska gugalnica: kako se rešite odvisnosti
    od hrane, spolnosti, dela, iger na srečo, nakupovanja in
    zadolževanja, sanjarjenja in televizije, duhovnosti ter
    odnosov.* Ljubljana, Slovenia: Mladinska Knjiga, 2007.

67. Rozman, Sanja. *Umirjenost*. Ljubljana, Slovenia: Založba Modrijan, 2013.

68. Rozman, Sanja. *Umirjenost: delovni zvezek*. Ljubljana, Slovenia: Založba Modrijan, 2014.

69. Sahithya, B.R. and Rithvik S. Kashyap. "Sexual Addiction Disorder—A Review With Recent Updates." *Journal of Psychosexual Health* 4, no. 2 (2022):95–101. doi: 10.1177/26318318221081080.

70. "Schedules Of Reinforcement." Burrhus Frederic (B.F.) Skinner. September 14, 2023. https://burrhusfredericskinner.weebly.com/schedules-of-reinforcement.html.

71. Shapiro, Francine. *Getting Past Your Past: Take Control of Your Life with Self-Help Techniques from EMDR Therapy*. Emmaus, PA: Rodale, 2014.

72. Shapiro, Francine. *Eye Movement Desensitization and Reprocessing (EMDR) Therapy: Basic Principles, Protocols and Procedures*. New York: Guilford Press, 2017.

73. Schulz, Matt. *2023 Credit Card Debt Statistics*. LendingTree. LendingTree, LLC, September 18, 2023. https://www.lendingtree.com/credit-cards/credit-card-debt-statistics.

74. Siegel, Daniel J. *Mindsight: The New Science of Personal Transformation*. New York: Bantam Books, 2011.

75. Siegel, Daniel J. *Pocket Guide to Interpersonal Neurobiology: An Integrative Handbook of the Mind*. New York: W. W. Norton, 2012.

76. Skynner, Robin, and John Cleese. *Families and How to Survive Them*. New York: Oxford University Press, 1984.

77. Steiner, Claude. *Scripts People Live: Transactional Analysis of Life Scripts*. New York: Grove Press, 1990.

78. Tolkien, J.R.R. *The Fellowship of the Ring*. London: HarperCollins, 1995.

79. Van Eeden, Annelies E., Daphne van Hoeken, and Hans W. Hoek. "Incidence, prevalence and mortality of anorexia nervosa and bulimia nervosa." *Current Opinion in Psychiatry* 34, no. 6 (2021): 515–524. doi: 10.1097/YCO.0000000000000739.

80. Wilde, Oscar. *The Picture of Dorian Gray*. Harlow, UK: Pearson Education, 2008.

81. Winfrey, Oprah. *What I Know for Sure*. New York: Flatiron Books, 2014.

Author Biography

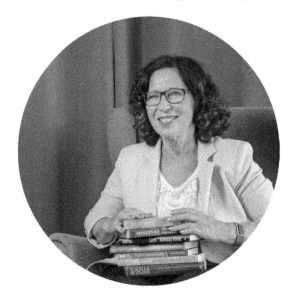

Photo: Tina Brinar

SANJA ROZMAN is a medical doctor and psychotherapist living in Slovenia, where she is known as a pioneer for her work speaking about behavioral addiction. Her many books about behavioral addictions discuss painful, complicated aspects of life like addiction and trauma in simple language with medical and psychotherapeutic accuracy, while her personal experience as the former wife of an addict allows her to approach the realities of addiction with honesty, compassion, and authenticity.

In her forty years of work as a medical doctor and thirty years as a psychotherapist, Rozman has listened to the testimonies of more than three thousand addicts and guided hundreds of her clients through many obstacles on the path to stable, long-term recovery. Their true stories testify to their resilience; and to the power of Rozman's original therapeutic model, described in this book.

www.ingramcontent.com/pod-product-compliance
Lightning Source LLC
Chambersburg PA
CBHW031715210125
20607CB00046B/880